PRINCIPLES AND PRACTICE OF
Electroconvulsive Therapy

PRINCIPLES AND PRACTICE OF
Electroconvulsive Therapy

Keith G. Rasmussen, M.D.

Professor, Department of Psychiatry and Psychology
Mayo Clinic, Rochester, Minnesota

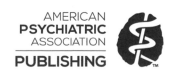

AMERICAN
PSYCHIATRIC
ASSOCIATION
PUBLISHING

If you wish to buy 50 or more copies of the same title, please go to www.appi.org/specialdiscounts for more information.

Copyright © 2019 American Psychiatric Association Publishing

ALL RIGHTS RESERVED

First Edition

Manufactured in the United States of America on acid-free paper
23 22 21 20 19   5 4 3 2 1

American Psychiatric Association Publishing
800 Maine Avenue SW
Suite 900
Washington, DC 20024-2812
www.appi.org

Library of Congress Cataloging-in-Publication Data
Names: Rasmussen, Keith G., author. | American Psychiatric Association Publishing, issuing body.
Title: Principles and practice of electroconvulsive therapy / Keith G. Rasmussen.
Description: First edition. | Washington, D.C. : American Psychiatric Association Publishing, [2019] | Includes bibliographical references and index.
Identifiers: LCCN 2018056193 (print) | LCCN 2018057526 (ebook) | ISBN 9781615372492 (ebook) | ISBN 9781615372416 (pbk. : alk. paper)
Subjects: | MESH: Electroconvulsive Therapy—methods | Electroconvulsive Therapy—history | History, 20th Century | Mental Disorders—therapy | Patient Care Management—methods
Classification: LCC RC485 (ebook) | LCC RC485 (print) | NLM WM 412 | DDC 616.89/122—dc23
LC record available at https://lccn.loc.gov/2018056193

British Library Cataloguing in Publication Data
A CIP record is available from the British Library.

Contents

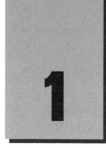

Introduction to ECT

Electroconvulsive therapy (ECT) is a topic of intense interest in the history of psychiatry. It has long been perhaps the most effective treatment for severe mental illness. Far from being effete or out of fashion, and definitely not supplanted by newer so-called neuropsychiatric brain stimulation methods, ECT is still used worldwide. Probably hundreds of thousands of people are treated with ECT each year, though precise data are lacking. To be competent to deliver ECT, a psychiatrist must be skilled at diagnosis as well as familiar with the techniques of treatment. The goal of this book is to teach psychiatric practitioners, whether in practice already or in training, how to be an ECT clinician. As such, the primary target audience naturally is psychiatrists or psychiatric residents. However, other mental health and medical professionals, and indeed anybody interested in mental health treatment, will find the book readable and comprehensible.

This introductory chapter is divided into four sections. The first is a capsule summary of what ECT is. This is intended for those readers who are new to this subject so that all subsequent chapters will make better sense. Next, a brief review of the history of ECT is presented. This is a very interesting topic for the history of psychiatry. This review is followed by a section outlining conceptualizations of the mechanism of action of ECT. The chapter ends with an outline of the remainder of the book.

What Is ECT?

ECT consists of the application of an electrical stimulus to the head to produce a seizure (convulsion) for therapeutic purposes. Thus, "electro" means use of an electrical stimulus, while "convulsive" means that a convulsion is induced, and "therapy" means it is done to help people with mental illness.

1

ECT is used to treat psychiatric patients who have been diagnosed with major depression, mania, catatonia, or schizophrenia. Usually, such patients' illnesses have been refractory to psychotropic medications or the patients are so severely ill that something quicker-acting must be used. This statement gets at the heart of why ECT is used in modern psychiatry: it works, it works very well, and it works faster than medications.

ECT is administered as a series of treatments. Once a psychiatrist has determined that ECT is appropriate for a patient, and the patient has agreed to proceed, a medical evaluation is undertaken to ensure ECT can be done safely and without complications. Each treatment session follows a standardized process. First, the patient is anesthetized to achieve unconsciousness. Thus, the patient is not aware when the electrical stimulus is applied. Next, muscle-paralyzing medication is given so that during the seizure, there is not much shaking of the limbs. This reduces the risk of bone fractures, which were common in the era when no such paralyzing medication was used during ECT. Because the patient cannot breathe after these anesthetic medications are given, oxygen is administered through a mask with a bag for ventilation. Heart rate, blood pressure, heart rhythm, and blood oxygen levels are all monitored throughout the procedure.

Once the patient is paralyzed, which is determined by the anesthesiologist in attendance, the psychiatrist and psychiatric nurse will apply two electrodes to the head. These are usually adhesive pads about the size and shape of a credit card. The electrodes are connected via thin cables to the ECT device. The amount of electricity to be given to the patient is set on the ECT machine, and then the button is pushed, and this sends an electrical current through the two electrodes and into the patient's brain, which causes a seizure. Small convulsive movements of the limbs can usually be appreciated, and an electroencephalogram records brain waves showing seizure activity. Usually, the seizure lasts a few seconds to a minute or so and stops on its own. A few minutes thereafter, the anesthetic medications wear off, the patient starts breathing, and a few minutes later awakening occurs. The patient is then transferred to a monitoring area known as the *post-anesthesia care unit* (PACU), where full return of alertness occurs over a few minutes to a half hour or so. The patient can then be taken back to the hospital unit where he or she is residing if an inpatient or go home accompanied by a responsible adult if an outpatient. Of note, it is quite common to deliver ECT to outpatients.

Treatments are repeated twice or thrice weekly until maximal improvement of the psychiatric condition occurs. This phase usually takes 2–4 weeks (thus, 6–12 treatments) for most patients. Once this acute-phase series of treatments is finished, patients may continue to receive treatments at spaced intervals, say once every week to once every 4 weeks, in order to prevent return of symptoms.

This so-called maintenance ECT phase may continue for a few months to a year or even longer depending on the chronicity of the patient's illness.

Side effects of ECT include muscle aches, headaches, nausea, and jaw ache. These are transient and easily treatable. Medical complications such as heart attack, stroke, or death are exceedingly rare. The most common bothersome side effect of ECT is memory difficulties.

There are three roles of the psychiatrist in ECT practice. The first is to recognize appropriate patients for this treatment. This may occur during an outpatient evaluation or with a hospitalized patient. The second role of the psychiatrist is to deliver the treatments in the ECT treatment area (known usually as the ECT suite). The third role is to follow the patient during a course of treatments and make decisions about electrode placement, treatment frequency, concomitant psychotropic medications, and when to stop the treatment course. These roles may be filled by three separate physicians. For example, a psychiatrist may recognize the need for ECT in an outpatient and then refer the patient for inpatient care to begin ECT if the clinical circumstances warrant inpatient admission. Then, another psychiatrist may actually follow the patient during the hospitalization, while a third actually performs the treatments. Alternatively, one or two physicians may fulfill these roles, depending on how staffing is arranged in a particular locale. It is important for these clinicians to sustain good communication with each other during a patient's ECT course.

This description of ECT is of course brief. All these topics and steps will be covered in much greater detail in the remaining chapters of this book. However, the previously ECT-naïve reader can now at least appreciate in general terms what happens during ECT.

History of ECT

The idea that a purposefully induced seizure could be a treatment for psychiatric disorders originated with Ladislas J. Meduna, a physician caring for mental patients in Budapest, Hungary, in the 1930s (Shorter and Healy 2007). Observing schizophrenic and epileptic patients clinically, as well as undertaking histological examinations of their brains at autopsy, Meduna concluded that the histological changes associated with epilepsy were not seen with schizophrenia. He hypothesized that there was some type of biologic antagonism between seizures and schizophrenia, with the attendant implication that inducing seizures in schizophrenia patients may cure that disease. His next step was to undertake clinical studies utilizing seizure-inducing chemical agents in psychotic patients. Starting in 1934 with the first such session, he used agents such as pentylenetetrazol (Metrazol, an intravenously administered drug) and flurothyl (Indoklon, an inhalational agent) to induce seizures. These treatments were dramatically effective, and the technique spread throughout the world rapidly. However, seizure induction with these chemical agents was not reliable and could take a long time to occur. Patient discomfort and anxiety were high.

Meanwhile, in Italy, two neuropsychiatric researchers, Ugo Cerletti and Luciano Bini, drew on their experiences inducing seizures electrically in lab animals and developed a device for doing so in humans via application of an electric shock to the head (Shorter and Healy 2007). Attempting this technique on a chronically catatonic patient in Rome in April 1938, they found that a series of induced seizures was effective and allowed the patient to be discharged from the hospital and return home. This new electrical method of inducing seizures rapidly replaced the chemical method and within a few years was used for seriously mentally ill patients the world over. Initially, the electrical stimuli were administered to conscious patients, obviously a frightening experience. Also, the fully expressed motor convulsions led to bone fractures frequently. The use of anesthetic agents to induce unconsciousness followed by paralytic agents to block motor movements was developed and is now the standard of care for ECT. This process is referred to as *modified ECT*.

Over the first couple of decades or so, psychiatrists learned what types of patients responded best to ECT: those with severe states of depression, mania, catatonia, and agitated schizophrenia. The use of ECT in both private and public hospitals was quite common in the 1940s and 1950s. The development of antipsychotic and antidepressant medications in the late 1950s led to waning use of ECT in subsequent decades, though it is still commonly used.

Along with the great popularity of ECT in the psychiatric profession, there have been those critical of its use. Some individuals and organizations in fact have been vehemently opposed to ECT. Anti-ECT sentiment is fueled probably mostly by two factors: involuntary usage of ECT and the cognitive side effects. In modern times in the United States as well as other countries, there are laws governing informed consent and provisions for using ECT involuntarily under some circumstances. However, this was not the case in decades past, when it was not uncommon for patients to be given ECT without their consent or any court proceedings to provide for authorization to administer the procedure involuntarily. This understandably led to anger.

Memory is affected by ECT. This was especially true in the early decades of ECT use, when high amounts of electrical current were used. ECT got a bit of a bad name in some circles as causing brain damage. Anti-ECT efforts in the 1960s through roughly the 1980s led to the establishment, at least in the United States, of laws in all states governing ECT usage that, even though mandating informed consent procedures, also affirm the benefits of and need for ECT as a medical procedure. ECT is not banned in any part of the United States. Thus, the legal status of ECT is well established. Those who have attempted to abolish ECT have failed. The interested reader is referred to the book by Shorter and Healy (2007), which is an excellent overview of the history of ECT.

Mechanism of Action of ECT

Throughout the history of ECT, there has been intense interest in the mechanism of action. There have been thousands of basic science investigations of brain changes associated with electroconvulsive shock (ECS) in animals as well as attempts to study mechanisms of ECT in humans. The scope and depth of this book preclude a thorough discussion of this area. However, some brief comments can give the reader an idea of the history of theories of ECT mechanisms and where current research is focused. It is important to note, however, that the mechanism of action of ECT is not known.

Undoubtedly, of the myriad biochemical and histological changes associated with electrically induced seizures in animal studies, most of the findings do not pertain to the mechanism of ECT in depression in humans. The likely action of ECT consists of a cascade of neurobiological events, beginning with the first induced seizure, involving molecules, cells, and neural circuits. There is no currently articulated theory of the mechanism of action of ECT that incorporates all of these levels. Furthermore, it is not necessary to be familiar with any theory of mechanism of action in order to practice ECT competently.

There have been several types of technology utilized to attempt to decipher ECT brain mechanims. These include single-photon emission computed tomography, positron emission tomography, functional magnetic resonance imaging (fMRI), computerized electroencephalography, magnetic resonance spectroscopy (MRS), and body fluid chemical analysis (blood, cerebrospinal fluid, and urine). In animals, histological analyses in brains of animals undergoing ECS have been done. The general types of theories can be categorized as neurotransmitter, neuroendocrine, anticonvulsant, neurotrophic, and neural connectivity hypotheses.

Early work revolved around psychoanalytic theories that were dominant in the early decades of ECT practice. Thus, Gordon (1948) briefly outlined no fewer than 50 theories, about half of which were what he called "somatogenic" (by which he meant neurobiological) and the other half "psychogenic." The discovery of neurotransmitters, such as dopamine, serotonin, and norepinephrine, led to theories revolving around monoamines (Bunney and Davis 1965; Schildkraut 1965). Studies involved measuring monoamine metabolite levels in various bodily fluids, such as cerebrospinal fluid, blood, and urine, and attempted to correlate changes over time with treatment response. Some data, such as those from MRS studies, have focused on enhancement of γ-aminobutyric acid (GABA) activity (Michael et al. 2003a; Sanacora et al. 2003) as a mechanism in ECT. Also, along with the current intense interest in ketamine in the treatment of mood disorders, there is interest in glutamatergic mechanisms in ECT action, though no specific supportive data exist.

As the 1970s and 1980s unfolded, biological psychiatry became enamored of neuroendocrine challenge tests, and ECT theories followed suit (Shorter and Fink 2010; Taylor and Fink 2006). For example, much attention focused on the dexamethasone suppression test as a possible correlate of ECT outcome and predictor of relapse (Shorter and Fink 2010). However, the sensitivity and specificity of this test were never good enough to justify its use in routine clinical care. Haskett (2014) reviews other neuroendocrine theories of ECT action, none of which has generated much enthusiasm.

The data of Sackeim et al. (1987b) showing that a course of ECT can have potent anticonvulsant effects, coupled with the then increasing use of antiepileptic drugs for mood disorders, led to hypotheses that the anticonvulsant effect of ECT was involved in the mechanism of action in depression. In one study, the degree of increase in seizure threshold over a course of treatments, which reflects the degree of anticonvulsant activity, did in fact correlate with antidepressant effects (Sackeim 1999). Theories along these lines focused on the effects of ECT on GABA, because that amino acid is the most widely disbursed inhibitory amino acid neurotransmitter in the brain. Some brain blood flow and electroencephalographic data also support not only an anticonvulsant effect of ECT but a correlation between the intensity of this effect and clinical response (Farzan et al. 2014).

The most recent conceptualizations of ECT mechanism of action focus on cellular changes within the brain, termed *neuroplasticity* or *neurotrophic* theories. This framework holds that morphological changes such as neurogenesis or gliogenesis, or alterations in dendritic arborization, are critical to ECT antidepressant effects (Bouckaert et al. 2014). Animal studies of ECS clearly and reliably demonstrate neurogenesis in the hippocampus and other structures thought to be involved in mood disorders, but whether these findings extend to humans awaits a technology capable of investigating such things in the intact human brain noninvasively. Preliminary data utilizing high-resolution magnetic resonance–based imaging have indeed demonstrated changes in regions at the limbic level, such as amygdala and hippocampus, with a course of ECT (Dukart et al. 2014; Joshi et al. 2016; Michael et al. 2003b; Nordanskog et al. 2010; Tendolkar et al. 2013).

The development of fMRI has allowed investigations of neural connectivity changes during ECT, which is the study of the manner in which various brain regions intercommunicate (Abbott et al. 2013; Beall et al. 2012; Christ et al. 2008; Perrin et al. 2012). However, these studies all involve very small sample sizes, and the results are not uniform or coherent. More definitive conclusions await further development of the technology of neural connectivity and large sample sizes.

In the early years of ECT practice, one theory of the mechanism of action of ECT was that by causing patients to forget their lives and the painful aspects, depression was removed. This is a relatively easily tested hypothesis. One merely needs to follow patients during ECT with ratings of psychopathology, such as depression, and careful assessments of memory function to see if there is a correlation. In fact, there is none, and this has been a robust finding in the literature. That is, the degree of retrograde or anterograde amnesia or postictal disorientation induced by ECT does not correlate with degree of antidepressant efficacy. (See Chapter 9 for further discussion of retrograde and anterograde amnesia as well as postictal disorientation and subjective memory function.) Thus, the neurobiological mechanisms underlying memory impairment and relief from psychopathology are dissociated in the brain.

What can be appreciated from this very brief review of conceptualizations of ECT mechanisms is that over the decades, there have been a variety of foci of theories, from neurotransmitters and neuroendocrine systems to cellular and neural circuitry changes. There is no one single comprehensive theory accounting for all data at all levels (molecules, cells, and circuits). However, the "good news" for the modern ECT practitioner is that, as fascinating as the subject of ECT mechanisms is, one does not need to know anything about any current theory in order to practice ECT competently. Thus, let us now proceed to what this book is about, which is how to practice ECT.

Organization of This Book

The purpose of this book is to teach the reader how to practice ECT. It is assumed that psychiatric trainees will have clinical skills verification at the hands of teachers in clinical rotations, so that this book is a supplement to clinical teaching, which of course is indispensable in learning a new clinical skill. The chapters will follow the typical course of ECT. Thus, Chapter 2 addresses the indications for ECT and how to select patients. Next, Chapter 3 provides an overview of informed consent procedures, which typically follow patient selection. Chapters 4 and 5 cover the pre-ECT medical evaluation and anesthesia for ECT, respectively. Chapter 6 then proceeds with a discussion of how to manage an individual ECT treatment. This is the only chapter of the book that is specific to ECT practitioners. All the other chapters include clinical activities that any general psychiatrist may participate in without actually delivering the treatments in the ECT suite. Chapter 7 covers managing the course of treatments. It is quite common for the psychiatrist in charge of a patient's care to manage the course of treatments without actually being in the suite delivering the treatments—thus, the separation of management of treatment into separate chapters (Chapters 6 and 7). Chapter 8 covers the very important topic of how to manage patients after a course of ECT treatments is finished, including the choice of delivering maintenance treatments to prevent relapse. Chapter 9 covers the effects of ECT on memory, which are the most important side effects of ECT, and how to assess for and manage them. Finally, Chapter 10 reviews other so-called neuropsychiatric stimulation therapies vis-à-vis ECT and how to choose among them.

Key Points

- ECT involves the application of an electrical stimulus to an anesthetized patient's head to induce a generalized seizure for therapeutic purposes.

- ECT has been used since 1938 and is safe and effective for depression, mania, catatonia, and schizophrenia.

- Modern ECT practice requires that the clinician be skilled in psychiatric diagnosis as well as all aspects of treatment technique and patient preparation.

- The mechanism of action of ECT in the brain is unknown.

2

Patient Selection for ECT

The first, and most important, step in electroconvulsive therapy (ECT) practice is patient selection. ECT is indicated for patients with depression, mania, catatonia, and schizophrenia, but ECT is not offered to every one of the patients with these diagnoses. Choosing among them those who need the intense treatment of ECT is the subject of this chapter.

Depression

Depression constitutes the most common psychopathological indication for ECT. Yet, choosing which patients from the large number of patients with depression should be offered ECT is probably the most challenging aspect of ECT practice. There are multiple sources of uncertainty that challenge ECT patient selection and outcome assessment for patients with depression. First, there is a lack of observable psychopathology in a large proportion of patients diagnosed with depression. It is not uncommon for a patient to endorse depressive symptoms but not "look" depressed, which means that outcome assessment is entirely dependent on what the patient tells the assessor. Such information is subject to capricious influences that may cloud confidence. Second, there is much temporal variability in signs and symptoms in depression. Depressed patients often tend to have variable and fluctuating symptoms on an hour-to-hour or day-to-day basis. The symptoms may be highly reactive to environmental events. Thus, it may be difficult over time deciding whether there has been sustained improvement. Third, there is much heterogeneity of clinical manifestations of depression. For example, there are psychotic depression, melancholic depression, bipolar depression, and atypical depression. The pathophysiology of depressive states is probably quite heterogeneous, and not all such entities respond equally to ECT. Outcome assessment is made more difficult by the lack of uniformity of the depressive syndromes. Fourth, many depressed patients have psychiatric comorbidity, the features of which may overlap with the core depressive features and confound outcome assessment. Finally, it must be kept in mind that all the research on patients with depression and ECT involves patients who were well enough to sign consent for research. Patients who are too ill to do so, because of psychotic ideations or profound psychomotor agitation or retardation with attendant information processing difficulties, are not represented in modern ECT research. Ironically, those are the patients who tend to respond most robustly to the treatment. Thus, research efforts on predictors of outcome are focused on the less ill patients, and the findings may not apply to depressed patients who are profoundly ill.

It bears emphasizing that the statement "ECT is effective for depression" refers to *major* depressive episodes, as opposed to the depressive symptoms associated with adjustment disorder with depressed mood, persistent depressive disorder (dysthymia), or other or unspecified depressive disorder (depressive disorder not otherwise specified). These are syndromes in which patients have depressed mood but their symptoms do not meet the criteria for a major depressive episode. Such patients may be suffering greatly and even be suicidal, but ECT is not indicated. The concept behind adjustment disorders is that a psychosocial stressor, such as financial losses, job uncertainty, or marital discord, is directly causing psychopathological features such as depression or anxiety. Furthermore, if the stressors are removed, the psychopathology disappears. This seems simple, but the relationship between life stress and psychopathology is complex and rarely falls unequivocally into "stress-induced" versus "autonomous." Nonetheless, a substantial portion of patients admitted to a psychiatric unit in a depressive-type crisis seem to have symptoms driven by identifiable stressors. Such patients may be suicidal and express hopelessness. They may already have been given medications and psychotherapy, and the clinician may be tempted to try ECT. The clinician must consider the possibility that an adjustment disorder does not better account for depressive symptoms than a primary, ECT-responsive major depressive episode, especially in patients whose psychosocial status is riddled with discord. In any case, if the clinician administers ECT to a depressed patient with an ongoing severe stressor, even though there may be symptomatic improvement with ECT, there must also be some strategy for helping the patient deal with the stressor; otherwise, there is a high relapse risk.

Additionally, some patients have substantial emotional distress but their symptoms are accounted for by labels such as persistent depressive disorder or other or unspecified depressive disorder. That is, a disciplined application of DSM depressive episode criteria finds that these patients, though suffering greatly, do not have presentations that meet such criteria. ECT is not appropriate in such circumstances.

Efficacy of ECT for Depression

ECT is highly efficacious for major depression and enhances quality of life (McCall et al. 2006). A recent epidemiological survey of a large number of patients in numerous hospitals in the United States found that 30-day readmission rates for patients who had been treated with ECT were approximately half as much as those for non-ECT-treated patients (Slade et al. 2017). However, the gold standard investigation for establishing the efficacy of a medical treatment is the randomized controlled trial, and such data are reviewed herein. Preferably, the control groups should include patients treated with placebo or other accepted modalities for the condition in question. In the case of ECT, randomized controlled trials fall into several categories: studies in which ECT is compared with "placebo ECT," a procedure known as "sham ECT" in the literature; studies in which ECT is compared with psychotropic medications; and studies in which various forms of ECT are compared with one another. Several well-conducted meta-analyses have all concluded that ECT is fundamentally effective for major depression (Kho et al. 2003; Janicak et al. 1985; Pagnin et al. 2004; UK ECT Review Group 2003). Of note, there are some comparison studies of ECT versus transcranial magnetic stimulation and magnetic seizure therapy, topics that will be covered in some detail in Chapter 10.

Sham ECT Studies

The purpose of a placebo-controlled trial is to establish that the treatment in question has inherent efficacy beyond that due to other factors, which include placebo effects, the natural history of the illness being treated, other therapeutic effects that might be operative in the trial (in the case of inpatient depression trials, this would include the therapeutic effects of the hospital milieu interventions), and any improvement in outcome measures that might be due to error in measurement (e.g., regression toward the mean). There have been a large number of ECT studies in which an actively treated group of patients with depression is compared with a group of patients who receive the so-called sham ECT, which is anesthesia induction without the concomitant seizure (Rasmussen 2009b). However, most of these studies were flawed by very small sample sizes, lack of randomization, nonsystematic outcome assessment, and diagnostic ambiguity.

Six of the sham studies, all conducted in Great Britain, are methodologically sound and do provide insight into ECT efficacy. The first was that of Lambourn and Gill (1978), who randomly assigned patients with "depressive psychosis" to receive either unilateral electrode placement ECT or sham treatments. Both groups of patients, blindly followed with the Hamilton Depression Scale (Hamilton 1960), enjoyed very large (23- to 25-point) reductions in scores. What is impressive about this study is the dramatic improvement in the sham-treated group. The improvement seen with sham treatment could be due to the incidental therapeutic effects of the inpatient hospital milieu, the placebo phenomenon, or perhaps bias on the part of the outcome assessors, who may have been blind to treatment group but who were not blind to stage of treatment (i.e., they knew whether a patient was pre- or posttreatment). Bias against a specific effect of ECT may have caused the outcome assessors to rate all patients as much improved. Of particular interest is the description of these patients as having "depressive psychosis." If in fact these patients were psychotic, then the dramatic improvement reported in the sham group is truly noteworthy. However, the investigators did not specify diagnostic criteria for their term "depressive psychosis," and it should be pointed out that decades ago the term "psychosis" was commonly used to describe any severely impaired psychiatric patient and was not necessarily reserved for those with delusions or hallucinations.

The next sham ECT study was reported by Freeman et al. (1978). In this interestingly designed study, depressed patients were randomly assigned to receive either four real twice-weekly ECT treatments or two sham treatments during the first week followed by two real treatments in the second week. At the end of the first week, the patients who had been given real treatments had lower depression rating scale scores in comparison to those who had received two sham treatments. Thus, if the study had ended there, the investigators would have concluded that real ECT is superior to sham ECT. However, at the end of the second week, both groups of patients had equally low scores, with the scores in both groups lower than those at the end of week one for the real ECT patients. This is an odd result, suggesting that two sham followed by two real treatments is just as therapeutic as four consecutive real treatments.

Johnstone et al. (1980) conducted a methodologically rigorous study in which endogenously depressed patients were randomly assigned to receive either real or sham treatments twice weekly over 4 weeks. For psychotically depressed patients, real ECT was more efficacious than sham ECT. However, for the nonpsychotic patients, there was no difference between real and sham ECT, with both groups enjoying robust improvements. This mirrors the Lambourn and Gill (1978) experience, in which sham-treated patients had excellent responses with ECT.

West (1981) randomly assigned depressed patients to receive 3 weeks of twice-weekly real versus sham ECT. In stark contrast to the three studies described above, the sham-treated group had no improvement in rating scale scores, while the group given real ECT had a dramatic improvement in outcome scores. Brandon et al. (1984) subtyped their depressed patients into delusional, psychomotorically retarded, or neurotic and assigned them to receive either eight real or sham treatments. Sham ECT was inferior in efficacy to real ECT for the delusional and psychomotorically retarded groups but not for the neurotic patients, who responded equally well to both sham and real ECT.

Finally, Gregory et al. (1985) randomly assigned depressed patients to receive either bilateral or unilateral real ECT or sham treatments. The two groups given real ECT enjoyed strong, robust improvements in depression, while the sham-treated patients had a relatively small, modest (and statistically significantly lower) reduction in depression ratings after six twice-weekly treatments.

It is interesting to try to glean clinically meaningful lessons from these sham ECT studies. Several meta-analyses of these studies have concluded that they provide strong evidence of the superiority of real over sham ECT (Janicak et al. 1985; Kho et al. 2003; Pagnin et al. 2004; UK ECT Review Group 2003). The two trials in which patients were separated by psychosis status (Brandon et al. 1984; Johnstone et al. 1980) both revealed superiority of real over sham treatments in psychotic patients. There is also the suggestion that nonpsychotic, "neurotically" depressed patients respond equally well to sham ECT as to real ECT (Brandon et al. 1984; Johnstone et al. 1980). It should be noted that just because patients did well in "placebo ECT" groups, it does not follow that it was the placebo effect that caused the improvement. The salutary effects of psychiatric hospitalization could have been, and probably were, at play to help such patients.

ECT Compared With Psychotropic Medication

There are numerous trials dating back several decades in which some form of ECT is compared with psychotropic medication for depression, and meta-analyses of these trials conclude that ECT is superior to medication (Rasmussen 2009a). Most of these trials suffer from various methodological flaws, including use of medications not usually considered antidepressant, nonblinded outcome assessment, outmoded ECT technique, inadequate dose and duration of antidepressant medication, outmoded diagnostic terms (or failure to provide needed information about depressive diagnosis), and combining of data from psychotic and nonpsychotic patients. Nonetheless, there is no signal from any of these trials that ECT is *inferior* to medications, so probably the most prudent conclusion from this literature is that ECT is at least as therapeutic as medications for depression. Two more recent studies with modern rigorously applied diagnostic and outcome criteria deserve mention. Folkerts et al. (1997) randomly assigned patients with treatment-resistant depression to receive either ECT or paroxetine therapy. The ECT group had a 59% reduction in depressive rating scale scores over 4 weeks versus a 29% reduction in the paroxetine group, a highly statistically significant difference. Another, more recent well-conducted study involved randomly assigning patients with medication-refractory bipolar depression to receive either ECT or an aggressive antidepressant pharmacotherapy regimen. Response rates (i.e., at least 50% reduction in depression scores) in the ECT group were almost twice as high as rates in the medication group (Schoeyen et al. 2015).

Methodological issues are difficult to overcome when comparing the efficacy of ECT with that of medications for depression. For example, if one simply randomly assigned patients to receive ECT or medication, then the patients would not be blind to treatment modality, and this might affect ratings on depression scales. It would also, in such a study, be difficult to blind the personnel who were making the ratings. The most methodologically sound ECT-versus-medication comparison would be to randomly assign patients to receive a combination of either real ECT and placebo medication or sham ECT and real medication. That way, the blinding of patients would be more effective and remove an important source of bias. One study did in fact utilize that methodology (Gangadhar et al. 1982) with sufficiently large sample sizes to make meaningful conclusions and found that depressed patients randomly assigned to receive 150 mg imipramine daily plus sham ECT fared equally well, though at a somewhat slower pace, by study end as patients randomly assigned to receive bilateral real ECT and placebo pill. It is a shame that more such studies have not been conducted. Two older studies utilizing this type of methodology (Harris and Robin 1960; Robin and Harris 1962), unfortunately, had extremely small sample sizes. Dinan and Barry (1989) randomly assigned depressed patients with inadequate response to a tricyclic antidepressant medication to receive either a course of bilateral ECT or lithium augmentation of the tricyclic. The groups fared equally well. It is important to reiterate that all these studies involved depressed patients sufficiently able to process information to enroll in a research study. Patients too impaired by psychotic ideations, psychomotor slowing, or the cognitive effects of severe depression (pseudodementia) were not enrolled in the studies—such patients probably respond better to ECT than to antidepressant medications.

Different Forms of ECT Compared With One Another

One option that is available to ECT researchers to establish the true biologically inherent efficacy of ECT for depression is to compare different forms of ECT with one another. If in fact differences in efficacy are found, then this constitutes evidence of the biologic efficacy of ECT, if one assumes that had there been a placebo (i.e., sham) group, those patients would have fared no better than the patients receiving the least efficacious form of ECT. In fact, there are several aspects of ECT technique that can be varied and that have been shown to influence efficacy, such as electrode placement, stimulus waveform, stimulus dosing, stimulus parameter configuration, and treatment frequency. Details of these will be presented in Chapter 7 on ECT technique. Suffice it to say here that many studies over the years have found efficacy differences among the various forms of ECT (Heshe et al.

1978; Sackeim et al. 1987a, 1993, 2000, 2008, 2009). It is these studies that probably constitute the best evidence for an inherent therapeutic effect of at least some
forms of ECT vis-à-vis other mechanisms of antidepressant action such as the placebo effect, the therapeutic effects of interpersonal interactions with study staff,
and the natural history of remission from depressive episodes in the untreated
state.

Predicting ECT Response in Depression

It was not long after the initial description of ECT in the 1930s that practitioners
realized that profound improvements in depressed patients could be achieved
with this new modality. However, it was also clear that not all depressed patients
responded so well. Thus, over the last approximately eight decades, there has
been an intense effort to elaborate which patients among the large group of patients
with depression respond positively to ECT (Rasmussen 2011a). In this section,
various potential predictor variables are reviewed that may assist the clinician
with patient selection. In general, putative predictors of ECT response in depression can be divided into four categories: demographics, longitudinal course of
illness variables, psychopathological features of the depressive episode, and comorbid psychopathology.

Demographics

Age. Tew et al. (1999) found excellent efficacy of ECT in very old patients.
O'Connor et al. (2001) found that patients over the age of 45 responded better
to ECT than did patients under the age of 45. Response rates were still quite good
in the latter group, however. Analyzing data from several ECT studies, Dombrovski
et al. (2005) did not find a correlation between age and ECT response. Damm et
al. (2010) also did not find age a predictor of ECT outcomes. Thus, the data are
mixed on this topic. A recent meta-analysis found a weak overall association between higher age and better ECT response (Haq et al. 2015). It should be noted
that these studies involved only adults. Probably the best summary statement is
that in adults, there is no reason to withhold ECT based on age, and there are
hints that middle-age and older adults might obtain greater benefits from ECT.

The particular challenges regarding age and ECT patient selection in depression revolve around children and adolescents. It is rare to treat adolescents with
ECT. The typical depressed adolescent treated with ECT has been chronically dysphoric, has been treated with a large number of antidepressant medications, has
had intensive efforts at psychotherapy, and is either suicidal or has dropped out
of school because of the depression. There are no controlled trials comparing
ECT with sham treatments or medications or different forms of ECT with one

another in this population. There are some reviews of open-label case series finding ECT to be associated with relatively high acute remission rates in depressed adolescents (Bloch et al. 2001; Consoli et al. 2010; Kutcher and Robertson 1995; Walter and Rey 2003). It is extremely rare to treat children with ECT. Most clinicians will not encounter children in their ECT practices.

Gender.   There is no evidence that gender affects ECT response (Haq et al. 2015; Kellner et al. 2006). Depression is more common in women than in men, and this probably accounts for the relative preponderance of women treated with ECT.

Other demographic variables.   There is no evidence that ethnicity or socioeconomic level affects ECT response (Williams et al. 2008). This is important because several data sets indicate ECT is less likely to be used in nonwhite compared with white patients (Euba 2012; Ona et al. 2014; Reid et al. 1998; Slade et al. 2017). The reasons for the differential rate of usage are not clear but are related either to a greater tendency to offer ECT to white than nonwhite patients or to a greater tendency of nonwhite patients to reject ECT that has been offered. It is likely that access to health insurance, which may distinguish white from nonwhite patients, affects ECT usage (Slade et al. 2017).

Longitudinal Course of Illness Variables

Duration of episode.   Though in one study, duration of episode was not associated with ECT response (Pluijms et al. 2006), it did correlate negatively with ECT response in several others (Dombrovski et al. 2005; Kho et al. 2005; Kindler et al. 1991; Kukopulos et al. 1977; Prudic et al. 1996). A recent meta-analysis of studies on the relationship between episode duration and acute response to ECT in depression found that shorter duration strongly correlated with better response (Haq et al. 2015). In other words, the longer the episode at the time of ECT, the lesser the antidepressant response. This argues in favor of treating earlier rather than later during a depressive episode with ECT, although it is possible that episode duration is a proxy for some other mechanism for poorer ECT response and that treating earlier will make no difference. In the Dombrovski et al. (2005) study, episode durations greater than 2 years were predictive of lesser ECT response. It is not known whether longer episode duration directly causes lesser ECT responsivity or whether there is something neurobiologically different about depressive episodes that last for prolonged periods that would render lesser ECT response even if the ECT was instituted earlier in the course of the episode.

Medication refractoriness.   Most ECT patients have used multiple psychotropics in the current depressive episode (Rasmussen et al. 2006a). Heijnen et al.

(2010), in a meta-analysis, found that the overall remission rate in patients with medication-refractory depression was 48.0% versus 64.9% in those without refractoriness. In another recent meta-analysis of this issue, Haq et al. (2015) found the respective response rates to be 58% and 70%. Similarly to the episode duration issue described in the previous subsection, it is not known whether patients with medication-refractory depression would have responded better to ECT had it been offered as first-line treatment or whether there is something inherent in the neurobiology of their illness, independent of but correlated with medication refractoriness, that limits their ECT response. Because all of these studies were observational (i.e., patients were not randomly assigned to receive medication first before ECT or ECT before medication), confounding factors such as psychosis status and duration of episode could be at play. Clearly, though, remission rates are sufficiently high even in medication-refractory patients to justify the treatment.

Several investigators have also found that patients with medication-refractory depression whose illness successfully remits acutely with an index course of ECT have higher relapse rates than patients with nonrefractory depression (Lerer et al. 1995; Rasmussen et al. 2009b; Sackeim et al. 1993, 2000, 2001, 2008). Post-index ECT patient management issues will be covered in Chapter 8.

Psychopathological Features of the Depressive Episode

In this subsection, the various subtypes of depression and depressive features as predictors of ECT responsivity are considered. A general principle is that psychopathological features predicting poor ECT outcome, such as hypochondriasis, are only such if they represent primary disorders. When such features are clearly secondary to a severe depressive episode, then ECT outcome will be excellent.

Psychotic depression. ECT is the treatment of choice for psychotic depression (Petrides et al. 2001). In the over eight-decade history of ECT at the time of this writing, there has never been any suggestion that psychotic depression does not respond exquisitely well to ECT. This has been a uniform finding in this line of research and clinical experience. In the older ECT literature, many of the patients described as having "involutional melancholia" would be diagnosed today with psychotic depression, and early authors extolled the virtues of ECT in such patients (Rasmussen 2011a). A recent meta-analysis found a weak association between psychotic depression and better response rates than in nonpsychotic depression, but heterogeneity among studies was high (Haq et al. 2015).

The pharmacology literature on the treatment of psychotic depression is not impressive. A well-controlled trial in which a large number of patients with psychotic depression were randomly assigned to treatment with the antipsychotic olanzapine in addition to either placebo or the antidepressant sertraline found abysmally low remission rates in both groups at 12 weeks (Meyers et al. 2009), though the double-medication group did do better. This argues in favor of ECT for such patients, because response rates for patients with psychotic depression treated with ECT routinely run in the 70%–90% range (Haq et al. 2015; Petrides et al. 2001).

A challenge is recognizing psychotic depression. A report from the group that conducted the large olanzapine study cited above showed a surprisingly high number of patients in whom structured, thorough questioning by research staff revealed psychotic ideations that had previously been missed (Andreescu et al. 2007). Thus, when interviewing depressed patients, the interviewer must ask explicit questions about psychotic phenomena, preferably of family members in addition to the patient.

Melancholic depression.   Of all the potential predictors of ECT response, none has been subjected to more contentious debate than the notion that patients with melancholic depression respond exquisitely better to ECT than do those with nonmelancholic depression (the latter variously described as having "neurotic" or "reactive" depression). Part of the problem has been the disparate and varying terminology used to describe different depressive states that are probably roughly synonymous with melancholia, such as "autonomous," "vital," and "endogenous" depression. All these have been taken by various authors to be synonymous with melancholia, but careful reading of the literature over the decades reveals that this may not be the case (Kendell 1976). Early large ECT case series reported that ECT was prominently helpful for "manic depressive" or "involutional melancholic" types of depressive episodes but not for "psychoneurotic" depressions (see Rasmussen 2011a for a review). One author in particular (Sands 1946), demonstrating prescience for later diagnostic conundrums, realized the diagnostic heterogeneity implied by the word *depression*. His is one of the earliest references in the ECT literature to the notion of differential responsivity of depressive subtypes. He emphasized that the diversity of nosological terms used in those days (e.g., melancholia, reactive/endogenous depression, psychotic, psychoneurotic, involutional) was a confounding factor in choosing the patients who best respond to ECT. In his case series, patients with primary depression responded to ECT much better than did patients with depression secondary to neurotic conditions such as anxiety disorders or somatization. There were early attempts to predict ECT response on the basis of positive and negative predictor psychopathological features (Carney and Sheffield 1972; Carney et al. 1965; Hobson 1953; Mendels 1965a, 1965b, 1967; Roberts 1959). Examples of the former included features roughly synonymous with modern melancholia signs, while examples of the latter included nonmelancholic depressive symptoms like hysterical attitude and high levels of neuroticism.

The modern concept of melancholia was wrought with DSM-III (American Psychiatric Association 1980), in which the vast number of depressive types were all combined into one category and the specifier "with melancholic features" was added as a qualifier to any depressive episode meeting the criteria. There has been some change in subsequent DSM editions, but the fundamental notion has remained intact—namely, that the core signs of melancholia include a dense, profound anhedonia with prominent mood nonreactivity. Of note, the latter term means not, as in prior decades, that the depressive episode occurred in response or reaction to external stressors, but rather that the patient's dysphoric mood is invariant and not responsive to environmental stimuli that might ordinarily brighten one's mood. Thus, modern DSM melancholia is seen primarily as a state of utter joylessness. Secondary features include guilty ideations, psychomotor changes, loss of weight or appetite, distinct quality of mood unlike normal sadness, early morning awakening, and diurnal variation with mood worse in the morning. Not all of these are needed to establish the melancholic diagnosis, and therein exists a source of rendering melancholia a nonspecific diagnosis, given that there are many combinations of signs or symptoms that can meet the criteria for melancholia. In one report of ECT in patients with well-defined DSM-III melancholia, no particular symptom or sign within the melancholia criteria was predictive of ECT outcome (Abrams and Vedak 1991).

In one report, Fink et al. (2007) found that DSM-IV (American Psychiatric Association 1994) melancholia status as assessed by structured interview was not associated with higher acute remission rates than in nonmelancholic depressed patients. Other groups using modern melancholia criteria have found similar results (see Rasmussen 2011a for a review). Thus, in the modern DSM-based era, there are no data indicating that patients with depression subtyped as melancholic respond better to ECT than those with depression subtyped as nonmelancholic. Patients with either subtype seem to respond quite well. It can confidently be stated that if a patient is diagnosed with a depressive episode according to modern DSM-based criteria, then teasing out melancholic signs (again according to DSM) seems to offer no more predictive power for ECT response as assessed by modern rating scales. What is not clear is whether more intense assessments of melancholia status, utilizing observational sources of information and longer-term outcome assessments of functional as well as symptomatic status, might detect differential ECT effects. This issue awaits further research.

Catatonic depression. This important topic will be discussed later in this chapter in the section "Catatonia."

Atypical depression.   Patients with atypical depression have the so-called reverse neurovegetative signs of increased appetite, excessive sleep, a feeling of heaviness in the limbs ("leaden paralysis"), and interpersonal rejection sensitivity. These patients tend to have high mood reactivity in day-to-day life, meaning that the mood is not constantly dysphoric, with euthymic mood states occurring at least temporarily in response to desirable external events such as interpersonal affirmations and other good news. In one large study, patients classified as having atypical depression did not differ from others in acute remission rates with ECT (Husain et al. 2008).

Bipolar depression.   As currently defined in DSM, "bipolar" means a history of at least one episode of mania, hypomania, or a mixed state. There are several relatively large data sets indicating that patients with bipolar depression have the same outcomes with index ECT as those with unipolar depression (Bailine et al. 2010; Daly et al. 2001; Grunhaus et al. 2002; Hallam et al. 2009; P. Sienaert et al. 2009c; Zornberg and Pope 1993), with one study showing lesser ECT responses in bipolar depression, especially bipolar I, than in unipolar depression (Medda et al. 2009). A meta-analysis found no evidence of differential ECT response in depression based on polarity (Haq et al. 2015). In general, no particular psychopathological features of bipolar versus unipolar depressive episodes have a bearing on suitability for ECT. The same criteria can be used in selecting ECT for unipolar and bipolar depressed groups. There are, however, certain treatment challenges applicable to bipolar depressed ECT patients, especially concerning concomitant psychotropic agents. These will be discussed in Chapter 7.

Psychomotor retardation or agitation.   In a study combining data from two sham-controlled ECT studies, Buchan et al. (1992) dichotomously classified patients according to the presence versus absence of delusions or psychomotor retardation. Among those with retardation, with or without concomitant delusions, ECT separated from sham ECT at 4 weeks. In the group with non–psychomotorically retarded delusional patients (a small group), ECT did not separate from sham. The addition of delusions to psychomotor retardation seemed to enhance specific ECT efficacy versus sham. Hickie et al. (1990) found in a sample of depressed ECT patients that degree of psychomotor abnormalities in psychomotorically retarded patients positively correlated with degree of improvement in depressive symptoms.

Depressed patients with the most severe degrees of psychomotor slowing or agitation often cannot engage in a sufficiently rational discussion to consent to participation in research studies. Such patients usually are elderly and psychotic and have prominent information processing difficulties. ECT consent often is substituted (i.e., provided by family members), and such patients are rarely enrolled in controlled ECT research. Thus, the true robustness of the predictability of psychomotor abnormalities for ECT response may be underestimated in the published research studies because the most severely affected patients are not represented therein.

Suicidality. It has been axiomatic for decades in the ECT literature and clinical lore that ECT is associated with excellent reductions in suicidal tendencies (Abrams 2002). Suicide ratings on depression rating scales drop substantially and predictably over a course of treatments (Kellner et al. 2005). Speed of response in depression treated with ECT is also faster than what is traditionally noted in depression treated with antidepressants (Husain et al. 2004). Additionally, there is evidence that the suicide reduction potential of ECT may extend beyond the acute course. Huston and Locher (1948a, 1948b), analyzing data from a large psychiatric hospital system before and after the introduction of ECT, found that on follow-up, suicide rates were diminished in discharged patients after the introduction of ECT. However, there are no data from randomized controlled trials of ECT versus other treatments documenting that ECT actually reduces suicide rates. Munk-Olsen et al. (2007), analyzing data from a very large cohort of psychiatric patients discharged from psychiatric hospitals in Sweden over a 25-year period, found an 18% reduction in all-cause mortality at long-term follow-up in ECT-treated versus non-ECT-treated patients. However, suicide rates were 20% *higher* in the ECT-treated patients, an effect that seemed to be true mostly in the 7-day period immediately after hospital discharge. There are multiple reasons why the ECT-treated patients may have had a higher suicide rate, probably mostly because they had more psychopathology to begin with.

The expression "not all suicidality is created equal" is probably the best way of getting across the point that suicidality in isolation is not an indication for ECT. That is, ECT does not have a "broad spectrum" anti-suicide action in the same way that aspirin has antipyretic activity regardless of the cause of the fever. Suicidal ideations secondary to uncontrolled physical discomfort or pain, a personality disorder (such as borderline personality disorder [BPD]), a crippling anxiety disorder, or the painful memories of posttraumatic stress disorder [PTSD], in the absence of meeting the criteria for a depressive episode, will not respond to ECT. In contrast, suicidality secondary to major depression is a strong indication for ECT.

Depressive pseudodementia. *Pseudodementia* refers to the syndrome, coined by the Australian psychiatrist Leslie Kiloh (1961), consisting of dense cognitive deficits, typically in the realm of information processing, that abate with remission of the depression. The syndrome is striking and usually occurs in elderly patients or younger patients who are deeply psychotic. One of the reasons that the syndrome as a predictive variable has not been discussed in the literature is that such patients cannot typically provide consent for research projects—they simply cannot process the information for the consent form, and, indeed, consent for ECT itself is often provided by a family member. Additionally, cognitive impairment does not appear specifically in any of the depressive subtypes in DSM, even though it probably should. The depressed patient with this clinical picture is an excellent candidate for ECT. One caveat, especially in the elderly, is that cognitive impairment may be partly or completely secondary to a neurodegenerative dementing syndrome, which of course will not improve with ECT. The depressive syndrome may abate nicely in dementia patients with ECT. The diagnostic distinction between dementia and pseudodementia can be difficult. If characteristic signs of a mood disorder are present along with psychomotor abnormalities and negativistic depressive cognitions (e.g., nihilism, suicidality), then a course of ECT is probably indicated, though one may over time appreciate emerging signs of dementia.

Comorbid Psychopathology

Many depressed patients, especially those with some modicum of chronicity in their picture, have psychiatric comorbidities that probably affect ECT responsivity. For example, Zorumski et al. (1986) found that patients with primary depression responded better to ECT than did patients whose depression was secondary to another psychopathological syndrome. This section will address some considerations in ECT patient selection for depressed patients with psychiatric comorbidity. Surprisingly, overall there is little research on the efficacy of ECT in treating depression and improving quality of life in patients with comorbid psychopathology. The lack of research is disappointing, given how common such comorbidity is in this population.

Anxiety disorders.   Primary anxiety disorders and symptoms will not respond to ECT. However, during depressive episodes, patients may develop secondary anxiety symptoms that may abate well with ECT. That is, severely depressed patients often develop panic attacks, generalized anxiety, phobic avoidance, social anxiety, obsessions, compulsions, or ruminations about past traumatic life events. Elucidating the longitudinal course of illness is critical in establishing whether the anxiety symptoms are due to an exacerbation of a chronic anxiety disorder or are related to a primary depressive episode. If the symptoms are secondary to the depressive episode, the clinician can expect resolution with ECT. The more difficult ECT-related decision is whether to treat a severe depressive episode that occurs supplementary to, or secondary to, a chronic anxiety disorder. Even with effective acute ECT response, rapid relapse rates can be expected if the primary anxiety disorder is not also treated effectively in some manner. A relatively common scenario is the patient who presents with what on first blush appear to be depressive symptoms, and even suicidality. However, on further investigation of the longitudinal course of illness, it may become apparent that the primary diagnosis is chronic generalized anxiety disorder, now with an acute worsening usually in the face of increasing psychosocial stressors. Even though the patient may be suicidal and have "neurovegetative" signs such as poor sleep and appetite, ECT is not likely to be dramatically effective because the depression is not primary. The astute clinician must be able to distinguish generalized anxiety disorder with acute worsening from primary depression. Patients with obsessive-compulsive disorder (OCD) may be disabled and subject to bouts of demoralization therein, but ECT does not generally help in such situations. The clinician must clearly differentiate major depressive symptoms from chronic OCD symptoms in order to elaborate whether ECT is worth pursuing. In patients with chronic, complex PTSD, a similar situation occurs, and ECT does not help that syndrome. Finally, hypochondriacal worry (i.e., anxiety about physical symptoms and illnesses) is common. If this is the primary psychopathology, in DSM-5 (American Psychiatric Association 2013) it is conceptualized as an anxiety disorder—namely, health anxiety. Such patients are not good ECT candidates because the primary psychopathological syndrome is an anxiety disorder. If, however, such symptoms only occur during depressive episodes, then ECT can help. Commonly, psychotically depressed patients or otherwise severely depressed patients with somatic ruminations will obtain dramatic relief of somatic symptoms with ECT.

Eating disorders.   Patients with eating disorders often become depressed. Patients with depression secondary to chronic anorexia rarely obtain meaningful, lasting relief from ECT. Patients with psychotic or melancholic depression often lose weight because of loss of appetite, and this condition, of course, must be differentiated from a true eating disorder. Psychotically depressed patients may have poor food intake due to delusions pertaining to their gastrointestinal tract or to the content of food, and in such patients this might be mistaken as anorexia, but good history taking will clarify whether the source of the weight loss is due to body image distortion. Individuals with bulimia tend to be young women and also get depressed, but again, their illness is usually not responsive to ECT. A lot of these young individuals with bulimia are not severely impaired and obtain their mental health care as outpatients, and the issue of ECT never arises. However, the ones who are admitted to the hospital tend to have a lot of psychiatric comorbidities, such as personality dysfunction, trauma-related symptoms, and suicidality. In this scenario, ECT may be brought up as an option. ECT is not indicated unless a clearly elucidated major depressive episode, as opposed to the other comorbidities, is present.

Personality disorders.   There is a fairly robust literature supporting the notion that patients with BPD either obtain less relief from acute ECT or have more rapid relapses after apparently successful index ECT (DeBattista and Mueller 2001; de Vreede et al. 2005; Feske et al. 2004; Prudic et al. 2004; Rasmussen 2015a). This literature ties in with the older attempts at predictive indices with ECT (Rasmussen 2011a). In those studies, some of the factors that fairly consistently predicted more negative outcomes with ECT seem similar to symptoms and signs in the modern DSM conceptualization of BPD, such as hypochondriasis, hysterical attitudes, neuroticism, emotional lability, and high mood reactivity. Capriciousness of mood reactivity and interpersonal relationships generally presages poor ECT outcome.

There are three reasons why a patient with BPD may not obtain as complete an antidepressant response to ECT as a depressed patient without this personality disorder. First, if the dysphoric and negativistic ideational features are all accounted for by the personality disorder, and there really is no separate major depressive episode, then ECT is not indicated. It is therefore incumbent on the clinician to perform a thorough diagnostic evaluation to clarify this issue. Second, there is substantial overlap between the features of BPD and major depression, so that even if there is a separate major depressive episode that responds well to ECT, the features of borderline personality, which do not respond to ECT, will cause the patient to have features that result in an elevated depression rating scale score. This may account for some research that shows that final depression rating scale scores are higher post-ECT in depressed patients with BPD (Feske et al. 2004). Finally, it is possible that there may be something neurobiologically in the brains of BPD patients that mitigates against the therapeutic mechanism of ECT for depression.

Of course, there is no reason why a patient with a personality disorder cannot suffer from an otherwise ECT-responsive syndrome, such as a DSM-defined major depressive episode or psychotic depression. However, once such patients are relieved of their depression, they can be expected to return to their usual personality-disordered selves with attendant interpersonal dysfunctions, which are not treated by ECT unless they are clearly secondary to the depression. Thus, what may be a good ECT outcome in terms of symptoms or signs such as ruminative thinking, blunted emotionality, or psychomotor slowing may be masked by return to excess emotionality or neuroticism with negative affect. One published case in particular (Flint and Hill-Johnes 2008) outlines in detail the behavioral and interpersonal challenges and difficulties in trying to conduct ECT in borderline patients. If a patient is diagnosed with BPD, the clinician must ensure that the criteria for a separate major depressive episode are met before considering ECT. In other words, if all the dysphoric symptoms are accounted for by the borderline personality, then ECT is not indicated.

Somatic symptom (somatoform) disorder, factitious disorder, and malingering. The fundamental psychological dynamic of patients with somatic symptom (somatoform) disorder is a subconscious need to assume the sick role. One can easily appreciate that for such patients, ongoing ECT helps meet that need. That is, the patient is treated by nursing and medical staff with "tender loving care," is allowed to be freed from responsibility for a while, and has the "legitimacy" of the medical patient. One must be on the lookout for such patients because they tend to report depressive symptoms, be refractory to everything else that is tried, and request ECT inappropriately (Rasmussen and Lineberry 2007). It is common sense that "patients" with self-induced (factitious) or overtly faked (malingering) psychopathology should not be given ECT. Scenarios in which these issues come to bear include patients in legal trouble who believe that a course of ECT will get them off the hook for their crimes or those pursuing disability status who also believe receiving ECT will aid their disability application. It is good practice for an ECT clinician to inquire about disability and legal issues as part of the pre-ECT evaluation.

Chronic pain, fibromyalgia, and chronic fatigue. Many depressed patients seen by psychiatrists complain of chronic pain. There are reports of some pain syndromes improving with ECT (Rasmussen 2003; Rasmussen and Rummans 2000, 2002). Depression secondary to chronic pain is unlikely to benefit from ECT. A particularly bad omen is the chronically angry, narcissistic pain patient. ECT should be avoided for such people. These are the patients who may seem depressed but are bitter, especially about disability and other legal issues that might be involved in their onset of pain. On the other hand, many psychotically or otherwise deeply depressed patients will have some bodily pain or other somatic complaint secondary to the depressive syndrome. Such patients respond exquisitely well to ECT, so the distinction between these two syndromes (i.e., primary pain with secondary depression versus primary depression with secondary pain) is important to make.

Chronic fatigue and fibromyalgia have enjoyed some stylishness as diagnostic entities. The syndromes are probably what was called "neurasthenia" in times past. Many patients, especially middle-age women, carry the diagnoses these days and suffer mood problems as well. It is a common differential diagnostic challenge in psychiatric practice to try to determine the "which came first?" issue— does the patient primarily suffer a depressive disorder with the attendant fatigue and sensitivity to pain, or is there a primary somatoform disorder with secondary dysphoria? If the patient identifies the fatigue or fibromyalgia as primary, and there is no compelling evidence from mental status examination that depression is causing these complaints, then ECT is not indicated. Chronic, long-standing duration of these somatic symptoms also presages poor ECT outcome.

Substance use disorders.   It is rare that a patient only abuses substances while depressed, even though many patients insist that the only reason they are using is because of depression. For the patient who has been recently actively abusing drugs such as cocaine, methamphetamine, alcohol, or marijuana in large quantities, ECT should be withheld unless there is a full depressive syndrome clearly associated with psychosis, profound debilitation, or suicidality. Some longtime alcoholics can become depressed, and their depression seems to be relatively refractory to medications. One can expect lesser ECT response rates than in non-alcoholics. Ordinarily, the active alcoholic should be placed in a treatment program geared toward sobriety. If, however, depression renders him or her incapable of participating, then a course of ECT may be indicated first. The ECT practitioner must not think that ECT will cure a patient's alcoholism; substance abuse treatment must still be part of the long-term plan.

Dementia.   Dementia is common in modern psychiatric practice, especially as the population ages. Many dementia patients and patients with mild cognitive impairment develop depression, and numerous case reports and case series attest that ECT can be helpful for such patients (Burgut and Kellner 2010; Burgut et al. 2010; Hausner et al. 2011; Rao and Lyketsos 2000; Rasmussen et al. 2003; Takahashi et al. 2009). These reports included a mix of patients with suspected Alzheimer, Lewy body, and vascular dementias. What is sorely needed in this literature are longer-term studies assessing the progression of cognitive impairment in patients with neurodegenerative dementias such as those due to Alzheimer's disease and Lewy body disease with concomitant depression who are treated with ECT versus medications. Another challenge in this patient group is trying to distinguish between cognitive impairment due entirely to depression (pseudodementia) and that due to a dementing syndrome such as Alzheimer's disease. The difficulties of attempting in-depth neuropsychological testing to resolve this differential diagnostic issue may preclude precise determination. The practitioner may simply need to treat the depression as aggressively as needed, such as with ECT, and assess cognition over time to pinpoint the cognitive status.

While it seems logical to use ECT in dementia patients who are suffering from depression, it is a bit more novel to use ECT strictly for the agitated, sometimes violent behaviors that such patients evince. Agitation is common in patients with severe dementia, and behavioral or pharmacological strategies often fail. There is a case report literature substantiating that such patients may be calmed with a course of ECT (Burgut and Kellner 2010; Grant and Mohan 2001; Sutor and Rasmussen 2008; Wu et al. 2010). ECT has also been reported to be effective in the screaming dementia patient (Bang et al. 2008; Carlyle et al. 1991; Roccaforte et al. 2000). If an acute, index series of treatments results in substantial improvement, which is typically reported by staff members at nursing homes or family members, then if ECT is stopped, quick relapse over the next couple of weeks or so is the rule. Thus, maintenance ECT is needed to sustain the gains. Maintenance ECT may yield challenges in terms of patient consent and transportation issues. Consent issues in dementia patients are covered in the next chapter. If patients are living at home, it is very important that there be adequate supervision of their activities so that wandering off or inadvertently dangerous behavior (e.g., leaving a stove on) does not happen and that the "nothing by mouth" status the mornings of ECT treatments is maintained.

A Suggested Approach for Selecting Depressed Patients for ECT

There are two overall steps in deciding whom to offer ECT among depressed patients. The first is ensuring that the patient's presentation meets criteria for a major depressive (or bipolar depressive) episode, as opposed to common similar-looking syndromes such as adjustment disorder with depressed mood, persistent depressive disorder (dysthymia), other specified and unspecified depressive disorder, or an exacerbation of chronic generalized anxiety disorder. Second, among patients for whom ECT is deemed a likely efficacious treatment, there must be an appropriate clinical level of severity or lack of availability of other treatments because of either medical safety issues or treatment resistance (American Psychiatric Association Committee on Electroconvulsive Therapy 2001). Additionally, patients who previously had a good response to ECT or who express a preference for ECT might be treated first with this modality (American Psychiatric Association Committee on Electroconvulsive Therapy 2001).

Some commonly encountered scenarios do bear mention. First, psychotic depression should prompt consideration of ECT as a first-line treatment. There is no source of data over the decades of ECT use indicating less than optimal responding in this population, and pharmacotherapy regimens, even aggressive combinations of antidepressant/antipsychotic, have proven to be of low efficacy (Meyers et al. 2009). A caveat, though, is that the clinician must be certain that the psychopathology is not better described as BPD or chronic, complex PTSD, given that both often present in younger, and especially female, patients with features that might superficially mimic psychotic depression, which is usually seen in middle-age and older patients. Another diagnostic challenge is distinguishing between psychotic depression and delusional disorder. In the latter case, a primary psychotic ideation, usually persecutory, dominates the clinical picture for a prolonged period of time, culminating in hospitalization. The patient may appear angry and dysphoric, but delusional disorder does not respond well to ECT. Depression in the context of catatonia should also be considered a first-line indication for ECT (see section "Catatonia" later in this chapter).

The highly neurotic BPD patient is unlikely to respond well to or sustain improvement beyond a few days with ECT. The non–psychotically depressed patient with prominent psychiatric comorbidities, especially if the comorbid conditions are chronic and account for much of the patient's suffering and functional impairment, should also not be considered a candidate for ECT as a first-line treatment. For those patients, other modalities, including psychological and medication therapies, should be maximally pursued first unless the patient is unequivocally profoundly impaired by the depressive episode and not the comorbid conditions. As mentioned earlier, the melancholia specifier in modern DSM editions has not proved to be a good predictor of differential response to ECT, although if that specifier is applicable, the patient should have a good ECT response. The point is that nonmelancholic depressions meeting DSM criteria for major depressive episodes also respond well to ECT.

Once the clinician has determined that the psychopathological picture favors good outcomes with ECT for depression, there must be sufficient reason for pursuing this high-intensity treatment over medications or psychotherapy. The decision to treat with ECT means the patient must take a leave of absence from work or school, and a responsible adult must take time off to undertake the transportation requirements (for outpatients). For ECT to be indicated, the depressive episode must be of sufficient severity and involve a high enough level of functional impairment that waiting for the time-consuming action of other modalities to take effect would be unsafe. Thus, patients hospitalized for depression are often considered candidates for ECT. Patients who have been incapacitated functionally usually are hospitalized, and ECT is a good option for them.

If a patient can be safely treated as an outpatient and is still able to function with daily responsibilities (e.g., work, school, child care), then the decision of when to offer ECT is a balance between the degree of suffering and the inconveniences, cost, or side effects anticipated with ECT. Treatment resistance to medications is often considered an indication for ECT. However, the literature does not support an algorithmic approach to this issue. That is, there is no fixed number of medication trials that should be undertaken before it is universally agreed that ECT is indicated. After a patient has had nonresponse to one medication trial, deciding whether to offer ECT as opposed to continuing on to other pharmacotherapy options depends on how much suffering the patient is experiencing versus how difficult ECT would be to initiate. For example, if the patient has substantial fears about cognitive impairment, then that would favor going further with medication trials. On the other hand, patients who have had ECT before or have family members or other acquaintances who have had it with good results may be more comfortable initiating ECT without pursuing extensive pharmacotherapy trials. Probably the biggest challenge in selecting depressed patients for ECT is when to offer a depressed outpatient ECT versus more medications, and as has been emphasized, there is no currently accepted algorithm for making that decision.

When patients have been essentially debilitated by their depression, ECT is indicated. The common debilitating signs and symptoms of depression include profound psychomotor abnormalities, cognitive impairment not due to dementia, ruminative ideations, and psychosis. Slowing (retardation) or agitation in severe forms precludes functioning at work. Cognitive disruption (pseudodementia) is also debilitating. When a patient's mind has been consumed with ruminative ideations—for example, worries about somatic symptoms, finances, jobs, or relationships—or by psychotic ideations, then normal daily functioning is usually quite impaired, and ECT is a recommended treatment. Ruminations have been considered a core feature of clinical depression (Nelson and Mazure 1985). There is even a rating scale to assess severity of ruminative thinking, the Ruminative Responses Scale (Treynor et al. 2003). However, this scale consists of questions that are asked of patients about how much they are thinking of certain topics and thus represents their subjectively reported ruminative *symptoms*. It is patients who manifest *signs* of rumination who are particularly ECT-responsive. These are patients in whom conversation is dominated by the worries they have—the interviewer cannot get them to talk about anything else. Ironically, such patients would have a hard time completing the Ruminative Responses Scale because they cannot defocus from their ruminations!

A particularly common dilemma for the practitioner is whether to administer ECT to patients who have been non–psychotically depressed for years and whose illness has been refractory to numerous psychotropic agents and psychotherapy. Such patients are common in modern mental health practice. They often have low functional levels—that is, they are not employed, enrolled in school, or taking care of children and tend to be a burden on family members or receiving disability payments. ECT outcomes in such patients tend to be subtle, and if improvement is noted, these patients are at high relapse risk if maintenance treatments are not undertaken. It may be worth attempting a course of ECT in such patients, but extended courses of maintenance treatment should be avoided unless there is clear evidence of functional improvement and not just subjectively reported symptomatic improvement.

The oft-listed indication of ECT being the medically safest treatment option (American Psychiatric Association Committee on Electroconvulsive Therapy 2001) would seem to be a bit dated in modern times considering the plethora of safe antidepressant medications available. In other words, even though a patient may have a medical contraindication for one class of antidepressant (e.g., heart block and tricyclics), there is almost always some other medication that could safely be used. If a patient has a previous history of good response to ECT, then a current episode can justifiably be treated first off with ECT, especially if the previous episode was highly medication refractory and if the patient expresses a preference for ECT. It must be noted that the ECT clinician should provide patients and their significant relations with information about what could be expected with a course of ECT in terms of antidepressant benefit as well as cognitive side effects, expense, and inconvenience vis-à-vis other treatments. In this way, the patients can participate in the choice of ECT versus continued use of medications. Pre-ECT education and consent issues will be further discussed in Chapter 3. Table 2–1 summarizes some of the factors to weigh when deciding whether to use ECT in depressed patients.

Mania

In stark contrast to the heterogeneous, evanescent, and often subjective nature of the various conditions constituting "depression" in modern psychiatric diagnosis, the syndrome of mania is quite distinct and easily recognized, especially in severely ill, hospitalized patients. Because of their usual good response to medications, the rarity of mania relative to depression, and the difficulty obtaining consent, manic patients are not often referred for ECT.

The literature on ECT in mania is not nearly as extensive as that in depression, but it is rather unanimous in its enthusiastic endorsement of the efficacy of ECT for this condition. It was recognized shortly after the introduction of ECT that dramatic improvements in mania could occur with this new modality (see, e.g., Schiele and Schneider 1949). Patients who formerly were managed largely with restraints or nonspecific sedatives while caregivers awaited spontaneous recovery or death from exhaustion could, after 1938, be treated to remission with ECT.

The first controlled trial appears to be that of Langsley et al. (1959), in which a large group of patients with "schizophrenic or manic reactions," the precise psychopathological features of which are unspecified, were randomly allocated to receive either ECT or chlorpromazine. The two groups fared about equally on a number of nonblinded outcome assessments. This study was weakened by the lack of precise criteria and the apparent combination of patients with schizophrenia and those with mania into one group. Nonetheless, ECT was revealed to be as efficacious as chlorpromazine for psychotic patients.

The first report providing quantitative estimates of the antimanic efficacy of ECT appears to be that of Oltman and Friedman (1950), who found that after the introduction of ECT into their hospital system, the average duration of admission for manic patients fell dramatically. Similar results were later reported by McCabe (1976) and McCabe and Norris (1977), who extended the scope to compare admission length among manic patients treated before ECT, during a time when only ECT was used, and after the introduction of chlorpromazine. In

---

TABLE 2–1. Choosing ECT for depressed patients

Factors favoring the use of ECT in depressed patients

1. Presence of psychotic or catatonic features

2. Debilitating ruminative thinking

3. Depression-related cognitive dysfunction (i.e., pseudodementia)

4. Profound psychomotor retardation or agitation

5. Refusal to eat

6. Suicidal drive secondary to the depression

7. Severe functional decline

Factors weighing against using ECT for depressed patients

1. Borderline personality disorder that accounts for the depressive features

2. Recent active substance abuse

3. Strong psychiatric comorbidity that represents the primary disorder

---

the latter report, both active treatments were superior to prior lack of active treatment, and chlorpromazine nonresponders did respond well to ECT. Thomas and Reddy (1982) also retrospectively reviewed experience in a prior era at their hospital and compared lengths of stay and time to readmission among patients with mania treated with lithium, chlorpromazine, or ECT. All three treatments had roughly equal outcomes, though ECT was given twice weekly for only 2 weeks (i.e., four treatments), which is probably too few for full remission in many manic patients. Small et al. (1985), Milstein et al. (1987), and Mukherjee et al. (1988) all commented on the relative efficacy of unilateral versus bilateral electrode placement in ECT, an issue that will be dealt with in more detail in Chapter 7, which addresses ECT technique.

Black et al. (1986), analyzing a large cohort of patients with either unipolar or bipolar depression or mania, found that manic patients responded just as well to ECT as the depressive patients, further bolstering the notion that ECT has good antimanic properties. In a further report from this group, analyzing the outcomes of all manic patients treated during the same time period, those treated with lithium had lower remission rates compared with those treated with ECT (Black et al. 1987). Other retrospective series and reviews reported good efficacy of ECT for mania as well (Alexander et al. 1988; Milstein et al. 1987; Mukherjee et al. 1994; Small 1985; Small et al. 1988b, 1991; Strömgren 1988). Some data indicated that prominent anger or suspiciousness in manic patients predicted lesser response with ECT, but the sample sizes were quite small in that series (Schnur et al. 1992).

There are several modern controlled trials of the use of ECT for mania. Mukherjee et al. (1988) randomly assigned patients with DSM-defined mania to receive right or left unilateral ECT, bilateral ECT, or combination haloperidol-lithium therapy. The sample sizes were quite small, so no definitive conclusions could be reached, but overall, ECT was associated with a 54% response rate. Barekatain et al. (2008), Mohan et al. (2009), and Hiremani et al. (2008) all randomly assigned manic patients to receive ECT with various different electrode placement or stimulus parameter combinations and found ECT to be highly effective. Issues pertaining to specific ECT technique in manic patients will be further discussed in Chapter 7.

Small et al. (1988a) randomly assigned 34 manic patients to receive either ECT or lithium (17 in each group) and found that mania ratings somewhat favored ECT patients at 8 weeks. Posttreatment follow-up showed no difference between the two groups in relapse rates over 2 years. Most of the manic patients in both groups stabilized sufficiently with their randomized treatment to be discharged. Concomitant antipsychotic medication on an as-needed basis was allowed in the study.

The best controlled study of ECT for manic patients, in the author's opinion, was performed by Sikdar et al. (1994). These investigators treated all manic patients in the study with 600 mg chlorpromazine daily and randomly allocated the patients to either real or sham ECT. After the end of eight thrice-weekly sessions, the patients treated with real ECT experienced an 80% remission rate versus a 6.7% remission rate among patients who received chlorpromazine plus sham treatment, the difference being highly statistically and clinically significant. Nonremitting patients were further treated with higher chlorpromazine doses, and most eventually achieved remission. Duration of the manic episode was cut in half by augmentation of chlorpromazine with ECT. This study mimics clinical practice, in which the majority of manic patients treated with ECT have been given a neuroleptic medication before and are given one during ECT.

Finally, regarding patients with mixed manic-depressive states, Medda et al. (2010, 2015) reported similar overall response rates with ECT for such patients as for those with bipolar depression. Several other groups have found similar response rates for bipolar mixed patients as for patients with depressions (Ciapparelli et al. 2001; Devanand et al. 2000; Gruber et al. 2000). Chanpattana (2000) reported that the combination of clozapine and ECT was safe and effective for otherwise treatment-resistant mania.

Typical manic patients considered for ECT are behaviorally disruptive and dysphoric and angry rather than euphoric, and spend a good deal of time in restraints or seclusion, the latter constituting the syndrome known as "delirious mania." Efforts at pharmacotherapy in these usually uncooperative patients consist of neuroleptic injections. Occasionally, a euphoric manic patient may be referred for ECT after aggressive pharmacotherapy attempts have proven unsuccessful. A particularly rare syndrome—namely, chronic mania—usually renders the patient hospitalized for prolonged periods. Such patients' illnesses are often refractory to medications, or the patients are unwilling to take them, and so the patients are referred for ECT. This may be quite helpful in restoring euthymia, but maintenance treatments will be needed in such patients to sustain the benefits.

Fever and autonomic fluctuations may accompany the fulminant behavioral disruption in mania. This is an urgent indication for ECT. It probably represents a form of malignant catatonia, and as such, neuroleptic medications may worsen rather than improve the clinical status. The presence of fever in a manic patient would contraindicate use of neuroleptics as antimanic therapy (assuming there is no medical or neurological cause of the fever, such as an infection), and ECT may promptly cause the fever to abate.

There is no issue with manic patients regarding concomitant disorders of personality, anxiety, substance abuse, or other interpersonal traits or demographic/longitudinal course-of-illness factors that would mitigate against the efficacy of ECT in the depressed patient. In other words, once the syndrome of mania is confidently diagnosed, one can correctly assume the patient is a psychopathologically good candidate for ECT. Of course, if a manic patient does have a baseline set of psychiatric comorbidities that normally do not respond to ECT, those traits will become evident once again after the mania has abated. The main challenges in choosing which manic patient to treat with ECT lie not in psychopathological elaboration of comorbidities, but rather in determining how medication refractory a patient's illness must be before ECT is tried and legally valid consent is obtained. This decision usually involves balancing how behaviorally disruptive the patient is with how intensive the medication trial has been and how compliant the patient has been with taking the medications. The more fulminant the behavioral severity, the more quickly one will pursue ECT, which is at the least equal to any currently available pharmacotherapy option for mania in terms of efficacy. Special consent issues with manic patients are covered in Chapter 3.

Schizophrenia and Schizoaffective Disorder

A depressed patient may be rendered nondepressed with ECT, and a manic patient can be similarly rendered nonmanic with this modality. In contrast, a schizophrenic patient will not be rendered "nonschizophrenic" with ECT, something pointed out long ago in an early review of ECT for schizophrenia (Salzman 1980). In fact, if a patient so diagnosed seems to enjoy complete psychopathological remission with ECT, then the disorder was probably a mood disorder misdiagnosed as schizophrenia. Nonetheless, ECT can make the difference between chronic hospitalization and community living for some patients with schizophrenia. Two editorials (Fink and Sackeim 1996; Van Valkenburg and Clayton 1985) and an early influential paper (Small 1985) support ECT for schizophrenia. Of note, in this section, schizoaffective disorder, closely related to schizophrenia, is included but not specifically mentioned for economy of word usage.

Early large case series indicated that ECT could be helpful in the management of patients with schizophrenia (Kalinowsky 1943; Lesse 1959; Palmer et al. 1951). Over the past several decades, the psychopathological characterization of schizophrenia, especially as it is differentiated from bipolar disorder, has undergone extensive changes, rendering the clinical utility of the early reports questionable. In all likelihood, some of the early "ECT in schizophrenia" case series were heavily represented by patients who would now be diagnosed with mania or psychotic depression.

In modern case series using currently utilized diagnostic criteria, there is a literature suggesting a synergistic effect of neuroleptics and ECT for patients with acute schizophrenic psychoses. Gujavarty et al. (1987) described in detail eight patients with schizophrenia diagnosed according to DSM-III criteria who had mostly positive symptoms and signs and whose illnesses were refractory to at least two adequate neuroleptic medication trials. Five of the patients had excellent recovery of function as well as symptomatic improvement with courses of ECT, which generally consisted of more treatments than the average depressed person would receive (a range of 5–23 treatments). Follow-up at 6 and 12 months, without intervening maintenance ECT, generally showed sustained improvement. Friedel (1986) reported on nine patients with DSM-III schizophrenia that was refractory to thiothixene trials with adequate blood levels and found excellent antipsychotic benefits with unilateral or bilateral ECT treatments, ranging from 8–25 treatments per patient. Benefits were sustained without maintenance ECT for several months in most of these patients. As was the case with the Gujavarty et al. (1987) report, no formal rating scales were used to assess psychopathology. In particular, only information on flagrant psychosis, and not negative signs of schizophrenia, was presented. It is likely that these patients continued to display the chronic negative signs of schizophrenia, such as amotivation or lack of emotional expression.

Childers and Therrien (1961) found that among neuroleptic nonresponders, about half enjoyed a seemingly good response when an aggressive course of ECT was added to the drug. Kales et al. (1999) added ECT to clozapine nonresponders and found at least temporary benefits in most of their group of five patients. Hustig and Onilov (2009) followed 27 schizophrenia patients who were given ECT for suboptimal medication response and found that most of these patients seemed to improve, and about one-third of them maintained the gains over a year. König and Glatter-Götz (1990) studied a series of patients with neuroleptic-unresponsive schizophrenia and found that about two-thirds responded favorably to ECT. Lewis (1982) also reported on a series of 29 schizophrenia patients whose illness was nonresponsive to neuroleptics and most of whom had good acute reductions in symptoms and signs with ECT. McNeill (1977) suggested that short courses of ECT may render previously medication-nonresponsive schizophrenia patients medication responsive. This interesting notion has not been followed up in a controlled trial. Rahman (1968) reported on a large number of schizophrenia patients treated in a tertiary care hospital. Most were given neuroleptic medications to begin with, and ECT was added if response was suboptimal. Rahman found that ECT combined with a neuroleptic resulted in remission of signs in all patients thus treated and felt that it was superior to neuroleptic treatment alone, at least acutely. Weinstein and Fischer (1971) reported several schizophrenia patients who responded well to the addition of ECT to neuroleptic medication. Witton (1962) reported on two schizophrenia patients who also responded well to the addition of ECT to medication. Kho et al. (2004) found that ECT added to clozapine was beneficial. Sajatovic and Meltzer (1993) also reported benefit of adding ECT to medication.

Ray (1962) randomly allocated schizophrenia patients to receive medication alone, ECT alone, or the combination and found the last-mentioned the most beneficial. Smith et al. (1967) randomly assigned schizophrenia patients to receive either chlorpromazine or chlorpromazine plus ECT and found more rapid reductions in signs, earlier discharge, and less likelihood of relapse in the combined treatment group. Taylor and Fleminger (1980) randomly assigned 10 schizophrenia patients each to receive active versus sham index ECT, with all patients receiving standard doses of neuroleptic medication, and found a clear acute advantage of real over sham ECT. By several months' follow-up, this advantage had disappeared.

May et al. (1976, 1981), in a long-term follow-up study, randomly allocated hospitalized schizophrenia patients to various treatments, including medications, ECT, or no biologic therapy and found that those treated with ECT had better posthospital outcomes than those given no treatments and about the same outcomes as those treated with medications.

Tharyan and Adams (2005), in a very thorough meta-analysis published in the Cochrane Database, concluded that there is good evidence that ECT combined with neuroleptics in patients with neuroleptic-nonresponsive schizophrenia has at least good short-term efficacy. In another meta-analysis, Matheson et al. (2010) also concluded that the evidence is strongly in favor of an at least short-term benefit of ECT in schizophrenia with or without concomitant neuroleptic therapy. A final meta-analysis, by Greenhalgh et al. (2005), supports the short-term efficacy of ECT for schizophrenia.

Childers (1964), in a controlled trial involving ECT, assigned patients sequentially (which is not exactly the same as randomly but probably close enough) to treatment with ECT alone, one of two antipsychotic medications alone (fluphenazine or chlorpromazine), or ECT plus chlorpromazine. The group receiving combined treatment experienced the best outcomes by a substantial margin, and ECT add-on to the regimen of nonresponders in the medication-alone groups resulted in high response rates as well.

Bagadia et al. (1983) conducted a well-controlled trial in 78 schizophrenia patients who were randomly assigned to receive either real ECT plus placebo pill or sham ECT plus chlorpromazine. After 6 sessions of real or sham ECT, the groups had similar reductions in psychosis scores.

Brandon et al. (1985), analyzing data from the Leicestershire sham ECT trial, found that among 19 schizophrenia patients randomly assigned to real or sham ECT, those who received eight real treatments had more marked reductions in psychosis scores than did those who received sham treatments over the same time period. However, at 12- and 28-week follow-up, with interval treatments not controlled, the scores had equalized, with the effect due both to an upward trend among the real ECT patients and to a downward trend in the sham-treated patients. The latter patients had not been aggressively treated with antipsychotic medications during the active phase of the trial (nor had the real ECT patients)—undoubtedly, during the follow-up phase these patients were given such medications, which probably accounted for their improvement over time. This underscores the need for aggressive treatment post–index ECT to sustain initial improvement.

Janakiramaiah et al. (1982) randomly assigned schizophrenia patients to receive low- or high-dose chlorpromazine, with or without concomitant ECT, and found that ECT augmented only the lower, but not the higher, dose of the drug.

More recently, there has been a series of excellent reports from Thailand in which patients with acute psychotic episodes diagnosed as schizophrenia by modern DSM criteria were randomly allocated to receive neuroleptic medication alone (fluphenazine in this study), ECT alone, or the combination. The last-mentioned group had the most acute improvement in psychosis, while follow-up continuation ECT studies by this group indicated that the addition of continuation ECT to maintenance pharmacotherapy resulted in better functioning than the use of medication alone for the 6-month period after acute remission (Chanpattana 1998; Chanpattana et al. 1999a, 1999c, 1999d). Finally, a recent well-described case series from Baeza et al. (2010) with in-depth psychopathological assessments of adolescents with schizophrenia spectrum disorders found that ECT was well tolerated and helpful especially in reducing the positive signs of psychosis and thought disorder in this age range.

Thirthalli et al. (2009a) compared the speed of response to ECT among a group of catatonic versus noncatatonic schizophrenia patients and found that the former responded faster—a result confirming the long-held belief that catatonia responds particularly robustly to ECT.

These studies point to a place for ECT in the treatment of schizophrenia patients, but clearly it is not feasible to treat *all* schizophrenia patients with ECT. Why? Many of them would not consent and would not meet criteria for involuntary court-authorized treatment. There is also the practical matter of the expense and inconvenience of extended courses of ECT for young people. Attempts at employment or educational rehabilitation would be hampered by ongoing frequent ECT sessions because of cognitive impairment.

So which schizophrenia patients should be given ECT? There are three general scenarios. The first and probably most common is when the patient has chronic positive symptom/sign psychopathology and is essentially living at a state hospital and his or her illness is refractory to aggressive medication trials. Such signs as disorganized or disruptive behavior, catatonia, formal thought disorder, and delusions or hallucinations can respond well enough to a course of ECT that the patient can be transitioned to community living. It is important to note that the patient will still probably have negative signs of schizophrenia and will require ongoing maintenance ECT to sustain the gains through index ECT. The second, somewhat related scenario for ECT in schizophrenia is when the patient has chronic or acute fulminant positive symptom/sign psychopathology and aggressive pharmacotherapy, such as with clozapine, is impossible because of noncompliance. A course of ECT may render such a patient cooperative with pharmacotherapy such that ongoing maintenance ECT may not be necessary. The third scenario for ECT in schizophrenia patients is when the patient has achieved some modicum of stability in a community setting, such as a group home or at home with parents, but experiences an acute episode or flare-up, usually because of noncompliance with medication, an intercurrent medical illness, or some other psychosocial stressor. An index course of treatments may render the patient in his or her usual mental state, and maintenance ECT probably would not be necessary. Specific issues regarding continuation and maintenance ECT are covered in more detail in Chapter 8.

Questions arise regarding psychopathological predictors of success in schizophrenia, such as subtype (e.g., catatonic, paranoid, disorganized, undifferentiated, residual) or positive-negative symptom distribution. Chanpattana and Sackeim

(2010) and Chanpattana and Chakrabhand (2001), analyzing data from the Thai studies, found that higher severity of negative signs of schizophrenia, as well as longer duration of illness, correlated with lower response rates. Dodwell and Goldberg (1989) found in their 17-patient series that predictors of good outcome in schizophrenia patients with ECT included short total duration of illness, short duration of current episode, and presence of perplexity, while negative predictors included presence of premorbid personality traits of schizoidia or paranoia. Salzman (1980), in his review of predictors of ECT response in schizophrenia, noted that the literature up to that date was scarce in terms of well-controlled trials and that, in general, chronic signs of illness tended not to respond well to ECT, whereas coexisting affective and catatonic signs did respond well.

Catatonia

The first patient treated with ECT was catatonic, and he enjoyed a dramatic improvement, with return to community living after having spent years in an asylum (Shorter and Healy 2007). Catatonia is a syndrome that occurs as part of mood disorder episodes (usually in bipolar patients), as part of schizophrenia, secondary to acute medical or neurological disorders or substances, and occasionally in isolation and not as part of any of these. All forms of catatonia respond exquisitely well to ECT. Use of the benzodiazepine lorazepam has been shown to lift a substantial proportion of patients with catatonia out of that state, and of course lorazepam is more immediately available and easily used than ECT, so it rightly constitutes a first-line treatment (American Psychiatric Association Committee on Electroconvulsive Therapy 2001). Oftentimes, however, even though lorazepam may cause the catatonic signs to abate, the patient is still left with underlying mood episodes or schizophrenic psychosis that requires other treatment. In such cases, ECT of course is a definitive treatment option. A particularly fulminant form of catatonia, with accompaning fever and autonomic instability, is termed *malignant catatonia*. This may be caused by neuroleptic medication (in which case it may be termed *neuroleptic malignant syndrome*)—again, ECT can be lifesaving for such patients. Occasional patients have had neurological illnesses such as viral encephalitis and are left with the acute phase of the illness abated but with continued catatonic signs, which may respond quite well to a course of ECT.

A series reported by van Waarde et al. (2010a) provides in-depth descriptions of a large (N=27 patients) cohort of catatonic patients, about half of whom had mood disorders or schizophrenia. Fifty-nine percent of the patients were felt to be improved with ECT. The patients were treated on average 2 months after the diagnosis of catatonia was made, indicating the need for prompt ECT treatment in this fulminantly ill population. In fact, among the 11 non-ECT-responding patients in this study, 3 died in the year of follow-up because of medical morbidities. Suzuki et al. (2004) painted a favorable picture of the 1-year outcomes in catatonic schizophrenia patients treated with ECT. The relative rarity of catatonia and the lack of patients' ability to consent to research have rendered the literature on this topic much smaller than that for depression.

ECT in Neurological Disorders

Given the profound and widespread neurometabolic changes that occur during seizures, it is not surprising that there are several neurological conditions that improve with ECT. While none of these would be considered a standard indication for this treatment, there is a literature supporting the occasional use of ECT for them.

Parkinsonism

It was not long after the discovery of ECT that some clinicians reported that signs of Parkinson's disease (i.e., tremor, bradykinesia, rigidity) improved with ECT (Fromm 1959). However, this potentially interesting and important early finding was rather ignored in the ECT literature until many years later, when numerous case reports and small case series rekindled interest in the possible antiparkinsonian benefit of ECT (for reviews, see Faber and Trimble 1991 and Rasmussen and Abrams 1991). In 1987, a somewhat landmark study was published out of Sweden in which a group of Parkinson's disease patients with well-quantified movement abnormalities were randomly assigned to receive either real or sham ECT (Andersen et al. 1987). Those patients receiving real ECT demonstrated significant improvements in motor functioning, specifically "on" time during the day, compared with the sham-treated patients. Other in-depth case series from Douyon et al. (1989), Balldin et al. (1981), and Ward et al. (1980) confirmed these findings. There seemed to be some enthusiasm brewing in the literature during this time (Abrams 1989; Fink 1988) that ECT might be used as a treatment for Parkinson's disease. However, the neurology community never embraced this idea. ECT is rarely used for the motor signs of parkinsonism, but authors still encourage more research (Popeo and Kellner 2009). Interestingly, ECT has been reported to abort neuroleptic-induced parkinsonism in patients co-treated with neuroleptic medication (Mukherjee and Debsikdar 1994).

Parkinson's disease patients frequently become depressed or psychotic, and ECT can be used for those syndromes. The ECT practitioner might expect that the motor symptoms of the disease may get better, and can even tell the patient this, but the reported experience is highly variable in terms of response. Even in those patients who do enjoy a substantial motor improvement with ECT, there may be a rapid relapse if no maintenance ECT is used, although some authors have reported long-lasting improvements in a few patients treated only with index ECT (Pridmore et al. 1995). Although Parkinson's disease is not a standard indication for ECT, it is justifiable as a treatment option if a patient is disabled and the informed consent process thoroughly emphasizes the experimental nature of ECT in that setting. Technical recommendations for treating Parkinson's patients with ECT will be covered in Chapter 7.

Tardive Dyskinesia ·

Tardive dyskinesia is a syndrome caused by long-term administration of neuroleptic medication in which mostly choreiform movements, usually of the mouth but sometimes affecting other body regions, occur. These can be permanent even if the offending medication is removed, and, indeed, there can even be worsening of the movements on medication discontinuation (a process termed *withdrawal dyskinesia*). Most such patients have psychotic conditions as the indication for the neuroleptic medication (e.g., schizophrenia or bipolar disorder), and so it is not surprising that ECT is occasionally offered. Case series on the use of ECT in patients with tardive dyskinesia are mixed in terms of the effect on the movement disorder, with some groups reporting improvement (Besson and Palin 1991; Chacko and Root 1983; Gosek and Weller 1988; Hay et al. 1990; Nobuhara et al. 2004; Price and Levin 1978) and others reporting either no change or worsening (Asnis and Leopold 1978; Holcomb et al. 1983). In two of the case series, the immediate reduction in dyskinetic movements was sustained on long-term follow-up over a year (Chacko and Root 1983; Gosek and Weller 1988). Interestingly, three epidemiological studies looking at the possible moderating effect of ECT on tardive dyskinesia prevalence have been published, with two finding that prevalence is lower in patients with a history of having had ECT (Go et al. 2009; Schwartz et al. 1993) and one showing ECT as an apparent risk factor for tardive dyskinesia (Struve 1985).

ECT is not indicated for tardive dyskinesia alone, although if a particular patient has a very severe, disabling case and no medications have helped, ECT can be broached as an experimental approach that might lead to worsening as well as benefit. An interesting series pertinent to this issue was reported by Sandyk (1990), who found among a group of bipolar patients, all of whom had tardive dyskinesia, that only those patients with orofacial involvement responded psychopathologically to ECT, as opposed to those with limb-axial involvement. There was no information given in this communication about the effects of ECT on the dyskinetic movements.

Dystonia

There are case reports of patients with either tardive dystonia (from neuroleptic usage) or idiopathic dystonia enjoying some benefit from ECT (Adityanjee et al. 1990; Garcia et al. 2009; Kwentus et al. 1984; Lauterbach and Moore 1990; Manteghi et al. 2009; Postolache et al. 1995; Sharma et al. 2007; Sienaert and Peuskens 2005), although ECT-induced worsening (Hanin et al. 1995) and no apparent effect (Sienaert et al. 2009a) have been reported as well. In several of these cases, the results were short-lived with index ECT. Thus for dystonia, as for tardive dyskinesia, ECT is an experimental intervention only used for a severe, disabling case of dystonia, with proper attention to adequate information being provided during the informed consent process. Additionally, if a particular dystonic patient otherwise has the psychopathological features indicating ECT, then the patient can be told that there may be improvement of the dystonia but there is also the possibility of worsening.

Neuroleptic Malignant Syndrome

Neuroleptic malignant syndrome is a fulminant, sometimes fatal neuroleptic-induced syndrome manifested by fever, rigidity, and autonomic instability (Strawn et al. 2007). Usual interventions consist of supportive care in an intensive care unit, and medications can include antipyretics, muscle relaxants, benzodiazepines, and dopamine agonists (Owens 2011). There are numerous case reports showing that ECT can cause the syndrome to abate (Trollor and Sachdev 1999). ECT is usually pursued after other measures have failed.

Delirium

Delirium is a syndrome manifested by diminution of consciousness with sharp fluctuations over the circadian cycle and hypoactive or hyperactive motor activity. Such patients can be quite agitated and require large doses of neuroleptic medication to calm down. There are many medical, neurological, and toxic causes of delirium, which usually clears with supportive care and treatment of the underlying condition. However, occasionally there is a patient with a fulminant, prolonged hyperactive delirium that persists after the underlying etiology is stabilized and that is refractory to neuroleptics. Relatively recently reported cases of neurologically induced deliria found ECT to be occasionally dramatically effective (Rasmussen et al. 2008b). These circumstances are quite rare, even at busy tertiary referral centers. The usual scenario involves a patient with documented viral encephalitis or autoimmune limbic encephalitis (e.g., anti–NMDA receptor antibody mediated) who is in a prolonged agitated state despite having received whatever treatment is available for the neurological condition. Such patients should be offered ECT, although as a nonstandard treatment. This fact should be broached as part of the informed consent process, which is undertaken with family members or other involved parties, as the patients typically cannot participate. Of historical interest, the syndrome of alcohol withdrawal delirium (*delirium tremens*) was once commonly treated with ECT, with good efficacy (Dudley and Williams 1972).

Epilepsy

Probably the most fascinating of the neurological conditions treated with ECT is epilepsy. How could one treat seizures with seizures? It was actually surprisingly early after the discovery of ECT, but before the era of anti-epileptic medications, that this new modality was found to help control spontaneous seizure frequency in epileptic patients (Shorter and Healy 2007). A series of electrically induced seizures has potent anticonvulsant properties, as manifested by ever-increasing amounts of electrical charge needed to induce a seizure over a course of treatments (Sackeim et al. 1987b). There are a few modern case studies in which ECT has been used to reduce spontaneous seizure frequency in patients with epilepsy with highly frequent uncontrolled seizures (Griesemer et al. 1997). However, the effects of an acute course of treatment would probably be short-lived, and such use is extremely rare with modern methods of epilepsy treatment. The potentially lethal syndrome of status epilepticus has been reported to be responsive to ECT in rare cases when all other routine measures have been exhausted (Kamel et al. 2010). Technical factors in delivering ECT to depressed, manic, or psychotic patients who happen to have epilepsy are covered in Chapter 7.

Key Points

- Proper patient selection is the most challenging aspect of ECT practice and is critical to avoid giving the treatment to those who will not respond and withholding it from those who would respond.

- Depression is the most common indication for ECT.

- Psychotically depressed patients respond exquisitely well to ECT.

- Patients with mania, schizophrenia, or catatonia also respond well to ECT.

3

Patient Education and Informed Consent for ECT

After patient selection is the education and informed consent process. This includes first broaching the procedure as an offered treatment, then educating the patient and significant others about it, and obtaining informed consent. In this chapter, these steps will be covered, with recommendations for handling various difficulties that occur. For the interested reader, Ottosson and Fink (2004) have published a monograph discussing various aspects of the ethics of electro convulsive therapy (ECT) administration and informed consent.

Broaching ECT With a Patient

A simple starting line can be the following: "I recommend a treatment known as electroconvulsive therapy, or ECT. Have you heard of this type of treatment?" The response helps the clinician understand what the patient's preexisting attitudes are, for this latter issue will decide how to proceed next. Sometimes the patient vigorously indicates a negative attitude toward ECT when the subject is first broached. The clinician can then acknowledge the patient's lack of desire to discuss ECT further but ask if the clinician can at least describe ECT—sometimes the patient will say no, but sometimes, even with preexisting hostility toward ECT, the patient is still willing to at least listen to what the clinician has to say. Exploring the basis for negative attitudes can be helpful. Such attitudes might be based on a previous bad experience either personally or in a family member or may stem from discussions with other patients or things the patient has heard from media sources (e.g., movies, news stories, internet content).

If the patient agrees to proceed with ECT discussion, the clinician can describe the process. The following can serve as a generic template for this initial description of ECT:

> ECT has been in use since 1938 and is used virtually all over the world. ECT involves a series of treatments, usually given twice or three times a week until the patient is well, and this usually takes 2–4 weeks. Each treatment consists of the use of an electrical current applied to the head to cause a seizure, performed under anesthesia. This does sound like a strange procedure, but the reason it has been used so long is that it is very helpful.
>
> Each treatment starts with an intravenous line in a vein, followed by some medication to cause sleep (i.e., anesthesia), and there is no awareness from that moment on until the procedure is finished. Next, muscle-paralyzing medication is given to dampen the shaking of the arms and legs that ordinarily would happen during a seizure. After the patient is asleep and the muscles are relaxed, two electrodes about the size of credit cards are placed on the head. They are like thick tape [NB: unless metal electrodes are used] and stick to the head. These electrodes are connected via a thin cable to the ECT machine. When the button on the machine is pressed, electricity is sent through the cables, into the electrodes, and from there into the head all the way to the brain, which causes a seizure. Normally during a seizure, the arms and legs shake, but because of the muscle-relaxing medication given a few minutes earlier, this does not happen, though there may be a little movement of the feet or hands. We also know the seizure is happening because we monitor brain waves through EEG [electroencephalography]. All this time, heart rate, blood pressure, heart rhythm, and blood oxygen are being monitored on the machine. Personnel at the head of the bed are giving oxygen through a mask. The seizure typically lasts about 20–60 seconds, sometimes more or less, and ends on its own. Then the anesthetic medications wear off and the patient resumes breathing. Next, the patient is moved to the recovery room for 30–45 minutes or so until awake and alert, and then he or she goes back to the hospital room if an inpatient or home if an outpatient. The whole procedure is repeated, usually every other day or twice weekly, until we determine that maximal improvement has occurred.
>
> This is a lot of information to absorb. Are there any questions thus far?

Of course, this suggested description of ECT will vary depending on geographic location, patient comprehension skills, psychopathological features, presence of other interested parties such as family members, and the patient's propensity to ask questions along the way. Also, some patients may not be able to process cognitively all this information, and the clinician can modify the description accordingly. Further description follows:

> ECT is highly effective, but of course improvement is not guaranteed. There are possible side effects, including muscle aches, headaches, and nausea or vomiting on the days of treatment. These may be uncomfortable but are not serious and are easily managed and treated. Medical complications such as heart attack, stroke, or death from treatment are extremely rare. We do a medical evaluation before treatments to ensure we are being as safe as possible in identifying medical issues.
>
> The main side effect that bothers people with ECT is memory impairment. This takes three forms. First, after the treatment it may take anywhere from a few minutes to several hours to feel alert and aware of what is going on. Patients need to be monitored by a responsible adult if an outpatient as there may be confusion as to directions and where to go and what is going on. Gentle reminders from others about what is going on are helpful during this time period.
>
> The second type of memory impairment from ECT is forgetting things that happened prior to the treatments. Usually, events happening during the few months prior to treatment are forgotten the most, say up to about 6 months or so, but there can be spotty forgetting of events going back years prior to the treatments. Some of these memories may come back after ECT is done, but some may not. Thus, ECT can cause a permanent loss of personal memories and knowledge, even events up to 1 or 2 weeks after the treatments are finished. The kinds of things that are forgotten include anything new learned during this time, such as the names of new acquaintances. If the patient is in school or employed, recent projects may be forgotten and may need to be relearned. This forgetting of personal life events is variable from person to person and hard to predict, and people react to it differently. Generally, we find that if patients successfully get out of their depression, they are less bothered by the memory impairment than if there is no improvement in the depression. The treatment team monitors memory throughout the course of treatments to assess for problems that may be occurring and can alter such things as how frequently the treatments are given or even stop the treatments if the memory loss is too bothersome. Some people are highly bothered by the ECT memory impairment.
>
> Finally, the third type of memory impairment with ECT is forgetting newly learned information. For example, during a course of treatments, the patient may watch a TV show one night and the next day forget he or she has done so. Thus, new memories become "slippery," so to speak. This type of memory impairment, though it can be bothersome, is not permanent. The ability to remember newly learned information goes back to normal within a few days to weeks of stopping ECT.
>
> Although these memory issues do happen with ECT, a lot of depressed people don't concentrate and focus well while depressed, and ECT can help this dramatically, so that after a course of treatments a lot of patients feel they are mentally sharper and more focused than before the treatments.

Patients who have never heard of ECT before may be a bit taken aback by this large amount of information and need time to process it and talk with relatives. Such conversations should be encouraged as well as the patient's taking time to think about ECT, review educational materials, come up with more questions, and talk with other trusted health providers (e.g., another psychiatrist, a primary care physician, nursing staff if an inpatient). The degree of detail may be modified depending on the patient's psychopathology. On one extreme is the highly agitated, hostile patient (usually a patient with mania, schizophrenia, or excited catatonia) with whom conversation may be virtually impossible. Consent in these cases is almost always substituted, though along the way attempts should be made to communicate the process to the patient as best as possible. On the other extreme is the patient who has researched ECT prior to the initial discussion or who has had ECT before. These may be patients referred specifically for ECT by another psychiatrist. Such patients may already be familiar with ECT technical details such as electrode placement and stimulus parameters. Conversations with such patients may be extensive.

This raises the very important question of whether issues of ECT technique (e.g., electrode placement, treatment frequency, stimulus parameter combinations) should be discussed with every patient. The American Psychiatric Association Committee on Electroconvulsive Therapy (2001) report recommends that electrode placement be discussed as part of the informed consent process. However, the thoughtful psychiatrist can tailor the discussion to the needs of the patient. Patients who inquire about the issue of electrode placement, of course, need to have their questions answered. However, some patients simply cannot process this type of information, whether because of agitation or because of information processing deficits of severe psychomotor retardation. It is not necessary to try to "review the literature" as a matter of routine with each patient. Ultimately, the informed consent process is basically founded on trust—it is impossible to make patients so knowledgeable about ECT that they can essentially pick their own technique like ordering from a restaurant menu. Patients agreeing to ECT ultimately should trust their doctors.

An interesting scenario is when a patient specifically requests a certain technique, such as right unilateral electrode placement, and will not consent to bitemporal. Should the practitioner treat the patient using the requested placement even if he or she disagrees about the placement? Individual practitioners must decide for themselves, but mostly in such circumstances it would be appropriate to document the conversation with the patient in the chart and proceed with the desired technique, with the notion that if it fails, eventually the patient may agree to changes. Another common clinical challenge occurs when a patient is receiving bitemporal ECT and, after several treatments, forgets what ECT is or does not remember having given consent earlier. In such cases, reminders need to be given, and the patient may need to be shown the consent document that was signed.

During the initial discussion phase of ECT consent, patients should not be badgered into agreeing to ECT. Under no circumstances should false information be given to inveigle a patient into consenting.

Educating Patients and Families About ECT

Educational documents are a good idea and come in two forms, either written brochures or videodiscs that are commercially available. Written brochures are relatively inexpensive for even modestly financially endowed hospitals to produce and have the advantage of being tailored to a specific hospital ECT service. Battersby et al. (1993) showed that educational videos enhance positive patient attitudes toward ECT. If possible, ECT services should produce their own educational videos that can also be tailored to local procedures. However, this is probably too expensive for smaller hospitals, in which case commercially available videos can be purchased. The ECT clinician pursuing this option is advised to view available videos first to screen them for suitability and accuracy.

Some patients may wish to read books about ECT. There are several written by people who have had ECT and have a favorable attitude toward this treatment (e.g., Dukakis and Tye 2007; Endler 1982; Manning 1995). Max Fink has written an educational book intended for patients and families (Fink 2009). Of course, highly motivated patients can read any one of the texts on ECT. Most patients do not have the time or inclination to read books, however, because of the effects of their depression on focus and concentration and because they trust their physician. It is likely that patients who read ECT-related books are doing so long after the treatments are finished to satisfy curiosity. It is unlikely that an ECT clinician will encounter a patient during the pre-ECT education process who desires to read a book before proceeding.

Another source of potentially educational material for patients is the internet. One need only go to a common search engine on the internet and type in "ECT" or a synonym, and up will pop countless links to web pages of all sorts. Some of them will appear serious and informative to ECT clinicians. Others will be mordantly anti-ECT and filled with horrible-sounding information. It is not uncommon for patients to have performed their own internet searches. Interestingly, patients who do this tend to grasp the questionable accuracy of the anti-ECT vitriol to be found.

Obtaining Informed Consent

Capacity to Consent to ECT

Patients can be divided into those who accept versus those who refuse ECT and, further, into those who have the capacity to consent versus those who do not. Thus, there are four combinations. Those who are deemed to have capacity to consent and accept ECT are given the treatment; those who are judged to have capacity to consent and refuse ECT are not given the treatment. Those who are deemed to lack capacity to consent should have substituted consent. The particulars of the latter depend on local laws governing ECT. For example, in some jurisdictions, ECT can be legally administered to an agreeable, or assenting, patient who lacks capacity if a responsible family member provides consent. In other jurisdictions, formal court procedures must be undertaken to appoint a substituted consenter.

The issue becomes clouded when we speak of "capacity" as a single, unitary phenomenon. Clearly there are patients who are mute, thought disordered, or so hostile that they simply cannot engage in conversation enough regarding consenting to ECT. These patients are deemed to lack capacity. On the other hand, some aspects of psychopathology render a patient's attitudes of questionable rationality, even if the patient can process basic information about diagnosis, ECT process and side effects, and possible alternative treatments. For example, a patient may be mentally sharp enough to understand ECT but so suicidal as to refuse because he or she wants to be left alone to die. Most physicians would favor petitioning for involuntary ECT in order to save a life. On the other hand, one would accept that patient's consent if he or she was willing to offer it. Capacity can be conceptualized as a set of abilities, including cognitive, emotional, behavioral, and ideational factors, any one of which may interfere with what physicians perceive as needed mental health care. From the cognitive standpoint, patients with dementia, delirium, developmental disorders or disabilities, or pseudodementia, or those who are extremely ruminative, might not be able to process information and understand ECT aspects. From an emotional standpoint, a patient may be so despairingly depressed or hostile that these factors interfere with the consent process. Agitated, violent patients may be behaviorally incapable of participating in conversation about ECT. Finally, from an ideational standpoint, delusional patients, who interestingly may be otherwise quite capable of all aspects of ECT consent, may refuse because of a psychotic belief—for example, that they really have a physical illness requiring more medical tests or interventions rather than a mental illness. Consent can generally be accepted from a patient who is able to participate in the ECT discussion. Obviously, there is a fine line here that does not lend itself to easy categorizations of those for whom to either accept refusal or petition for involuntary ECT. The pragmatic psychiatrist will take into account family preferences and of course may wish to consult with an attorney for clarification of local laws in difficult-to-decide cases.

The MacArthur Competency Assessment Tool (MacCAT-T) for treatment provides a good explanation of the fundamental elements of competence (Grisso et al. 1997). These are divided into four dimensions: a) understanding of various aspects of the decision to be made regarding treatment (e.g., the proposed treatment, expected benefits or side effects, and alternatives); b) reasoning, or the ability to apply logic to the understanding to reach a decision considering alternatives and pros and cons of those as well as the offered treatment; c) appreciation that the treatment in question applies to the patient and that there is the possibility of benefit; and d) expression of choice in treatment. Delusional patients typically are the ones who fall short on appreciation (e.g., the psychotically depressed patient who believes he or she has a physical illness in spite of medical testing). Of note, in the Grisso et al. (1997) case series testing the MacCAT-T, approximately one-fourth of psychotic patients on an inpatient unit could not even participate in the interview process because of cognitive impairment or behavioral agitation. Lapid et al. (2003) demonstrated that most patients undergoing ECT, even the elderly, have capacity to provide informed consent. Furthermore, the usual educational initiatives to help such patients result in improved scores on the MacCAT-T. Martin and Bean (1992) suggested that a few questions be asked of the patient to aid in determining capacity, pertaining to whether the patient is aware of being asked to make a decision about ECT, whether the patient is having trouble making the decision, and whether the patient wishes to make the decision or have someone else do that.

If during the course of the ECT decision-making process the clinician assesses the patient and determines that the patient lacks capacity to consent, what next? Such patients deserve ECT, of course, just like patients with capacity. The ECT clinician will need to be guided by local laws and hospital policies. In general, there will be substituted consent obtained from a next of kin, from a person with formal power of attorney or a guardian, or from a judge in a court of law, depending again on local statutes. A further factor to consider in this regard is the urgency of need for ECT: contrast the nonsuicidal outpatient with the mute, stuporous catatonic patient with a feeding tube. For the former, the treatment can wait until substituted consent is obtained according to local regulations; for the latter, it may not be suitable to wait, depending on how long the process will take. Consideration for undertaking emergency ECT before formal court proceedings will depend on whether such is allowable by local statutes. If not, and if there is no provision for signature of consent by next of kin, and there is no guardian, then the court system may be the only recourse. Another scenario is the patient who is proclaimed to not have capacity to consent (e.g., patients with schizophrenia, patients in manic episode) but who is assenting, as opposed to consenting, to ECT. Typically, in these cases, there is a guardian who is expressly given authority to provide consent, but the patient is usually assenting, or agreeable to ECT. ECT in this case does not constitute involuntary treatment, as the patient is agreeable. Just because somebody has been found not to have capacity to consent does not mean he or she cannot at least participate in discussions about his or her care or offer opinions. The thoughtful psychiatrist faced with the dilemma of the psychotic patient who has been judged to lack ability to provide informed consent but who would benefit from ECT is well advised to take a broad view, taking into account the expressed wishes of the patient, the threat to health caused by the psychopathology, and the opinions of interested family members or guardian.

The Informed Consent Document

There is a tendency to conflate signing an informed consent document with the educational process preceding it. The educational process, including provision of written and video materials, is where the details of ECT should be described. The informed consent document does not need to be multiple pages. The signing of an informed consent document is required in most jurisdictions and by most hospitals. Sample consent forms are available elsewhere (Abrams 2002; American Psychiatric Association Committee on Electroconvulsive Therapy 2001). The American Psychiatric Association sample, in the author's opinion, is too long and detailed. A consent form should not be so long that most patients undoubtedly will not read the whole thing and will simply go to the end and sign. In fact, many of the best ECT candidates, such as the severely psychomotorically retarded or psychotically depressed patient, will have a hard time processing extensive documents. The information on an ECT consent form can easily cover no more than the front side of one standard piece of paper, with a place for signatures by the patient and the physician. Some might also recommend a signature from a witness not involved in the patient's care to provide testimony that the patient really did sign the form. This is unnecessary unless required by local laws. For patients receiving ongoing maintenance ECT, the informed consent process should be repeated periodically—for example, once every 6 months.

ECT services are encouraged to develop their own consent forms so as to tailor them to the needs of local patients. It is important for the clinician undertaking the patient education and informed consent process to document in the patient's record the discussions that have taken place. In particular, if the patient expresses concern about technical aspects of ECT, such as electrode placement, the clinician should document the rationale for whatever technique will be used.

Finally, it is important to remind patients and families of consent issues as the course of ECT proceeds. Some patients may forget that the procedure is voluntary and must be reminded that they can refuse at any time. This issue can be particularly difficult in the elderly patient receiving bilateral ECT who forgets not only the consent but the ECT procedure itself and maybe even that he or she was ill to begin with. Ongoing reminders of why and with what procedure they are being treated, enlisting family member assistance, will help vulnerable patients in their understanding of ECT.

Involuntary ECT

The decision to procure court authorization (or guardian/conservator authorization if allowed by local law) against a patient's specified wishes is not easy. Local statutes must be followed. Decisions about issues of capacity and urgency of need for ECT, which are in many cases the deciding factors in determining whether involuntary ECT is authorized, are often subject to interpretation.

Substituted consent does not mean that the resultant ECT is performed involuntarily. Many chronically psychotic or demented patients will clearly benefit from ECT and are in no position to render consent but do not object to being given the treatments after the proper legal steps have been taken. ECT under those circumstances is not involuntary (Dare and Rasmussen 2015).

The typical scenario for involuntary ECT is a patient who is psychotic and cannot care for self. Medications have been tried, but to no avail. ECT is an option that is felt to be able to render the patient stable to pursue community living, rather than being chronically hospitalized. Such patients tend to be hostile in all interpersonal situations. Oftentimes, food and fluid intake are suboptimal. There may be acts of violence directed against self or others. An overall view of such patients' care is that without ECT, death will occur from malnutrition, hospitalization will become chronic, or there will be a risk of committing suicide or violence toward others. Depending on local laws, if such patients already have a legally appointed conservator or guardian, that person may consent to ECT. Alternatively, there may be court proceedings required, in which case a judge is petitioned. While such a scenario seems fraught with negative, hostile emotions, many patients, typically those with medication-refractory mania, elderly patients with psychotic depression, or schizophrenia patients in acute severe decompensations, recover with ECT and render positive attitudes toward having received it (Dare and Rasmussen 2015).

A more thorough discussion of the ethics of involuntary ECT can be found in the monograph by Ottosson and Fink (2004).

Special Topics in the ECT Consent Process

Psychosis

The presence of psychotic features does not automatically render a patient incapacitated for ECT consent. The scenarios in which psychotic features do interfere with capacity typically revolve around failure to comprehend that one has an illness that can respond to ECT. For example, psychotically depressed patients who are so preoccupied with the idea of having physical medical problems and the presumed need for more medical tests may not understand they are depressed. Of note, it is rare to encounter a patient with persecutory delusions who cannot comprehend the illness at hand, which seems counterintuitive. Most patients with schizophrenia who lack consenting capacity lack capacity not because of delusions but rather because of thought disorganization. Psychosis itself surprisingly often does not interfere with discussions about the process of ECT, expected risks and benefits, and alternative treatments.

Mania

As indicated in Chapter 1, most manic patients do not need ECT. It is usually the severely behaviorally disruptive manic patients for whom ECT is being considered, and such patients often do not cooperate with the consent discussion process. Involuntary ECT is commonly needed for such patients because of the risk of harm to self or others.

A special scenario in this regard is the patient with a bipolar disorder, either known or unknown, who is depressed and consents to ECT but who becomes manic during the course of ECT. Some practitioners in this scenario recommend continuing with the ECT course, but the formerly consenting depressed patient may now be a refusing manic patient, in which case severity of the mania and its impairment will determine whether involuntary ECT should be pursued. Specific recommendations for managing mania-prone patients during ECT are covered in Chapter 7.

Catatonia

Patients with the milder signs of catatonia, such as automatic obedience, echolalia, echopraxia, and motor or verbal stereotypies, can usually participate in a rational discussion of ECT consent procedures. However, those with mutism and stupor cannot, so arrangements for substituted consent need to be made. Some catatonic patients respond well to lorazepam. Consent for ECT in catatonic patients should not be obtained from the patient when under the influence of a sedative medication. Such patients should have substituted consent pursuant to local laws governing such procedures.

The Elderly

When elderly people are depressed, decision-making functions such as attention, concentration, self-confidence, and the ability to consider alternative options can be impaired because of depression-related cognitive dysfunction, otherwise known as *pseudodementia* (Kiloh 1961). Depressed elderly patients are often psychotic or have profound ruminations dominating their minds, which also impair the consent process for ECT. Psychotic ideations related to negativism, pessimism, and nihilism render such patients so cynical that they may not be able to participate in discussions regarding their care. However, the irony is that these psychopathological features presage excellent recovery with ECT. The approach to such patients during the consent process should include concerned family members to assist with decision making regarding ECT. Information about ECT will often need to be repeated several times to reinforce the basic principles. The communications to the patients should not be coercive or threatening—for example, by saying that refusal to accept ECT will result in dismissal from the hospital. On the other hand, if the clinician is confident that medications have been ineffective and ECT presents the best option, persistence in discussing ECT without forcing the issue is appropriate practice. Some patients are simply too ill to read and cognitively process the consent form for ECT. Laws vary on the topic of substituted consent. In some locales, it is legal to accept the patient's passive assent to ECT while a close family member actually signs the consent form. In most jurisdictions, if the patient actively refuses ECT, then some type of court order must be obtained unless there is a guardian authorized to override the patient's expressed wishes.

Pediatric Patients

The patient education and informed consent process for adolescents is remarkably similar to that for adults, except that consent must be obtained from a guardian. The American Psychiatric Association Committee on Electroconvulsive Therapy (2001) report recommends that two child/adolescent psychiatrists document the need for ECT in such cases. If an adolescent refuses ECT but the parents or guardian wishes to proceed, the clinician must decide if the clinical circumstances are so dire as to override the patient's wishes, assuming that local laws allow such practice. Usually, if an adolescent refuses ECT, then the treatment is not done. Somewhat more common are cases in which an adolescent is quite psychotic, manic, or catatonic and cannot participate in the consent process but may not be actively refusing, in which case proceeding with ECT with the guardian's consent is appropriate if allowed by local statute. Most practitioners will not encounter children needing ECT in their careers.

Pregnant Patients

Aspects of ECT care for pregnant women will be discussed in later chapters. In brief, though, the consent process will involve conveyance of information about the risk of ECT to the developing fetus. It is rare for pregnant women to be treated with ECT. Usually, the psychopathology is either catatonia or severe mania, conditions typically requiring substituted consent.

Family Refusal of ECT

An occasional scenario in ECT practice occurs when the patient is willing to sign consent for ECT but one or more closely involved family members strongly reject ECT. Theoretically, if the patient is providing consent, then it does not matter what family members say. In practice, however, ECT should be delayed until at least some type of family meeting is held for all interested parties to vent their opinions and concerns. It is especially important that if the patient decides to go against family advice and proceed with ECT, the family members need to hear this verbalized by the patient in order to reduce any probability later on that the family can accuse the physician of coercing consent from the patient. A scenario to be avoided is obtaining consent from a frail, usually elderly patient without discussing the situation with any family members, proceeding with ECT, and then having angry relatives proclaiming that ECT should not have been done.

Maintenance ECT

The conceptual difference between acute, or index, ECT treatments and continuation/maintenance treatments is that the former are designed to reduce current symptoms and signs, while the latter are designed to prevent the return of such symptoms and signs. In practice, the two can blend together. For example, a patient whose depression is freshly remitted with index treatments can be enrolled in weekly maintenance treatments, only to have a mild return of symptoms along the way and receive one or more extra "booster" treatments during a particular week.

Do these treatments constitute a return to index ECT and necessitate another signing of consent? ECT practitioners differ in their response to this question. What is more critical than having the patient sign another consent form is good communication between doctor and patient about the goals of continued treatments and the expected extra memory impairment that may accrue. Some institutions utilize the same consent form for index and maintenance ECT. The American Psychiatric Association Committee on Electroconvulsive Therapy (2001) report suggests obtaining a separate consent form once maintenance treatments begin.

Anti-ECT Sentiment

There is plenty of hostility directed against ECT. One need only look on the internet for a while to appreciate this, as discussed earlier in this chapter. This occasionally impacts the consent process, and of course the ECT practitioner wishes to avoid having angry patients down the road, so a question arises as to how to deal with anti-ECT hostility as part of consent and how to prevent it from happening. Professor Richard Abrams, a psychiatrist who has contributed greatly to the theory and practice of ECT for many decades, mentions that in a National Institute of Mental Health–sponsored public conference on ECT held in 1985, the two main things ex-ECT patients were angry about were not having been informed of risks (mainly, memory issues) and having been given ECT against their will (Abrams 2002, p. 230). If good attention is paid to proper patient education and informed consent, then later patient anger is rare. The bedrock of preventing conflictual relationships with ECT patients is the establishment a priori of a positive, trusting doctor-patient relationship before ECT is commenced. Even though modern psychiatrists are under pressure with inpatients to proceed quickly and shorten lengths of stay, the ECT practitioner must simply resist the temptation to start quickly with ECT treatments and not skip the various steps outlined in this chapter. It is well worth some extra days in the hospital to make sure all consent-related loose ends have been tied up before the treatments are begun.

Key Points

- Pre-ECT informed consent is a standard part of ECT practice.

- Formal informed consent documents to be signed by the patient or legal representative can be developed according to local customs and legal requirements.

- Patient and family education is a critical aspect of the consent process and can be supplemented with educational materials or videos.

- Occasionally, ECT is delivered to patients involuntarily or to patients deemed to lack ability to provide informed consent according to court procedures established by local laws.

4

The Pre-ECT Medical Workup

Aſter patient selection and consent, the next step in an electroconvulsive therapy (ECT) course is pretreatment medical evaluation. Although ECT is very safe, with extremely low serious morbidity or mortality (Nuttall et al. 2004; Watts et al. 2011), one must ensure a thorough medical examination and attention to special needs of patients with various medical illnesses in order to lower adverse event risks. Additionally, because many patients take a multitude of medications, attention must be paid to selection of those to administer in the mornings just prior to ECT treatments. This chapter provides advice on the management of medical issues pertinent to making ECT as safe as possible. First, a review of the medical physiology of ECT is appropriate to provide a context for the recommendations for practice. Of note, ECT anesthesia is covered in Chapter 5.

As a patient is being prepared for ECT, there likely will be involvement of the ECT clinician, referring psychiatrist (if separate from the ECT clinician), anesthesiologist, and internal medicine clinicians. The ECT clinician should be aware of involvement of these various personnel and any medical issues being investigated. Good communication among these clinicians is critical for safe ECT, especially in medically complicated patients.

Medical Physiology of ECT

Cardiovascular

Shortly after the presentation of the electrical stimulus used to induce a seizure, there is a brief but intense parasympathetic nervous system outflow, causing bradycardia or brief periods of asystole. This parasympathetic phase is rapidly replaced by intense sympathetic nervous system stimulation that causes heart rate and blood pressure elevation. If the electrical stimulus is subthreshold—that is, insufficient to result in a seizure—there is no sympathetic phase. The unopposed parasympathetic phase can then cause a somewhat prolonged period of bradycardia or asystole (Rasmussen et al. 1999). The rapid rise of blood pressure and heart rate during the seizure causes an increase in myocardial oxygen consumption. This may last until several minutes after the seizure. Thus, the seizure acts as a "stress test" of sorts on the heart, with implications for those with coronary artery disease (CAD), congestive heart failure (CHF), or cardiac arrhythmias. The rise in blood pressure and pulse are quite variable, with some patients having little rise at all and other patients experiencing systolic blood pressures of 150–200 mmHg or so, diastolic blood pressures of 100–130 mmHg or so, and pulse rates of 150 beats per minute or more.

Electrocardiographic studies conducted during and after ECT seizures have noted common changes, including premature atrial and ventricular beats as well as ST and T wave changes suggestive of brief ischemia (Rasmussen et al. 2007a). Additionally, echocardiographic studies have documented equally brief periods of ventricular wall motion abnormalities during ECT seizures in some patients (McCully et al. 2003). Finally, one study of troponin values taken serially during ECT courses found that a few patients show laboratory evidence of myocardial ischemia during ECT (Martinez et al. 2011). In spite of these known cardiac physiological changes during ECT, cardiac complications are quite uncommon (Nuttall et al. 2004). The ECT clinician and anesthesiologist must be knowledgeable about a patient's cardiac status and history in order to render the treatment maximally safe from a cardiac standpoint. Specific risk reduction strategies are discussed in the section "Specific Illnesses."

Neurological

A seizure is a profound neurometabolic event, with rapid depolarization of neurons and release of numerous neurotransmitters (Abrams 2002, Chapter 11). During the seizure itself, there is a rapid rise of cerebral blood flow, followed postictally by an abrupt fall in cerebral blood flow below baseline levels, with the flow eventually returning to baseline (Abrams 2002, Chapter 4). Additionally, intracranial pressure rises in accordance with the increased cerebral blood flow, and this is normally not worrisome but might be for the patient with preexisting increased intracranial pressure—for example, from a brain tumor or other mass effect. Concomitantly with the increased cerebral perfusion during the seizure, there is a sharp increase in cerebral oxygen and glucose consumption. Electroencephalographic studies have consistently shown, in addition to the obvious ictal patterns, a postictal pattern of diffuse slow wave activity, maximal over the stimulated hemisphere(s), which progressively disappears to basal frequencies within days to weeks of the end of the ECT course (Abrams 2002, Chapter 4). However, none of all these types of findings have implications for the pre-ECT workup.

Coffey et al. (1991) conducted a magnetic resonance imaging (MRI) study before, during, and after ECT courses with follow-up several months later and found no MRI evidence of adverse effects of ECT. Of course, nobody has or ever will (probably) conduct brain biopsy studies in ECT patients to determine if histological changes occur, either positive or negative, with ECT, but animal studies in primates conclusively show no evidence of "brain damage" in animals given electroconvulsive shock in a manner that mimics human ECT (Abrams 2002, Chapter 4).

The question of whether ECT causes epilepsy has been broached in the literature. Generally, with a routine course of treatments, ECT has anticonvulsant activity. However, with prolonged courses of maintenance ECT, it is possible that epilepsy can be induced (Lunde et al. 2006; Rasmussen and Lunde 2007).

Pulmonary

Shortly after the administration of anesthetic medication, the patient stops breathing. Thus, positive pressure ventilation must be administered throughout the procedure until resumption of spontaneous respirations after the seizure is finished. Competent airway management during ECT treatments is critical.

Endocrinological/Metabolic/Hematological

An ECT treatment causes a brief, approximately 9% increase in blood sugar levels (Rasmussen et al. 2005, 2006b). Such an increase is not usually clinically significant, though patients with diabetes should have blood sugar monitoring by finger stick before treatments to ensure absence of hypoglycemia or excessive hyperglycemia.

The hypothalamic and pituitary hormones secreted acutely during ECT seizures do not have clinical significance for the medical safety of ECT. The succinylcholine used to paralyze muscles during ECT seizures does cause a brief rise in serum potassium, which in the patient who is already hyperkalemic may predispose to cardiac arrhythmias. Other laboratory parameters that are typically assessed prior to ECT, such as other electrolytes, blood counts, and renal and liver tests, are unaffected by ECT treatments.

Musculoskeletal

Tonic-clonic seizures, which are the seizure type induced during ECT, obviously cause vigorous shaking of all four extremities. This neuromuscular effect is blocked by the administration of a muscle-paralyzing agent such as succinylcholine, so the risk of bone fractures is vastly reduced from times past, when no muscle blockade was used. Myalgias, on the other hand, are quite common with ECT (Rasmussen et al. 2008d), especially after the first treatment. The etiology of this is obscure and does not correlate with degree of muscle shaking or fasciculation induced by succinylcholine (Rasmussen et al. 2008d).

Ocular

ECT seizures cause an acute, temporary rise in intraocular pressure (Good et al. 2004). Patients with glaucoma should have intraocular pressures checked before commencement of an ECT course if not done recently.

Gastrointestinal

Even though muscle paralysis has been achieved with succinylcholine, the passage of electrical current through the head to induce the seizure does directly stimulate jaw muscles to contract. Thus, there is a risk of tooth or dental appliance fracture or loss and tongue, cheek, or lip laceration. Careful oral exam prior to ECT to inspect for loose teeth and removal of removable dental appliances, coupled with proper use of a bite-block during electrical stimulation, can prevent these oral complications.

Upon anesthesia administration, there is a loss of gag reflexes and stomach contents may regurgitate. Thus, there must be an empty stomach during ECT treatments. There may also be bowel or bladder incontinence during seizures, so voiding of each is recommended prior to treatments. Nausea is also quite common with ECT.

Urogenital

Urinary incontinence can also happen during seizures, so voiding of bladder is recommended prior to each treatment. With the strong Valsalva that can occur during the tonic phase of a seizure, there may be a sharp increase in intra-abdominal pressure with attendant theoretical risk of bladder rupture. However, with proper muscle relaxation, this is an extremely remote risk. If an anticholinergic agent is used before anesthesia (see Chapter 5 for a more detailed discussion), then a day or so of uncomfortable urinary hesitancy may follow, especially in elderly men with prostate hypertrophy. Such medications are generally not mandatory during ECT.

Dermatological

Piloerection occurs during seizures as well as flushing from sympathetic stimulation. Flushing of the face from the sympathetic outflow during a seizure, which may be unilateral across the face in unilateral ECT and which may include the conjunctivae, may be quite prominent shortly after the seizure but lasts only a few minutes or so.

Medical Complications of ECT

ECT is a remarkably safe procedure. Deaths due to treatment are extremely rare (Nuttall et al. 2004; Watts et al. 2011). The low mortality rate due to ECT is all the more impressive considering the medical comorbidity of the many patients now treated with this modality. Complications due to ECT, defined as medical events of sufficient severity to warrant emergent resuscitation, evaluation by a specialist physician, or transfer to a medical service, are also rare with ECT. Usually, these consist of cardiac arrhythmias, evidence of myocardial ischemia, or respiratory events such as breathing difficulties. Strokes due to ECT are extremely rare in spite of the spikes in blood pressure that commonly occur during and shortly after the seizures. The main issue in preventing medical complications during ECT is thorough medical review and stabilization prior to treatments as well as proper anesthesiologic vigilance during the treatments.

Basic Pre-ECT Workup

The most important aspect of the pre-ECT medical workup is a complete medical history, review of systems, and physical exam. Further testing, such as cardiac tests, radiological studies, and blood work, can be tailored to the needs of individual patients. It is rare that a patient is found outright to be too medically sick to have ECT. Most patients can proceed with no further investigations beyond a good medical review, physical exam, and some basic testing as per below. Some patients should have specialist consultations and tests depending on medical morbidities, and even then most patients either can proceed afterward to ECT or can do so after some time is spent on medical stabilization. The pre-ECT medical evaluation can be completed by any practitioner competent to do so, with specialist consultations depending on what is found.

When taking the medical history, the ECT clinician should particularly inquire about cardiovascular, respiratory, and neurological disorders. This history should include any diagnoses given to the patient and the workups and treatments administered over time. For example, the patient with a history of CAD, which of course is common, should be asked about any procedures for revascularization, such as surgery or stent placement, and about whether any diagnostic testing has been done and, if so, how recently. If possible, the results of such testing, such as echocardiograms or other cardiac imaging scans, should be reviewed. Patients with known arrhythmias, most commonly atrial fibrillation (AF), should be asked about treatments given, such as medications, cardioversion, or ablation. Symptomatic status can be reviewed with questions about shortness of breath and exercise tolerance. Cardiological evaluation prior to ECT is advised for any patient who has significant cardiac disease. This may lead to a recommendation for a stress echocardiogram.

A neurological history is important to identify conditions that might conceivably worsen during ECT, such as multiple sclerosis or dementia. Other common neurological disorders, such as Parkinson's disease and epilepsy, do have implications for how ECT is managed, as covered in the subsection "Neurological Disorders." The results of recent neurological diagnostic tests, such as electroencephalograms or neuroimaging scans, should also be reviewed to establish baseline status with which to compare any posttreatment tests that might be ordered. Any significant neurological illness should prompt evaluation by either a neurologist or a general medical physician prior to ECT unless a recent evaluation has been performed.

Respiratory status is critical to evaluate prior to ECT, because this has implications for how anesthetic management proceeds during the course of treatments. Patients with any active, ongoing respiratory condition, such as chronic obstructive pulmonary disease (COPD), asthma, pneumonia, or pulmonary edema due to less than optimally controlled CHF, should have these conditions evaluated by medical specialists for maximal stabilization prior to ECT.

A pre-ECT chest X-ray is not routinely needed, because the patient without known respiratory problems who has a normal chest exam coupled with lack of respiratory symptoms such as shortness of breath is unlikely to have something significant for ECT detected by a routine chest X-ray. An electrocardiogram is recommended by the American Psychiatric Association Committee on Electroconvulsive Therapy (2001), but rarely does this show something significant for ECT in a patient with no cardiac history. As far as blood laboratory tests go, at a minimum, sodium and potassium levels should be checked, with the latter being particularly important because of the potassium-raising effects of the neuromuscular blocking agent succinylcholine. Liver function, renal function, and hematological tests are often ordered but are unlikely to yield information useful specifically for ECT, though they may be helpful as part of a patient's overall care. Table 4–1 summarizes aspects of the pre-ECT medical workup.

TABLE 4–1. **Elements of the pre-ECT medical workup**

Routine

1. Medical history and review of systems

2. Physical examination

3. Blood potassium

4. Electrocardiogram

In selected patients

1. Chest X-ray (e.g., recent pneumonia, chronic obstructive pulmonary disease, congestive heart failure)

2. Brain imaging (known or suspected intracerebral mass or structural abnormality)

3. Stress echocardiogram (e.g., congestive heart failure, coronary artery disease, valvular disease)

4. Specialist consultation (e.g., cardiology, neurology)

Concomitant Medication Issues

Patients are to be kept nothing-by-mouth prior to ECT treatments to ensure an empty stomach to prevent reflux and tracheal aspiration of gastric contents. However, some medications should be administered with a small amount of water, as discussed below. In the modern era, most ECT patients take a large number of medications, both for psychiatric conditions and for medical illnesses. Nonpsychotropic medication issues are covered herein, while those associated with psychotropics are covered in Chapter 7.

Antihypertensives

Patients should be given their routine morning doses of antihypertensive medication with a small amount of water the mornings of ECT. This will help mitigate the hypertensive effects of the ECT treatment and will have no negative impact on ECT efficacy. An older literature implied that beta-blockers such as labetalol and esmolol, which are available intravenously and are commonly used during the treatments to dampen blood pressure and tachycardia (see Chapter 5), may shorten seizure length (Howie et al. 1990; McCall et al. 1991), but there is no evidence this compromises efficacy. Patients should be given prescribed diuretics the morning of ECT with the opportunity to void the bladder right before the treatment to prevent urinary incontinence.

Antidysrhythmics

Medication for AF, the most common cardiac dysrhythmia encountered in ECT patients, should be administered the mornings of ECT if that is the usual time of administration for a given patient.

Inhalers

Patients with asthma or COPD often use inhalers on a regular, daily basis. If a patient receives a routine morning dose of an inhaler, it should be administered at the normal time prior to ECT, in order to prevent bronchospasm during the treatments. For a patient with asthma who uses inhalers only as needed (typically beta-agonists), it is usually not necessary to administer the inhaled medication before ECT unless there is felt to be a risk of precipitation of wheezing during ECT.

Eyedrops

Antiglaucoma drops should be administered prior to treatments for those patients taking them. Long-acting anticholinesterase inhibitor eyedrops such as echothiophate could conceivably prolong the action of succinylcholine but are rarely used anymore.

Insulin

Diabetes mellitus is common among ECT patients. For the patient with type 1 diabetes, in whom there is an absolute dependence on insulin and in whom blood sugars are brittle, close attention must be paid to blood sugars around the time of each treatment. Ideally, such a patient should be treated promptly in the morning (i.e., not at the end of the morning after prolonged fasting without insulin). One strategy is to administer half the usual morning insulin dose, treat promptly with ECT, and then administer the second half along with juice or breakfast. Another strategy is to hold off on insulin entirely until after the treatment is over. In either case, there should be finger-stick blood sugar testing just prior to ECT. If the blood sugar levels are hovering in the hypoglycemic range, a glucose IV can be started cautiously to raise blood sugar before anesthesia induction. Close attention to blood sugars must be paid.

In patients with type 2 diabetes, blood sugars are not as brittle. The same half-dose or no-dose insulin strategy can be employed as above until after the treatment if the patient is taking insulin. For patients with type 2 diabetes who are taking oral agents to control blood sugar, these agents need not be taken until after the treatment.

For all patients with diabetes, it would be ideal to check finger-stick blood sugars in the recovery room after treatment, but this is not mandatory unless the patient is known to have unpredictable blood sugars.

Antiepileptics

Common sense would indicate that the presence of antiepileptic medication makes inducing a seizure at the time of ECT more difficult. However, if these medications have clearly been effective for the patient's seizure disorder, maintaining them at the current dose and treating with ECT is recommended, with the exception of holding morning doses until after the treatment. Most of the time, therapeutically effective seizures occur (Lunde et al. 2006). If not, then switching from an anticonvulsant anesthetic (e.g., a barbiturate or propofol) to etomidate, and hyperventilating before seizure induction, might help prolong seizure duration. If this does not work, then consultation with the patient's neurologist, or whoever has been managing the antiepileptic medication, about cautiously lowering the dose is indicated. Lowering the dose can help ECT seizures, but spontaneous epileptic seizures are a risk.

Antiparkinsonian Medications

Dopamine-enhancing medications have been associated with excess cognitive impairment (namely, delirium) during ECT as well as the occurrence of dyskinetic movements (Douyon et al. 1989), likely reflecting dopaminergic toxicity related to the pro-dopaminergic activity of ECT. However, abruptly lowering or stopping a patient's antiparkinsonian medications, particularly levodopa/carbidopa, can be dangerous and cause a syndrome identical to neuroleptic malignant syndrome. A cautious stance is recommended, in the form of keeping such medications at their current effective doses and carefully observing for the appearance of dyskinetic movements during the ECT course and of course also for delirium. If these become a problem, then with neurologist consultation, a lowering of the levodopa/carbidopa doses can be attempted. After the ECT course is finished, the doses may need to be raised again to the former level. It is prudent to administer the usual morning dose with a small amount of water prior to the scheduled ECT treatment.

Glucocorticoid Hormones

The anesthesia field has taught that patients taking glucocorticoid hormones, most commonly prednisone, on a chronic basis have poor stress-response reserves and must be given "stress doses" of intravenous glucocorticoid medication prior to any procedure involving general anesthesia. However, the stress of an ECT treatment seems so minimal and short-lived that not giving such extra doses seems prudent, especially since such drugs could have side effects and adverse effects of their own, especially if given thrice weekly for several weeks. A relatively large series of cases in which ECT patients were prescribed ongoing steroid medications and did not receive "stress doses" prior to treatments revealed no evidence of complications (Albin and Rasmussen 2007; Rasmussen et al. 2008a).

Theophylline

Theophylline used to be used quite commonly for patients with COPD but is rarely encountered in modern practice. A methylxanthine compound similar to caffeine, theophylline prolongs seizure duration and was implicated in several cases of status epilepticus during ECT (Rasmussen and Zorumski 1993). If it is used, regular blood levels should be obtained to ensure there is no toxicity, the lowest effective blood levels should be a goal, and caffeine should not be used as a seizure-enhancement measure.

Gastric Acid Modulators

Gastric acid modulators, which include H_2 blockers and proton pump inhibitors, are commonly used for patients with peptic ulcer disease as well as those with gastroesophageal reflux disease or non-ulcer dyspepsia. If a patient is prescribed such a medication for morning dosage, it should be administered with a small amount of water on the days of ECT before treatment, to reduce the likelihood of gastric reflux during ECT.

Anticoagulants

The question of anticoagulation and ECT is oft discussed. It is recommended that patients be continued on whatever "blood thinner" they are prescribed, with regular monitoring of the relevant coagulation parameter (e.g., international normalized ratio [INR], partial thromboplastin time) (American Psychiatric Association Committee on Electroconvulsive Therapy 2001). If such indices are normal, that is obviously ideal. The question, though, is what to do if the coagulation parameter is too low or too high. The former puts the patient at risk of thrombosis, and the latter places the patient at risk of bleeding. Does the ECT procedure present greater-than-average danger of either of these two eventualities? This is an issue that has not been the focus of research. It is hard to see, if the INR is too low, how the ECT treatment itself would cause greater risk of thrombosis, unless the patient has a tendency toward atrial fibrillation, in which case a thrombus may form in the atrium. If the INR is too high, then one might expect that the blood pressure surge might place the patient at greater risk of bleeding. Unfortunately, confident limits of the safe use of ECT for coagulation parameters cannot be given. The most conservative stance would simply be to insist on a therapeutic INR level for every treatment. There should be some flexibility, however, because there does tend to be fluctuation of the INR even in patients taking stable doses of warfarin. One must balance the reason for use of warfarin, and the expected risk of thrombosis or bleeding with a too-low or too-high INR, respectively, with the urgency of the need for ECT. For example, in a non–acutely suicidal cooperative patient, one could take a more conservative stance and insist on a therapeutic INR for each treatment. However, in a stuporous, mute patient with catatonia in an extreme state of psychopathology unresponsive to other measures, one can be more liberal in use of ECT even if prescribed warfarin is not resulting in a precisely therapeutic INR on a particular ECT day; but of course, attempts must be made to make it therapeutic henceforth. Newer blood thinners not requiring monitoring should be continued during ECT if they are medically indicated.

Miscellaneous Medications

Of course, there are a lot of medications in the modern medical pharmacopoeia. Some that come to mind are skin preparations, cancer chemotherapy agents, antibiotics, antihyperlipidemics, anti-rejection compounds for organ transplant recipients, anti-inflammatory agents, and immune modulators for connective tissue and autoimmune diseases. None of these are contraindicated in ECT patients, and they can be given at their usual doses and times, except that oral morning doses can be held until after the day's ECT treatment.

Specific Illnesses

The psychiatric clinician will need to use his or her judgment about when to request specialist consultation, such as with a cardiologist or neurologist, before commencing ECT. Commonly, at least in the United States, a general internist is the first physician to be consulted, and further specialty consultations occur at the discretion of that practitioner.

Congestive Heart Failure

Of all the various medical conditions typically seen in an ECT-treated population, CHF presents one of the most substantial increased risks of medical complications during ECT. The failing heart may be unable to tolerate the increased myocardial oxygen demand that occurs during the intense sympathetic phase of the ECT seizure. There have been several case series of ECT patients with CHF published over the years. Gerring and Shields (1982) reported four patients with known CHF who received ECT. Only one received ECT without complication. Among the other three, one had AF after one treatment, leading to a decompensation of the CHF. On stabilization, this patient went on to receive further treatments without complication. Another patient had a cardiac arrest 45 minutes after a treatment and died. The fourth had transient atrial and ventricular dysrhythmias after several of her treatments, which she otherwise tolerated well.

In the Zielinski et al. (1993) series with 12 CHF patients given ECT, none died but most had noted transient electrocardiographic changes consisting usually of arrhythmias at the time of the ECT seizures. Goldberg and Badger (1993) reported on two patients with CHF and implantable cardioverter-defibrillators (ICDs), one of whom had a decompensation of cardiac pump function leading to death after one of the ECT treatments. Petrides and Fink (1996) reported on two patients with CHF and AF who tolerated ECT well but who in one case converted to sinus rhythm and in the other case fluctuated between AF and sinus rhythm. Stern et al. (1997) reported on three CHF patients undergoing ECT without complication. They used pre- and afterload reductive agents (nitroglycerin, nifedipine, labetalol) to reduce risk. Rivera et al. (2011) reported on a series of 35 patients with CHF treated with ECT who had a mean baseline cardiac ejection fraction of 30%; more than 500 treatments were assessed without serious complications or death. The authors suggested that use of beta-blockers, such as labetalol, esmolol, or metoprolol, during treatments to control heart rate is a safe and effective intervention to reduce risks of cardiac decompensation. They also suggested that a baseline pre-ECT workup be conducted to include electrocardiography, echocardiography, and complete blood count, liver and kidney function testing, and electrolytes.

The patient with known CHF who is being prepared for ECT must have optimal stabilization of the CHF prior to each ECT treatment. This stabilization should be supervised by a physician familiar with the management of this condition. Once ECT is to be commenced, the patient's cardiac medications should be administered at their usual times, even on the days of ECT. Diuretics, such as furosemide, should not be withheld. CHF patients often teeter on the balance between compensation and decompensation of their cardiac function, and missing diuretic doses, combined with the stress of a seizure, may precipitate acute worsening of cardiac output. The ECT clinician should be familiar with the particulars of the CHF patient's exercise tolerance, general appearance, and breathing characteristics, as well as the results of the patient's lung exam, prior to treatments so that should significant changes occur during the course of treatments, these will not be missed. It is particularly important in the CHF patient that if early signs of a decompensation occur, they be recognized early so that further treatments are held pending restabilization. Thus, during the course of ECT treatments, there should be daily assessment of the patient's CHF status.

Coronary Artery Disease

It is not uncommon to encounter a patient needing ECT who has a known history of CAD or a myocardial infarction. Such patients often have had either a coronary artery bypass graft or an intravascular stent placed and tend to be taking cardiac medications. Prior to beginning ECT, the patient should be evaluated by a cardiologist or internist familiar with CAD as well as ECT cardiac physiology. Patients without known CAD who nonetheless evince signs or symptoms suggestive of such during the pre-ECT medical evaluation should be evaluated by a cardiologist before proceeding.

If a known CAD patient is not having any chest pain episodes, has good exercise tolerance, or has had recent cardiac imaging showing relatively normal left ventricular function, then no further cardiac testing need be ordered in anticipation of ECT. However, if the patient is having active cardiac symptoms, such as shortness of breath, poor exercise tolerance, or anginal episodes, then further testing (such as a stress echocardiogram) or cardiac medication adjustment may be indicated in the hands of a cardiologist.

There are several case series documenting that ECT can be given safely to patients with known CAD (Gerring and Shields 1982; Magid et al. 2005; Petrides and Fink 1996; Rice et al. 1994; Ruwitch et al. 1994; Zielinski et al. 1993). However, it is also known from echocardiographic studies performed during ECT that left ventricular wall motion abnormalities occasionally occur during the seizures (Ruwitch et al. 1994), but these are temporary. From a pre-ECT workup standpoint, the major teaching issue is that a careful pretreatment evaluation will determine whether further workup or medication adjustments are needed. It is important to administer ongoing cardiac medications in the mornings of treatments with a small amount of water if that is the usual time. As is the case with CHF patients, cardiac medications for CAD patients that normally are administered in the morning should be given on days of ECT treatments. Anesthesiologists commonly administer beta-blockers such as labetalol at the time of ECT for CAD patients to lessen the strain on the heart (Albin et al. 2007; Rasmussen et al. 2008c).

Dysrhythmias, Pacemakers, and Implantable Cardioverter-Defibrillators

AF is a common dysrhythmia in ECT patients. If a patient is known to have AF prior to ECT, then evaluation by a physician knowledgeable of its management should be undertaken to determine if further rate control or defibrillation should be undertaken. Considerations will include the patient's current heart rate, left ventricular function, and presence of any worrisome symptoms such as chest pain, shortness of breath, poor exercise tolerance, or other cardiac morbidities such as CHF. Care should be taken to correct metabolic abnormalities such as thyroid or electrolyte disturbances. The patient in chronic AF whose rate is well controlled and who is symptomatically stable will probably not need further cardiac studies and should receive his or her usual cardiac medications on the mornings of treatments (including warfarin if ordered).

If the AF patient's rate is not well controlled prior to ECT, then the internist or cardiologist will decide on a strategy to control the heart rate, usually consisting of medication adjustments in the patient with chronic AF. If the patient has had a recent acute onset of AF, then the primary physician may decide on electrical cardioversion. A case series of patients with AF during ECT showed that fluctuation between normal sinus rhythm and AF is relatively common in these patients during ECT treatments (Petrides and Fink 1996). Attention should also be paid to reducing or discontinuing medications that may prolong the QTc interval, with the assumption that they are not otherwise needed, as prolonged QTc is common in ECT patients and may predispose to dysrhythmias (Dodd et al. 2008; Rasmussen et al. 2007a). However, reassuringly, other studies have shown that patients with prolonged QTc did not have a higher rate of complications during ECT than those with normal QTc intervals (Pullen et al. 2011) and that courses of ECT had no lasting effect on cardiac rhythm (Rasmussen et al. 2004).

Patients with pacemakers are also commonly encountered in modern ECT practice. A large case series found that ECT did not cause any particular problems relative to pacemaker function or heart rhythm during ECT (Dolenc et al. 2004a). Modern pacemakers are so well constructed as to be electrically isolated from the ECT electrical stimulus. A prudent measure in pacemaker patients is to have the device interrogated prior to commencing ECT. More important than the pacemaker itself, though, is the cardiac comorbidity such as CHF or CAD, both of which require pre-ECT evaluation as noted earlier. There is no evidence to support the old recommendation of placing a magnet over the chest above the pacemaker site to convert a demand mode pacemaker to fixed mode. With modern pacemakers, ECT can proceed as usual without any magnets (Dolenc et al. 2004a).

ICDs are devices capable of detecting abnormal rhythms and providing a defibrillating shock if needed. If a patient with an ICD is slated to receive ECT, then personnel competent in the management of these devices should be present in the ECT suite, turn it off while the patient is on a cardiac monitor, and turn it back on after the treatment is completed. As with pacemaker patients, the key issue is any cardiac comorbidity and proper pre-ECT evaluation of that, rather than the presence of the ICD itself.

Aneurysms

There is presumably a risk of rupture of aneurysms due to the blood pressure spike during ECT treatments. There are several case series of safe use of ECT in patients known to have aneurysms (Mueller et al. 2009; Porquez et al. 2003), and undoubtedly it is actually fairly common to give ECT to patients with aneurysms that have not been detected because of the relative frequency of these vascular abnormalities in the population at large. Even though the risk of rupture is quite small during ECT, if a patient is known to have an aneurysm, it is prudent to have a vascular surgeon evaluate the acuity before ECT, especially for aortic aneurysms. A decision would then be made about whether the aneurysm should be repaired prior to ECT. There are no empirical data to provide a confident recommendation, so this situation has to be managed on a case-by-case basis balancing the stability of the aneurysm and the acuteness of the need for ECT. If a patient is known to have an intracerebral aneurysm, then consultation with a neurosurgeon or vascular neurologist would be ideal prior to ECT.

Hypertension

As part of the pre-ECT evaluation, it is common to encounter the patient with high blood pressure, which is the most common cardiovascular condition in ECT patients. Stroke at the time of ECT is undoubtedly extremely rare. Indeed, there are only two case reports of spontaneous intracerebral hemorrhage in ECT (Rikher et al. 1997; Weisberg et al. 1991), and neither patient was hypertensive. Albin et al. (2007) showed that hypertensive patients do not experience a sustained rise in blood pressure during a course of ECT. A review article on the pre-ECT evaluation recommended not treating a patient with blood pressure greater than 140/90 mmHg (Tess and Smetana 2009). However, many ECT patients have difficult-to-control blood pressure, and so insisting on limits that tight may effectively eliminate them from the treatment or at the very least cause undue delays in starting treatments. Of course, it makes intuitive sense that it would be ideal to have good blood pressure control before starting ECT, but one need not wait more than a day or so to lower a hypertensive patient's blood pressures before commencing ECT, unless there is extremely high pressure and/or the presence of very unstable cardiovascular disease. The pressures can always be managed effectively in the ECT suite (see Chapter 5).

Valvular Abnormalities and Heart Transplants

If a patient has had valvular replacement surgery successfully and is taking an anticoagulant at an adequate dosage, ECT should not be any riskier than normal if it is assumed that no other significant cardiac abnormality, such as CHF, is present. However, if a patient is known to have a significant valvular abnormality (most commonly aortic stenosis in ECT patients), then this should be evaluated before ECT by either a cardiac surgeon or cardiologist (Mueller et al. 2007; Rasmussen 1997; Sutor et al. 2008). With aortic stenosis, the cardiac output is exquisitely sensitive to increased myocardial workload and requires expert management during the procedure. As with the patient with significant aneurysms, a decision must be made as to whether ECT should proceed before valve replacement or vice versa. The psychotic, catatonic, or deeply functionally impaired depressed patient is not necessarily a good surgical candidate, so the best course of action may very well be to do ECT first followed by cardiac surgery, though of course a case-by-case decision has to be made considering all aspects of the patient's status.

Regarding heart transplant recipients, consultation with the patient's cardiologist should be undertaken before ECT is started. Whatever anti-transplant-rejection medications the patient takes should be administered at the usual times, even if in the morning, to avoid fluctuations in blood levels.

Neurological Disorders

In contrast to the cardiac system, for which there are a variety of physiological tests and cardioprotective procedures and medications, there is no "neuroprotective" strategy that protects the brain during ECT. Perhaps in the future there will be medication that reliably reduces the cognitive effects of ECT, which is the major neurological side effect of this treatment.

For the dementia patient, there is no particular pre-ECT testing that needs to be conducted. Common sense would predict that such patients will be sensitive to the cognitive side effects of ECT, but as of this writing, there has been no randomized prospective study comparing cognitive outcomes in ECT-treated versus non-ECT-treated dementia patients. In particular, neither in-depth neuropsychological testing nor brain imaging, as a matter of routine, is helpful in pre-ECT management, and these procedures only add cost and delay. Besides, if the patient is severely depressed or behaviorally disturbed (the two most common reasons for doing ECT in patients with dementia), then these tests may be difficult to complete.

The interesting case of Parkinson's disease and ECT was discussed in Chapter 2. In preparation for ECT, the Parkinson's patient should have as much simplification of the antiparkinsonian regimen as possible. Such medications, if taken in the morning, should be administered prior to ECT as normally scheduled to avoid precipitating an abrupt onset of motor stiffness ("off" time). Dose reduction of levodopa/carbidopa should only be considered, in consultation with a neurologist, if the patient experiences undue cognitive disturbance or onset of dyskinesias during ECT. Issues related to electrode placement and treatment frequency will be discussed in later chapters. Thus far, three patients with deep brain stimulators, something increasingly used for Parkinson's patients, have been described as receiving ECT without complications (Bailine et al. 2008; Chou et al. 2005; Moscarillo and Annunziata 2000). In all three of these patients, the generator was turned off during ECT.

Patients with a history of stroke can be safely treated with ECT (Weintraub and Lippmann 2000). A prudent recommendation, though, is not to treat with ECT in a patient with a recent stroke unless there is an unequivocal need for ECT. A history of hemorrhagic stroke would seem to be particularly risky for ECT, given the blood pressure spikes during the seizures. Pretreatment blood pressure control in this population would be a reason to delay ECT if needed. In some patients with cerebrovascular disease, internists do not necessarily insist on a "normal" blood pressure range of around 120/80 mmHg, as the cerebral vasculature in patients with chronic hypertension may not be able to sustain good blood flow at pressures this low. Thus, the ECT clinician must ensure that an internist or neurologist has provided an opinion about an optimal blood pressure goal in such patients. If the poststroke patient is taking an anticoagulant, then the ECT clinician should ensure that the parameters such as INR are in the prescribed range for the patient.

Patients with epilepsy should be evaluated by a neurologist before ECT to ensure optimal control of seizures with current medications. ECT has anticonvulsant activity, and in the years before anti-epileptic medications were available, ECT was actually used to control spontaneous seizure frequency in patients with epilepsy (Regenold et al. 1998). This is only of historical interest now, however, but this does provide reassurance that ECT probably will not cause increased frequency of an epileptic patient's spontaneous seizures. As noted earlier, the issue of obtaining adequate seizures may be a problem requiring judicious lowering of the patient's anti-epileptic medication during ECT if such lowering is felt to be safe by a neurologist. Routine neuroimaging or electroencephalography is not needed in epileptic patients specifically for ECT. Occasionally, a patient receiving long-term maintenance ECT will develop epilepsy, which may complicate ongoing seizure efficacy (Rasmussen and Lunde 2007).

It is exceedingly rare for a patient with a malignant brain tumor to be referred for ECT. More common is a patient with a meningioma, and this probably does not substantially increase ECT risk if there is no mass effect, surrounding edema, or associated focal neurological signs (Rasmussen et al. 2007d). If such worrisome signs do exist in the prospective ECT patient, consultation with either a neurologist or a neurosurgeon to discuss strategies to reduce intracranial pressure is indicated. ECT should be considered a very high-risk procedure under those circumstances. Other intracranial masses include arachnoid cysts, which probably do not increase ECT risks (Perry et al. 2007). Vascular abnormalities such as hemangiomas also are probably safe for ECT, unless there is evidence of a rapid rate of growth (Rasmussen and Flemming 2006).

A static, chronic neurological condition such as cerebral palsy probably does not present an increased risk of complications due to ECT (Rasmussen et al. 1993). ECT has been utilized safely in patients with multiple sclerosis, although if recent MRI reveals gadolinium-enhancing lesions, there may be increased risk of their worsening during ECT (Rasmussen and Keegan 2007).

Diabetes Mellitus

Blood sugars rise a few percentage points on average within a few minutes after ECT seizures, both in persons with diabetes and in endocrinologically healthy individuals (Rasmussen and Ryan 2005; Rasmussen et al. 2006b). Thus, blood sugar levels should ideally be checked by finger stick just before and after the treatments, although the latter is not mandatory. Over the course of treatments, patients with type 2 diabetes mellitus, which is very sensitive to weight, exercise, and diet, may experience improvements in their blood sugars as their depression improves and they take better care of themselves in terms of diet and psychomotor activity (Netzel et al. 2002). Patients with type 1 diabetes mellitus tend to have brittle blood sugars and should be treated as early in the morning as possible, with either no insulin or a half dose of insulin just prior to the treatment. The remainder of the dose can be administered after the treatment along with juice or breakfast. Patients with type 2 diabetes who take insulin do not tend to have brittle blood sugars and can get by with insulin withheld until after the treatment as well as oral agents for diabetes. Occasionally patients with diabetes have very low blood sugars prior to ECT. The sugar should be raised—for example, with a glucose IV—before treatment is started. In the absence of scientific data establishing a safe upper limit for blood glucose in ECT, generally one would not treat the patient if the blood sugar level is greater than 250 mg/dL. If the treatment is felt to be urgent, then insulin can be given carefully to bring down the value in a safe manner prior to treatment.

Pulmonary Disorders

Patients with asthma or COPD should receive any routine prescribed inhalers prior to treatments. The patient with occasional asthmatic attacks probably does not need any special pretreatment workup beyond the routine, but if asthmatic attacks are regular, then consultation with a physician familiar with asthma treatment should be undertaken to achieve maximal stability prior to commencing ECT. The same is true of COPD patients. Large case series of asthma patients and COPD patients reveal that ECT is generally safe in these patients (Mueller et al. 2006; Schak et al. 2008).

If a patient is known to have pneumonia, one must balance the presumed pulmonary risks of ECT with the urgency of the need for ECT. Common sense would dictate waiting until the pneumonia has cleared before starting ECT, but in severe cases of psychopathology, the patient may need to be treated. Patients with pulmonary hypertension should be considered at increased risk of complications with ECT and should be seen by a pulmonologist before considering ECT.

Miscellaneous Medical Issues

Various abnormalities may show up on pre-ECT blood work. Mild sodium abnormalities do not correlate with seizure length in ECT and probably present no increased risk of complications (Rasmussen et al. 2007c). Potassium rises during treatment with succinylcholine, so preexisting hyperkalemia needs to be addressed prior to commencing ECT. Laboratory evidence of renal or hepatic impairment probably does not increase ECT risks, though patients in frank liver or renal failure obviously need attention to those issues. Likewise, anemia per se does not contraindicate ECT. Mild thyroid abnormalities are common in psychiatric patients and should not preclude ECT either, though, again, further workup is probably needed if such abnormalities are found anew.

Patients with severe osteoporosis might be at heightened risk of bone fractures with ECT, so assurance at time of anesthesia should be made of adequate muscular paralysis, preferably with the aid of a peripheral nerve stimulator. Occasionally, patients post–orthopedic surgery or in casts because of bone fractures are treated with ECT and also need assurance of good muscular blockade.

Occasionally in ECT practice a pregnant woman is encountered who may be considered for treatment. Ordinarily, "biological" treatments such as ECT or medications are avoided if possible during pregnancy so as to minimize risk to mother or fetus. However, in cases of severe psychopathology, usually catatonia, mania, or profound depression, some treatment must be given. In these cases, ECT is probably at least as safe an option as psychotropic medications. Minimization of medical risk during ECT in pregnancy will be covered in Chapter 5. Postpartum psychotic and manic states are exquisitely responsive to ECT.

A typical dilemma arises when a pregnant patient is depressed and requires more than psychotherapy. Should one choose medications or ECT? If the patient is being treated as an outpatient, which usually means she is not suicidal and is eating properly, and is able to cooperate, then probably pharmacotherapy will be the treatment of choice, though by no means is there universal agreement that psychotropic medications are safe during pregnancy. Consultation with an obstetrician is of course desirable. However, if the depression is so severe as to warrant inpatient hospitalization, then ECT should be given serious consideration insofar as it is quickly effective. Pregnant patients who are psychotically depressed, catatonic, or manic or who are in the throes of a schizophrenic decompensation affecting bodily functioning should be treated with ECT.

Monitoring Medical Issues Through the Course of Treatments

It is likely that an internist or other general medical physician, plus specialists when indicated, will provide pre-ECT consultation and guidance as part of the pre-ECT workup. Additionally, the anesthesiologist will manage within-treatment medical issues. However, over the course of treatments, the psychiatrist caring for the ECT patient will likely be the only physician providing regular assessments of the patient's status and thus will need to be familiar with the patient's medical problems and how to assess for anything requiring re-consultation with another physician. It cannot be overemphasized that even though a medically ill patient may be deemed "cleared for ECT" at baseline, there may be changes in that patient's status over the course of treatments that necessitate further assessment, and the psychiatrist is responsible for detecting them. Good, thorough ongoing physical assessments, including physical examinations and proper history taking, are thus essential aspects of the ECT clinician's responsibilities in managing patients over the course of treatments.

Patients undergoing ECT should of course have regular vital sign assessments, to include pulse and blood pressure, before each treatment. Such assessments are not required daily, as many patients are treated as outpatients and of course will not have daily visits. Before each treatment, there should be some questions about any new-onset symptoms such as shortness of breath, chest pain, or other bodily discomforts since the last treatment. There should also be an examination focusing on heart, lungs, and sensorium before each treatment. The clinician should be familiar with the pre-ECT status of the patient in terms of these symptoms and signs so as to be able to detect any apparent new-onset findings that occur during the course of treatments. Significant new vital sign changes, symptoms, or physical examination findings should prompt consideration of cancellation of that day's treatment and reassessment by a general medical physician or specialist.

Key Points

- ECT is a very safe procedure associated with rare medical complications and extremely rare mortality.

- Complication risk can be reduced with a thorough pre-ECT medical evaluation.

- The most important elements of the pre-ECT medical evaluation are history and physical examination.

- Specialty consultation and testing are appropriate for patients with certain medical conditions, most commonly cardiological.

5

Anesthesia for ECT

Electroconvulsive therapy (ECT) is a procedure performed after the induction of general anesthesia, which is referred to as *modified ECT*. Originally, ECT was conducted unmodified by anesthesia. In those days, the treatment electrodes were placed on the patient's head, a bite block was placed in the patient's mouth, and usually several attendants would grip the extremities firmly, and then the electrical stimulus was presented, with the resultant seizure being a fully expressed tonic-clonic (formerly "grand mal") convulsion. Holding down the extremities was a way to attempt to prevent bone fractures, which were quite common before anesthesia and muscle relaxation were introduced. Bennett (1940), in what has become a classic ECT paper, introduced curare muscle paralysis as an effective method to reduce bone fracture incidence. The problem with using muscle paralytics alone is that an awake patient, while paralyzed, experiences the extreme fright of not being able to breathe. This is an intolerable sensation. General anesthesia was introduced into ECT practice to render the patient unconscious before paralysis is induced, to avoid awareness of paralysis. Of course, when anesthesia and muscle paralysis are induced, spontaneous breathing ceases, necessitating administration of ventilations to the patient. Thus, the three critical aspects of ECT anesthesia practice consist of general anesthesia induction, muscular paralysis, and airway management. Each of these topics will be covered in separate sections below.

Additionally, the anesthesia staff will need to monitor vital signs (e.g., cardiac rhythm, blood pressure, pulse oximetry readings), address treatment-emergent medical issues such as cardiac dysrhythmias or extremes of blood pressure or pulse, and assist with recovery assessment. Because of the rapid and profound autonomic changes during ECT seizures, the anesthetist will occasionally utilize medications to control heart rate, blood pressure, or ECT rhythm. Additionally, side effects such as headache, myalgia, nausea, or postictal agitation will occasionally prompt use of other medications. These issues will be discussed in the section on adjunctive pharmacological agents for ECT anesthesia later in this chapter. Discussion of a few miscellaneous anesthetic considerations and implications of specific medical illnesses will round out the chapter.

Of course, the practice of anesthesia requires proper training and competence. In modern ECT practice there is typically, at least in the United States, an anesthesiologist or nurse anesthetist in attendance to supervise administration of anesthetic and adjunctive medications; assess the patient for unconsciousness so that muscular paralysis can be induced; monitor physiological functions such as cardiac activity, blood pressure, and pulse oximetry; and ensure proper ventilation. The last mentioned is typically directly performed by a second person, usually a respiratory therapist or nurse anesthetist. In this chapter, the expression *anesthesia staff* or *anesthetist* will be used when referring to the various practitioners providing these services.

The psychiatrist should be familiar with ECT anesthesia to ensure proper integration of administration of the electrical stimulus with the other activities in the suite as well as communication with patients, families, and other involved medical personnel, because the ECT clinician is most often the focal point of communication in this system of concerned parties. Additionally, there are certain aspects of anesthetic practice in ECT that have a direct impact on ECT efficacy and tolerability, and the psychiatrist should be aware of these. This chapter will review *what* is done for ECT anesthesia. There is a difference between *what* is done and *how* to do it. The author is not trained in anesthesia, and this chapter is to be construed solely as an introduction intended for psychiatric personnel and not as instruction on how anesthesia services are to be provided for ECT. Additionally, recognition and management of emergent medical conditions at the time of ECT treatments, such as malignant cardiac dysrhythmias or respiratory distress, also fall under the responsibility of the anesthesia staff but will not be discussed in this chapter.

General Issues

Relationship Between the Psychiatrist and the Anesthetist in the ECT Suite

The personnel present in an ECT suite during the treatments include the psychiatrist, anesthetist (anesthesiologist or nurse anesthetist), psychiatric nurse or other assistant, and somebody to ventilate the patient. These people work as a team, of course, but there are situations occurring during ECT treatments when one person is responsible for making final management decisions. The psychiatrist chooses electrode placement and stimulus dosing and determines seizure onset and termination. In contrast, the anesthetist will supervise the anesthetic induction method, muscle paralysis, management of heart rate, blood pressure, and electrocardiographic rhythm, and oxygenation. Most of the time, these functions do not intersect and events progress harmoniously. Occasionally, however, there may be issues of concern to the psychiatrist that might have an impact on anesthetic issues, in which case a good working relationship between the two is needed. For example, the ECT clinician is obviously concerned about inducing an adequate seizure for therapeutic purposes. Some anesthetic agents have potent anticonvulsant activity, as discussed later in this chapter, and the psychiatrist may wish to ask the anesthetist not to use, for example, a barbiturate but rather to use etomidate, which is associated with longer seizures. There may be a request to the anesthetist to withhold anticholinergic medication prior to treatment in the patient who has had urinary hesitancy. Yet another example in which the psychiatrist (or nursing staff) may wish to provide input is when the patient has postictal agitation, which may be managed with sedating medication that is usually prescribed at the hands of the anesthetist.

Occasionally, there may be anesthesia staff who are not particularly familiar with ECT anesthesia and who may be receptive to a few suggestions by the psychiatrist, usually involving which anesthetic agent to use to minimize possible deleterious effects on seizure expression. The importance of a good working relationship among all the ECT staff cannot be overemphasized, and it is key for the ECT psychiatrist to help facilitate this rapport and mutual respect.

American Society of Anesthesiologists' Physical Status Classification System

The American Society of Anesthesiologists (ASA) has developed a physical status classification system to evaluate degree of medical morbidity prior to procedures requiring general anesthesia (Mak et al. 2002). The anesthetist performing an assessment of a provisional ECT patient will rate the patient on this scale. There are five levels relevant to ECT patients. ASA I consists of healthy patients. ASA levels II and III consist of patients with mild and severe systemic disease, respectively, while ASA IV consists of patients with severe systemic disease that is a constant threat to life. ASA V consists of patients who are moribund and who are not expected to live without the surgical procedure in question. In ECT practice, most patients will be rated ASA levels I–IV. ECT patients who are rated as ASA level V might theoretically include those who will commit suicide or die of complications of profound catatonia without treatment, interesting scenarios not anticipated by the original framers of the ASA physical status assessment system. However, if the medical status of such patients is otherwise stable, they will probably not be given such a high rating. The ASA system was developed as a method of rating morbidity prior to surgery and not ECT. Whether this classification system accurately predicts risks specific to ECT, and, more importantly, whether it leads to any specific preventive action to lessen risk, has never been investigated in the ECT literature. What has proven to be far more practical as a method to alleviate medical risks of ECT is assessment of disease-specific strategies rather than relying on the ASA score. Aspects of anesthetic management of specific diseases will be covered later in this chapter.

Anesthetic Induction

As indicated earlier, the purpose of inducing general anesthesia in ECT is to render the patient unconscious for muscular paralysis. This process renders the patient without the usual gag reflex, so there is a risk of aspiration if there is reflux of any gastric contents. Thus, patients should have nothing by mouth for several hours prior to ECT. The anesthesiologist will confirm this prior to inducing anesthesia. Since ECT is usually conducted in the morning, the typical order is for nothing by mouth from midnight the night before treatments. Exceptions to this include necessary morning medications with a small amount of water.

The ideal ECT anesthetic agent would cause no pain on injection, induce anesthesia quickly, involve little if any effect on cardiovascular parameters (heart rate, blood pressure), have a rapid offset of action (so as not to have lingering effects into the recovery process), not interfere with the efficacy of the seizure, not worsen ECT-induced cognitive dysfunction, and not cause any posttreatment side effects such as nausea. None of the currently available general anesthetic agents for ECT are ideal on all of these parameters. The available agents include the intravenously administered anesthetics thiopental, methohexital, propofol, etomidate, and ketamine. Additionally, anesthesia can be induced with the inhalational agents, the most common of which is sevoflurane. Finally, occasional ECT teams have used high-potency narcotic agents, such as alfentanil or remifentanil, in combination with a barbiturate, the latter at lower doses than usual, as a strategy to prolong seizure length on the theory that longer seizures produce better antidepressant efficacy. All these agents will be discussed in the subsections below. Over the years, there have been occasional availability problems with methohexital and thiopental. The most commonly used agent at the time of this writing is methohexital. Table 5–1 summarizes common medications and doses for ECT anesthesia.

Pain on Injection

All intravenously administered anesthetic agents can cause pain on injection, which is termed *angialgia*. Etomidate and propofol seem to be the biggest offend-

---

TABLE 5–1. **Common anesthetic medications and dosing in ECT[a]**

Anticholinergics

Glycopyrrolate	0.2–0.4 mg IV
Atropine	0.4 mg IV

General anesthetics

Thiopental	2.0–4.0 mg/kg IV
Methohexital	1.0–1.5 mg/kg IV
Etomidate	0.3 mg/kg IV
Ketamine	1.0–2.0 mg/kg IV
Propofol	1.0–2.0 mg/kg IV
Sevoflurane	0.5%–3.0% inhaled

Muscle paralytics

Succinylcholine	1.0–1.5 mg/kg IV
Nondepolarizers[b]	Variable

Note. IV = intravenously.
[a]Doses cited are typical but may be higher or lower for individual patients.
[b]The most frequently used nondepolarizers in the author's experience are atracurium, cisatracurium, and rocuronium.

ers in this regard, followed by methohexital and then thiopental and ketamine, the latter two rarely causing injection pain (Rasmussen and Ritter 2014a). A small dose of lidocaine, a local anesthetic, into the intravenous (IV) site, with blockage of blood flow from that vein a few inches downstream from the site of injection, which causes the lidocaine to stay in the area around the injection site and block nerve endings, can help prevent angialgia when this is followed by the anesthetic. Of note, one would not want to give too much lidocaine because it has anticonvulsant properties and in older studies reduced antidepressant efficacy (Cronholm and Ottosson 1963a). Typical doses of lidocaine for angialgia prevention would be 10–30 mg or so. Use of a large bore vein for the IV site, such as an antecubital, has been shown to lessen angialgia (Jalota et al. 2011). For patients who are afraid to pursue further ECT because of excessively painful angialgia with intravenous agents, anesthesia induction with sevoflurane can be much more comfortable.

Rapid Onset of Unconsciousness

All the intravenous and inhalational anesthetic methods listed above cause a rapid anesthesia. The differences among them are clinically insignificant, so there are no grounds for choosing differentially based on this issue. Usually, if an effective dose is given, then unconsciousness occurs within about 30 seconds of administration. The personnel administering ventilations will check for loss of an eyelid reflex as a sign of deep enough anesthesia to administer the paralytic agent without awareness of paralysis. There are occasional patients who are a bit agitated as they fall unconscious. Fortunately, such patients do not tend to recall this apparently uncomfortable phase of their anesthesia experience. Note should be made that etomidate commonly causes myoclonic jerks as anesthesia descends on the patient. These adventitious movements involve the whole body sometimes and may make evaluation of loss of lid reflex and determination of depth of anesthesia more difficult than with the other anesthesia agents.

Cardiovascular Effects of Anesthetics

The ECT seizure is associated with a sharp spike in pulse and blood pressure that typically lasts for several minutes after seizure termination (Rasmussen et al. 1999). Ketamine, in anesthetic doses, causes a rise in blood pressure (Erdil et al. 2015; Rasmussen et al. 1996). Because the seizure itself causes a sharp rise in blood pressure and heart rate, the relatively subtle effects of the different anesthetics tend to be less prominent or clinically relevant. Propofol, which in numerous studies has been associated with less ictal rise in pulse and blood pressure than other anesthetics (Rasmussen 2014), may allow the anesthesiologist to use less antihypertensive medication such as beta-blockers or eliminate it altogether. There does not appear to be a strong differential effect of the available anesthetic agents on cardiovascular parameters beyond the first 10 minutes or so during recovery, as by that time the hemodynamic effects of these agents have largely disappeared.

Another cardiovascular parameter of interest is cardiac dysrhythmias that commonly occur during and shortly after ECT seizures, including premature ventricular contractions, premature atrial contractions, very short runs of ventricular tachycardia (i.e., just a few beats or so without compromise of cardiac output), and, especially at the end of the seizure when parasympathetic stimulation predominates, junctional rhythms. These rhythm disturbances, which by and large are temporary and quite benign, are mostly caused by the intense autonomic nervous system changes induced by the seizure (i.e., an initial short-lived parasympathetic phase, followed by a sympathetic phase, followed at the end of the seizure by another parasympathetic phase). In general, the differential effects of the various anesthetic agents on cardiac rhythm independent of those caused by the seizure itself are small. Choice of anesthetic in ECT is generally not made on the basis of dysrhythmic potential.

Effect on Seizure Duration and Antidepressant Efficacy

Of course, the therapeutic element of ECT is the seizure. It is ironic that several of the anesthetic induction agents used in a procedure designed to induce a seizure are themselves potent anticonvulsant agents (mainly the barbiturates and propofol). However, it is clear from controlled ECT trials that ECT can be highly effective when barbiturates or propofol is used as the anesthetic.

That being said, the ECT clinician wants the fullest expression of seizure efficacy. Determining seizure efficacy will be discussed in more detail in Chapter 6. Suffice it to say here that seizure duration and electroencephalographic (EEG) indices are the two main proxies for seizure efficacy that can be assessed at the time of the treatment. Of course, the only way to determine efficacy over the course of treatments is to assess clinical response. Researchers over the decades have speculated that seizure duration might correlate with efficacy, and barbiturate anesthetics may result in shorter seizures than when etomidate or ketamine is used. Propofol results in the shortest seizures, yet several controlled trials demonstrate no compromise in antidepressant efficacy when this agent is used (Rasmussen 2014). However, occasionally there may be failure to elicit a seizure outright, or ultrashort seizures occur, and one cannot help but worry about a lack of efficacy with, say, single-digit-duration seizures (less than 10 seconds). In such circumstances, it is quite easy to switch from a barbiturate or propofol to etomidate, or to use a lower dose of the original anesthetic and supplement with a high-potency narcotic like remifentanil or alfentanil (Akcaboy et al. 2005; Chen 2011; Nguyen et al. 1997; Nishikawa et al. 2011; Vishne et al. 2005). The benefit of these high-potency opiate compounds in enhancing seizure duration is mediated not by exerting a direct proconvulsant effect, however, but by allowing lower doses of anticonvulsant anesthetics to be used (Rasmussen et al. 2009a; van den Broek et al. 2004).

There has been recent excitement in psychiatry at the prospect that ketamine may have independent antidepressant properties. Ketamine has been shown in numerous controlled and open-label trials to have potent and rapid antidepressant activity (Rasmussen et al. 2013). ECT clinicians have been understandably curious as to whether anesthesia with ketamine may hasten or augment the already good antidepressant activity of ECT. Some studies have indeed shown that ketamine anesthesia in ECT (or at least ketamine supplementation of another anesthetic) can hasten the antidepressant activity of ECT without affecting the ultimate remission rates (Bryson et al. 2014; Kranaster et al. 2011; Loo et al. 2012a; Okamoto et al. 2010; Wang et al. 2012), while other studies have failed to find such a beneficial effect (Abdallah et al. 2012; Järventausta et al. 2013; Rasmussen et al. 2014; Yen et al. 2015). A recent meta-analysis concluded that there was currently no evidence to support an antidepressant-enhancing effect of ketamine when used in ECT for major depression (McGirr et al. 2015).

Concerns have also been pointed out about poor tolerability of ketamine when this agent is used as an ECT anesthetic (Rasmussen and Ritter 2014b). Most commonly, vestibular effects such as headache, vertigo, and dizziness occur and can last for much of the day. Also, psychotomimetic effects such as emergence agitation or dissociative experiences (e.g., out-of-body phenomena) can be quite traumatic to some patients. At this time, in this author's opinion, ketamine is not to be recommended for routine use as an ECT anesthetic or anesthetic supplement. It should be reserved for situations in which adequate seizures cannot be elicited with other means. Etomidate or the combination of low-dose barbiturate or low-dose propofol with high-potency opiates is a preferable alternative to ketamine. If ketamine is used, then probably a benzodiazepine such as midazolam or diazepam should be administered after the seizure has stopped but before conscious awareness is regained in order to prevent psychotomimetic reactions (Rasmussen and Ritter 2014b). Most studies have used racemic ketamine. There are observational data from a group in Germany utilizing the enantiomer esketamine purporting to show good tolerability of this agent when it is used in ECT (Hoyer et al. 2014; Janke et al. 2015; Kranaster et al. 2014; Sartorius et al. 2015). Data comparing esketamine with racemic ketamine would be welcome and are currently not available.

Etomidate is associated with no shortening of seizure duration (Hoyer et al. 2014) and would thus seem to be the ideal anesthetic for ECT. However, concerns in the anesthesiology literature about adrenal suppression and increased mortality in the operative setting when etomidate is used versus other anesthetic agents have limited its use by some anesthesiologists (Lebowitz 2014). There are data from an ECT study indicating mild suppression of adrenal activity, but not to levels below normal (Wang et al. 2011). Also, there are data indicating that etomidate anesthesia in ECT is not associated with any compromise of antidepressant activity (Abdollahi et al. 2012; Ayhan et al. 2015; Canbek et al. 2015; Graveland et al. 2013; Janouschek et al. 2013). For the purposes of this chapter, the ECT clinician needs to be aware that some anesthesiologists hesitate to use etomidate, even though from the psychiatric standpoint it has good qualities for ECT usage.

There have been several EEG markers implicated in correlations with ECT outcome (e.g., EEG amplitude, regularity of spike and wave complexes, degree of postictal suppression), a topic that is discussed further in Chapter 6. As far as these so-called EEG indices are concerned, however, none as yet have been shown to correlate consistently with particular anesthetic agents. Thus, if the ECT clinician is paying close attention to ictal EEG quality, anesthetic manipulations are not likely to have a clinically relevant impact.

Duration of Anesthesia

As the purpose of ECT anesthesia is to prevent awareness of muscular paralysis, one would obviously want the duration of the anesthetic agent to exceed that of the succinylcholine. Occasionally, after the seizure is complete, some patients start to wake up and are still paralyzed. The sensation is intensely uncomfortable for patients and quite frightening. The heart rate typically spikes to very highly tachycardic levels, the patient demonstrates rudimentary but not effective attempts to breathe, and occasionally the patient will groan. A repeat dose of anesthetic is indicated in this situation.

Beyond the point of wearing off of succinylcholine, a rapid recovery (i.e., return to breathing and consciousness) is desirable. Among the available anesthetics, thiopental has a particularly long duration of action. All the other agents have roughly similar durations of action. It is important for the psychiatrist to be aware that the period from seizure termination until resumption of spontaneous respirations constitutes a vulnerable time for the patient's airway, and expert management at the hands of the person handling the ventilation is mandatory. Once the patient can breathe without assistance, and blood pressure, heart rate, and cardiac activity are stable, the patient can be safely discharged from the ECT suite to the recovery room. The psychiatrist should be aware that on recovery from anesthesia after the seizure, shivering (especially associated with barbiturates) may occur and must not be confused with recurrent seizure activity.

Post-anesthesia Side Effects

The recovery room time consists of special attention to the patient's regaining conscious awareness. During this time, which typically lasts 15–30 minutes or so, the patient is monitored via electrocardiography with regular blood pressure checks and continuous pulse oximetry. The airway, which should initially be supported with supplemental oxygen, is still vulnerable, especially in patients with obstructive sleep apnea. Such patients should ideally have whatever device they use for nighttime airway assistance available to use in the ECT recovery situation. Occasionally, heart rate and blood pressure rise as the patient awakens, and the anesthetist may wish to supplement with a beta-blocker such as labetalol. If the blood pressure is high and the pulse rate is relatively low, then a vasodilator such as hydralazine may be used to lower the blood pressure without causing further reduction in heart rate.

Some uncomfortable aspects of recovery include nausea/vomiting, agitation, headache, myalgia, and subjective confusion. Overall, there is no compelling evidence that the different anesthetic agents are associated with substantial differences in any of these parameters (Rasmussen 2014). Exceptions include the propensity of ketamine to cause prolonged vestibular side effects (Rasmussen and Ritter 2014b). Additionally, propofol may be associated with less posttreatment nausea (Rasmussen 2014). Nausea and even vomiting later in the day (i.e., several hours posttreatment) are somewhat common in ECT practice, but by that time, the cause is probably the seizure itself, because anesthetic medications have worn off.

Ketamine has been associated with emergence reactions when used for surgical anesthesia (Rasmussen and Ritter 2014b). These reactions typically consist of perceptual distortions such as visual hallucinations and can be quite vivid and disturbing. Additionally, dissociative reactions, which may be described by patients as "out of body" experiences, can be quite traumatic. If ketamine is used for ECT anesthesia, it probably would be prudent to add a benzodiazepine (midazolam or diazepam) at the end of the seizure to reduce emergence discomfort with this agent.

Inhalational Anesthesia for ECT

Inhalational anesthesia is rarely used for ECT but is available as an option. These agents flow through the oxygen mask used to ventilate the patient and can effect a fairly rapid, comfortable state of unconsciousness sufficient for muscular paralysis. However, some patients find the use of the mask to cover the face uncomfortable and prefer not to have inhalational anesthesia.

The most commonly used inhalational agent is sevoflurane, which has been compared to a variety of the intravenous agents in ECT and found to have a comparable tolerability and cardiovascular profile (Calarge et al. 2003; Hodgson et al. 2004; Loughnan et al. 2004; Rasmussen et al. 2007b; Toprak et al. 2005; Wajima et al. 2003). This type of anesthesia induction may prove convenient for the patient with a severe needle phobia, allowing unconsciousness to be reached so that the intravenous needle can be inserted without causing pain. Additionally, the patient who is severely agitated prior to ECT can be effectively anesthetized with sevoflurane, allowing an easier time getting the IV line placed (Rasmussen et al. 2005). Of course, if the patient is so agitated that a mask cannot be fit well over the mouth, then intramuscular ketamine may present the first step in calming the patient down for IV access. Also, for patients with highly distressing angialgia with intravenous agents, inhalational anesthesia may prove more comfortable. Finally, sevoflurane has a vasodilating effect, making IV access easier in patients who have very difficult veins to access.

Muscular Paralysis

The original procedure in ECT practice consisted of an awake, unanesthetized, unparalyzed patient having an electrical stimulus passed through the head. The resultant unmodified convulsion caused a significant risk of bone fractures, which was actually the main adverse effect of ECT in decades past. After the groundbreaking report by Bennett on the use of curare in ECT (Bennett 1940), the risk of bone fractures has been almost eliminated with the use of effective muscular paralysis during ECT seizures. The standard neuromuscular blocking agent in ECT today is succinylcholine (also called suxamethonium in some countries outside the United States). This agent is a depolarizing muscular paralytic, the effects of which are achieved by occupation of acetylcholine receptors on the neuromuscular junction causing depolarization of the membrane. Continuous depolarization eventually paralyzes the muscle. Succinylcholine is the standard neuromuscular blocking agent around the world and is used in the vast majority of ECT treatments.

As succinylcholine takes effect, fasciculations of the limb muscles can be appreciated. When these disappear, usually within 60–90 seconds or so from the time of administration, then the patient is paralyzed. Typical doses of succinylcholine are 1.0 mg/kg or thereabouts. Some anesthesiologists prefer to use a nerve stimulator to confirm muscular paralysis. Of note, direct muscular stimulation by an electrical current bypasses the paralysis induced by the succinylcholine, so that when the button is pushed on the ECT machine, and the electricity passes through the head and stimulates muscles of mastication, there will be a sharp clenching of the jaw. Thus, a bite block should be placed in the mouth prior to this in order to protect oral structures. When succinylcholine is used, the first muscles to be paralyzed are upper airway muscles and the last are the muscles of the diaphragm. Later, the first muscle to regain use is the diaphragm and the last muscles to recover are those of the upper airway, so the patient might be trying to breathe but have obstruction of the airway. Whoever is managing the airway should be aware of this, and the patient may experience air hunger, which is uncomfortable and frightening. An extra dose of anesthetic may help at this juncture if the patient appears panicky.

Succinylcholine has been associated with causing malignant hyperthermia (MH), a potentially fatal condition characterized by high spiking fever and fulminant tachycardia. It is usually inherited as an autosomal dominant gene. Thus, patients with a family history of MH should not be given succinylcholine but rather should be administered a nondepolarizing neuromuscular blocking agent. Volatile anesthetics have also been associated with MH and should not be used in susceptible patients. There is no test for MH prior to ECT other than muscle biopsy, which is not routinely indicated. Of note, the anesthetist may elect not to use succinylcholine in patients with a history of neuroleptic malignant syndrome (NMS), on the theory that there may be some pathophysiological similarity between that and MH. While NMS and MH would seem to be separate entities with separate risk factors, data on use of succinylcholine safely in NMS patients are scarce, and it is true that safe alternatives to succinylcholine exist.

Succinylcholine causes an abrupt release of potassium into the extracellular space. This may put the patient with already elevated potassium levels at risk for hyperkalemia-induced cardiac dysrhythmias. Neurological conditions causing motor neuron abnormalities increase the risk of succinylcholine-induced hyperkalemia. There is much variability in the threshold used by anesthetists in choosing when to avoid succinylcholine and use a nondepolarizing agent in patients with histories of neurological illnesses such as cerebral palsy and stroke. Some anesthetists will not use succinylcholine in patients with virtually any neurological history—the psychiatrist should be aware that practice among anesthetists varies, and nondepolarizing paralytic agents may be used in some of their patients. Recent history of NMS is sometimes considered a risk for this phenomenon as well, so some anesthetists prefer to use nondepolarizing neuromuscular blocking agents in these patients.

A contraindication for succinylcholine is deficiency of pseudocholinesterase, the plasma enzyme responsible for metabolizing succinylcholine. This manifests in paralysis prolonged beyond the usual few minutes that occurs for people with normal pseudocholinesterase activity. Genetic variants of this enzyme, either the heterozygous variant or the more sinister homozygous variant, can cause prolonged paralysis with succinylcholine. If a patient has prolonged paralysis at the first ECT session, the anesthesiologist may elect to order a test such as pseudocholinesterase blood levels or the dibucaine number. Dibucaine is a local anesthetic that is known to inhibit activity of normal pseudocholinesterase but not hetero- or homozygous atypical variants of that enzyme. In laboratory assays, the dibucaine number is expressed as a percentage of inhibition by dibucaine—larger values (say, 80%–100% inhibition) reflect normal pseudocholinesterase activity, while values about 30%–70% reflect heterozygote mutant enzyme activity, and values below 30% inhibition reflect homozygote mutant enzyme activity. Homozygote mutant pseudocholinesterase activity will result in much more prolonged paralysis than the heterozygote activity. If abnormal results occur, then a nondepolarizing neuromuscular compound (none of these compounds except mivacurium are metabolized by pseudocholinesterase) would be used at subsequent ECT treatments. There are also some nongenetic causes of abnormal pseudocholinesterase activity, such as malignancy, liver disease, pregnancy, and inanition.

In these scenarios in which succinylcholine is deemed unsafe to use, the anesthetist will undertake muscular paralysis with a nondepolarizing neuromuscular blocking drug. These agents occupy the acetylcholine binding site at the neuromuscular junction, without causing depolarization, and prevent it from being stimulated, thus directly causing paralysis without depolarizing the membrane. There are no fasciculations seen when these agents are used. Because they all take a longer time for onset and have a longer duration of activity than succinylcholine, these agents are only used when there is a contraindication for succinylcholine. When nondepolarizing agents are used in ECT, the anesthesiologist may, after the seizure is over, utilize a "reversal" agent such as neostigmine or edrophonium, which are cholinesterase inhibitors that prolong the action of endogenous acetylcholine, to hasten the end of paralysis. Since these latter agents could cause bradycardia based on cholinergic stimulation of the heart, they are typically administered with an anticholinergic agent such as glycopyrrolate or atropine to prevent that action. If rocuronium or vecuronium is used as the nondepolarizing neuromuscular blocking agent, a specific reversal agent—namely, sugammadex—is used that chemically attaches to the rocuronium molecule and irreversibly inhibits it, allowing for a fairly rapid reversal of activity and a shorter time to breathing after the ECT seizure is done.

There are two types of nondepolarizing neuromuscular blocking agents: benzylisoquinolines (those ending in "urium," such as atracurium, cisatracurium, and mivacurium) and steroidal compounds (those ending in "onium," such as vecuronium, pancuronium, and rocuronium). These agents differ from one another by speed of onset and total duration of paralysis. Mivacurium, with its relatively fast onset and short duration, showed initial promise as an alternative to succinylcholine but was found to cause symptomatic histamine-mediated reactions, and it is metabolized by pseudocholinesterase like succinylcholine and thus would not be appropriate with deficiency of that enzyme. As of this writing, it is not available in the United States but is still used in other countries. None of the remaining nondepolarizing agents are ideal for all parameters. Anesthetists use atracurium, cisatracurium, and rocuronium with some regularity. They all have a much longer duration of paralysis than succinylcholine. Thus, it is likely that the patient given such medication will awaken while still paralyzed, necessitating repeat doses of anesthetic to prevent awareness of paralysis. A new development in this regard is a medication known as sugammadex, which when administered intravenously after nondepolarizer paralysis with either rocuronium or vecuronium binds the paralytic agent and, in turn, prevents it from occupying its receptors at the neuromuscular junction. The complexes are excreted, and spontaneous breathing occurs much faster than if the paralytic is excreted on its own.

Ventilation

It is rather obvious that proper ventilation is critical in ECT practice. Pulse oximetry assists the person doing the ventilating, who may be an anesthesiologist, nurse practitioner, or respiratory therapist in the United States. Other countries have their own type of specially trained personnel to perform this vital function. The bite block must be placed carefully in the mouth prior to electrical stimulus delivery because the jaw will contract tightly, thus making it necessary for the mouth to be held shut during stimulus delivery to prevent biting of the tongue, lips, or cheek or breaking off of a tooth or dental appliance. There should be nothing metal, like wristbands or watches, on the person doing the ventilations that could touch the stimulus electrodes during stimulus delivery.

Once the baseline pulse oximetry reading is established, and the blood pressure, heart rate, and ECG rhythm have also been assessed, general anesthesia is induced, during which time breathing stops. The person performing the ventilations must be aware of this and commence with positive pressure ventilations using a bag valve mask (Ambu bag) and 100% oxygen and will be able to assess adequacy of ventilations by observing chest rise with each ventilation and pulse oximetry readings. Endotracheal intubation is not routinely used in ECT anesthesia. Such a procedure presents significant risks and discomforts, and performing this procedure three times a week for a few weeks or so would cause discomfort to a patient (e.g., sore throats) and unnecessary buildup of intubation risks. Situations in which intubation may be needed include extreme obesity, severe cases of gastroesophageal reflux disease, and the later stages of pregnancy, all situations in which the anesthetist would be concerned about the risk of reflux and consequent pulmonary complications. Also, occasionally a patient will develop laryngospasm (i.e., spasm of the vocal cords) or some other acute ventilation difficulty after anesthesia is induced, necessitating rapid intubation. Thus, the presence of equipment and personnel competent to manage such situations is critical in the ECT suite.

Ventilations usually proceed quite smoothly, however, and are given at a pace of one ventilation every few seconds or so throughout the procedure until the seizure stops and the anesthetic and muscle relaxant medications wear off. The psychiatrist may notice that as these medications lose their effect, the patient may appear to struggle at first with breathing, so the person doing the ventilations must be attentive to assisting just enough until the patient is fully capable of breathing independently. Only at this point can the patient be dismissed from the treatment suite to the recovery area. Sometimes, the general anesthetic agent wears off faster than the paralytic agent, leading to a state after the seizure in which the patient is gaining some awareness of paralysis, which as discussed earlier is to be avoided because of the intolerable sensation of not being able to breathe. In such cases, one may be able to deduce that this is happening by a rapid escalation of heart rate and the "fish flop," a type of movement in which the patient struggles to move but is only capable of gross truncal movements. The patient may also groan in a manner communicating distress. Readministration of a dose of anesthetic agent is appropriate, as is trying to reassure the patient that he or she is not suffocating.

Another issue pertaining to ventilation, one that the psychiatrist will be more involved with, is whether to undertake hyperventilation prior to seizure induction as a method of seizure prolongation. The relationship between seizure length and clinical outcome is unclear; however, markedly short seizures do occasionally occur during a course of ECT, and the psychiatrist may be concerned that maximal efficacy is not being achieved. The issue of seizure augmentation strategies, including hyperventilation, is discussed more fully in Chapter 6.

Adjunctive Pharmacological Agents for ECT Anesthesia

Anticholinergics

Because of the profound autonomic changes during ECT treatments, there may be other medications chosen by the anesthesiologist to help control blood pressure, heart rate, or ECG abnormalities. Anticholinergic agents, such as glycopyrrolate or atropine, can be given prior to the treatment, usually intravenously, to prevent the bradycardia that can occur right after presentation of the electrical stimulus (i.e., the initial parasympathetic phase). Normally, this would not be necessary, because this phase is rapidly replaced by the intense sympathetic phase associated with the seizure with its attendant tachycardia. However, if the electrical stimulus fails to elicit a seizure, then the parasympathetically mediated bradycardia may go unopposed, resulting in occasional disconcertingly long periods of asystole. There have also been case reports of prolonged asystole when a nonconvulsive stimulus is given in the face of prior beta-blocker administration, an effect that would obviously enhance any tendency toward bradycardia (Wells et al. 1988; Wulfson et al. 1984). For these reasons, most anesthesiologists prefer to administer an anticholinergic. Glycopyrrolate is used for this purpose in a typical dose of 0.2 mg. Alternatively, atropine in a dose of 0.4 mg could also be used. High-dose atropine (0.8 mg IV) may be necessary to prevent prolonged asystole in rare cases (Robinson and Lighthall 2004). Intravenous administration of these drugs is appropriate before anesthesia induction. Another purpose of the anticholinergic agents is to dry up oral secretions that cause ventilation to be compromised. Use of these drugs intramuscularly 30 minutes or more before anesthesia in order to allow the antisialogogue effect to reach full intensity leads to greater patient discomfort with the dry mouth and of course involves yet another needle stick. Intramuscular administration of anticholinergic medications pre-ECT should be avoided in favor of the intravenous route.

Anticholinergics can cause difficulties, such as prolonged tachycardia even after the treatment is over, as well as urinary hesitancy, especially in elderly men with prostate hypertrophy. If either of these two problems occurs, further anticholinergic medications prior to ECT should be withheld for patient comfort. The problem of bradycardia in the face of subconvulsive seizures should be quite unlikely after the first treatment establishing seizure threshold; with further treatments, there is very high confidence that a seizure will occur. For the occasional patient with profuse oral secretions during ECT, making ventilations difficult, a double dose of anticholinergic (e.g., glycopyrrolate 0.4 mg IV) helps dry up the secretions. Of course, the downside of this will be a higher-than-usual heart rate, a posttreatment sensation of dry mouth, and possibly urinary hesitancy for at least the rest of the day.

Antihypertensives

The blood pressure spikes during ECT seizures can be high, prompting some anesthesiologists to administer an antihypertensive medication to dampen this tendency. However, the duration of the elevation in blood pressures is short, on the order of a few minutes to perhaps 15–20 minutes or so after the seizure is over (Rasmussen et al. 1999). There is no study in which use of medications to blunt the blood pressure rise in ECT has been shown to result in a lower incidence of major adverse cardiovascular events such as cerebrovascular accidents, dangerous dysrhythmias, or myocardial infarctions. The incidence of those conditions is extremely small for ECT, so any prospective controlled trial would have to be inordinately large to be sufficiently statistically powered to detect a protective effect. However, it seems to be prudent to use such medications in ECT in situations involving high cardiac risk. The most commonly used one has been labetalol, which has alpha- as well as beta-blockade and can thus control tachycardia as well as blood pressure. Esmolol, an ultra-short-acting (i.e., half-life of approximately 9 minutes) pure beta-blocker, has also been used. In a comparative study of these two beta-blockers, esmolol was most effective at blunting the blood pressure and heart rate elevation in the first 3–5 minutes or so after the end of the seizure, while labetalol was more effective in the 5–10 minutes after the seizure, findings reflective of the differing half-lives of these two drugs (Shrestha et al. 2007). An early literature cautioned that beta-blockers might shorten seizure length in ECT (McCall et al. 1997; van den Broek et al. 1999; Weinger et al. 1991). Such effects were of small magnitude (typically a few seconds) and not consistently found (Blanch et al. 2001; Kovac et al. 1990, 1991; O'Flaherty et al. 1992). There has been no study that randomly assigned patients to receive either esmolol or labetalol versus placebo for the entire course of treatments and assessed antidepressant outcome. Such a study would be welcome. The anesthetic propofol has a definite seizure-shortening effect without compromising ECT efficacy, according to several controlled trials (Rasmussen 2014). Thus, it is unlikely the small seizure-shortening effect of beta-blockers is clinically significant.

There are other antihypertensive medications used for blood pressure control during ECT. Hydralazine, for example, is a vasodilator that can cause reflex tachycardia and so is rarely used except when there is bradycardia to begin with, in which case a beta-blocker might not be optimal. Finally, calcium channel blockade with verapamil, diltiazem, or others may be preferred by some anesthesia practitioners.

Antiemetics

Nausea and vomiting are common after ECT treatments. Preventive measures include medications such as prochlorperazine (2.5–10 mg IV), metoclopramide (10–20 mg IV), and ondansetron (4 mg IV), the last mentioned being the preferred treatment given the dopamine blockade–induced akathisia potential of the first two agents. Usually, antiemetic medication is administered before subsequent treatments after a patient experiences nausea or vomiting after the first one.

Analgesics

Post-ECT headaches, muscle aches (myalgia), and jaw pain are common. Myalgias and jaw pain usually are worst after the first treatment and then abate substantially with further treatments (Rasmussen et al. 2008d). Headaches may occur after each treatment. Preventive measures include oral acetaminophen or ibuprofen before the treatment or intravenous ketorolac, a nonsteroidal anti-inflammatory drug (NSAID). The latter may inhibit platelet formation and renal function, so these parameters should be followed in patients receiving that drug regularly. Ketorolac is not needed at the first treatment session; rather, its use should be reserved for subsequent treatments in those patients who experience troublesome headache after the first treatment (Rasmussen 2013). Opiate compounds for post-ECT headache are not recommended because tolerance tends to build up rapidly to their effect.

The patient with temporomandibular joint disease (TMJ) may complain of much jaw pain both before and after ECT treatments. Making sure the jaw is tightly closed with a bite block before electrical stimulation is important to lessen the effects of jaw contraction. Use of high doses of succinylcholine under the presumption that it might lessen the degree of clamping of the jaw during electrical stimulation, and thus lessen ECT-induced pain, is unlikely to help, because the electrical stimulation directly causes contraction of the jaw muscles, thus bypassing any effect of succinylcholine at the neuromuscular junction. TMJ patients may benefit from pretreatment with NSAIDs such as ketorolac IV or ibuprofen by mouth.

Miscellaneous

Occasionally there is hypotension during or after the seizure, in which case a pressor agent such as ephedrine may be used to raise the pressure. Ventricular ectopy may indicate use of lidocaine. Patients receiving ongoing glucocorticoid medications such as prednisone are often prescribed "stress steroid" doses prior to surgical procedures. A recent report indicates no need for use of such medications, which may have deleterious effects such as hyperglycemia, before ECT (Rasmussen et al. 2008a).

Miscellaneous ECT Anesthesia Issues

Difficult IV Sticks

Patients typically receive 6–10 or more ECT treatments per index course and obviously more if maintenance ECT is done. This adds up to a lot of IV sticks, the pain of which is almost unbearable for some patients, especially those in a fragile emotional state. Some patients in addition have difficult-to-access veins, making it necessary to perform multiple sticks per session. One solution, especially for the patient expected to receive long-term maintenance ECT, is an implantable IV access port, such as a Port-a-Cath. A percutaneous intraluminal central catheter (PICC line) is another option, especially for inpatients. Another option, for short-term use, is to leave the IV catheter in place in between treatments. This is acceptable only if the patient is behaviorally stable enough not to manipulate the IV site. Yet another option is to anesthetize the patient first with the inhalational agent sevoflurane and then place the IV access. Sevoflurane has the added advantage of causing some venodilation, making access easier. The sevoflurane method may also be useful for the highly agitated patient, in whom it may be quite difficult to obtain an IV access site because of behavioral uncooperativeness (Rasmussen et al. 2005). Intramuscular ketamine may also cause sufficient sedation to render the patient behaviorally calm for IV access in such situations.

Oral Care During ECT Anesthesia

There is a sharp contraction of jaw muscles during presentation of the electrical stimulus. This contraction occurs because the electrical stimulus directly stimulates the jaw muscles, bypassing the paralysis caused by succinylcholine. Thus, there must be attentive placement of a bite block to prevent dental complications or cuts to the lips, cheeks, or tongue. Before treatments, there should be inspection of the oral cavity, with the examining staff looking especially for loose teeth or dental fixtures such as caps. Dentures should be removed (assuming they are removable) prior to treatment, as should any dental appliance that is removable, such as a bridge. If there are any loose teeth, they should ideally be removed prior to treatment. However, in the interest of not delaying treatments, good placement of a bite block can help prevent a loose tooth from falling out during the treatment. Of course, it can be highly problematic if a tooth falls out of place and goes down the trachea.

Specific Medical Conditions and ECT Anesthesia

Congestive Heart Failure

Once the patient with congestive heart failure (CHF) is prepared to begin ECT treatments, it is important to assess baseline oxygenation levels prior to anesthesia administration to have a basis for comparison after the treatment is finished. Adequate preoxygenation is important as well. Time to onset of anesthesia will be increased and muscular paralysis will take longer than usual because of low cardiac output. The decision of whether to administer an anticholinergic agent depends on a variety of factors, such as baseline heart rate and whether the patient is taking a beta-blocker, as the latter may predispose the patient to prolonged asystole in the case of nonconvulsive stimulations. Also, because patients with CHF tend to be elderly, there may be uncomfortable urinary hesitancy as well. It probably is prudent to administer an anticholinergic at the first treatment session and assess for heart rate response as well as urinary symptoms later in the day before determining whether to use it again for subsequent treatments. Blood pressure control during the treatments may be achieved with judicious use of beta-blockers such as labetalol, with caution regarding depression of myocardial function as a possibility. Doses of such medication are typically low. Arrhythmias are common during ECT in CHF patients and can be effectively prevented most of the time with adequate preoxygenation.

Coronary Artery Disease

Anesthetists tend to be aggressive in using medication to lessen myocardial workload during ECT in coronary artery disease (CAD) patients. Most commonly, beta-blockade with labetalol is used to lessen the rise in heart rate and blood pressure. This is usually administered around the same time as anesthesia. Esmolol is less commonly used because it has such a short half-life (i.e., approximately 9 minutes) that repeated doses are needed for a more sustained effect. As is the case with CHF patients, good preoxygenation before anesthesia will probably help prevent ischemic changes on the electrocardiogram.

Several studies have shown that beta-blockers lower the rise in heart rate and blood pressure during ECT, but several studies looking at ECG evidence of ischemic changes showed no effects of these medications (Castelli et al. 1995; O'Connor et al. 1996; Zvara et al. 1997). However, it certainly seems reasonable to use these medications, given their proven cardioprotective effect in CAD patients in other settings. Concern about orthostatic hypotension later in the day with labetalol, which has a relatively long half-life, is allayed by a report showing that use of this drug was not associated with drops in blood pressure the afternoons of treatments (Rasmussen et al. 2008c).

Dysrhythmias and Pacemakers/Implantable Cardioverter Defibrillators

There is no need to use a magnet over a pacemaker in modern ECT practice. These devices are electrically isolated from the ECT electrical stimulus. Use of anticholinergic premedication is probably unnecessary, because the pacemaker will prevent asystoles, unless there is profuse sialorrhea making ventilation difficult, in which case an anticholinergic can help.

Implantable cardioverter defibrillators (ICDs) should be turned off by a competent cardiac electrophysiology nurse (or other trained technician) only after the patient has been placed on the ECG monitor with resuscitation equipment readily available. The ECG monitor should be left on at least until the ICD is turned back on after the seizure is completed.

It is a bit of a quandary to determine how to handle atrial fibrillation (AF) during ECT treatments. Even if the patient with known AF is rate controlled prior to treatments, it is not uncommon for him or her to go into a prolonged rapid rate during treatments. Beta-blockers can be quite helpful in this scenario. The patient in AF who converts to sinus rhythm should have evaluation by an internist for initiation of anticoagulation if the patient is not already taking such medication. If a rate-controlled AF patient goes into a prolonged rapid rate unresponsive to initial beta-blockade, then the patient should have emergent evaluation by a cardiologist to determine management. If the patient is already taking an anticoagulant, it is ideal that the relevant parameter, such as international normalized ratio (INR), be checked regularly throughout the ECT course to ensure it is therapeutic.

Aneurysms

For the patient with a known aneurysm, the anesthetist will probably give a medication that lessens heart rate and blood pressure. Labetalol is ideal for this purpose and will probably lessen the probability of aneurysm leak or rupture during ECT. If the aneurysm is abdominal, then the clinician will be well advised to examine for evidence of increase in size after the treatment and will want to pay close attention to blood pressure, looking for an abrupt drop as a potential sign of aneurysm rupture. In such patients, ECT should probably be performed in a general hospital with access to emergency surgical services should emergent aneurysm repair be necessary.

Hypertension

In spite of intense efforts to obtain good control of hypertensive patients' blood pressure before coming to the ECT suite, it is quite common for such patients to have high pressures before anesthesia is administered. Undoubtedly, this is largely due to the stress-inducing aspects of receiving ECT in emotionally fragile patients. The anesthetist can administer any one of a number of agents to lower blood pressure. Labetalol is used most frequently.

Valvular Abnormalities and Heart Transplants

Aortic stenosis is the most common significant valvular abnormality in ECT patients. This condition renders the patient exquisitely sensitive to both increases in preload or afterload and increases or decreases in blood pressure. Thus, while one would want to prevent high blood pressure spikes, one must equally avoid drops in pressure as well lest there be a precipitous drop in cardiac output. Striking this delicate balance requires skill on the anesthetist's part.

Patients with a heart transplant have a denervated heart, so one might theorize that there would be lesser blood pressure and heart rate changes during ECT treatments. Nevertheless, the anesthetist will be especially watchful of cardiac parameters during ECT treatments in this rare population.

Anticoagulation

Ongoing anticoagulation is typically arranged for patients with a history of deep venous thrombosis, AF, or valvular abnormality/replacement. The INR should be monitored regularly throughout a course of treatments in patients taking coumadin. A dilemma concerns what to do if the current INR is out of the desired range. For example, in ECT practice, is there a greater than usual risk of clotting events in patients with a subtherapeutic INR or of bleeding events in those with a supratherapeutic INR? Unfortunately, there is no published evidence-based literature guiding clinical action in ECT. The most prudent strategy is to cancel ECT until the INR is in the therapeutic range. However, in severely ill patients—for example, those with malignant catatonia or manic delirium—the decision to delay treatments may pose greater risk than treating with a suboptimal INR. Decisions should be made on a case-by-case basis involving good communication between the ECT psychiatrist and anesthesiologist.

Pregnancy

Pregnant women are occasionally encountered on an ECT service. Once the patient is evaluated pretreatment, including by an obstetrician to establish risk factors, a decision must be made where to deliver ECT. Some pregnant women are treated safely in the ECT suite, with noninvasive fetal monitoring easily utilized. At other times, a request is made either by the anesthesiology staff or by the obstetrician to undertake ECT in the labor and delivery operating area so as to be able to handle an emergency. The anesthesiologist will pay close attention to blood pressure control to avoid complications such as placental rupture or premature delivery. If the stage of pregnancy is sufficiently advanced, noninvasive fetal monitoring will be undertaken.

Key Points

- The presence of competent anesthesia personnel and equipment has rendered ECT much safer, especially in medically ill patients.

- The use of general anesthesia, muscular paralysis, and continuous ventilation is standard practice in modern ECT.

- Choice of anesthetic agent does have an impact on psychiatric outcome, so the ECT clinician must be knowledgeable enough to discuss this with the anesthesia provider.

6

ECT Technique, Part I: Managing the Individual Treatment

The responsibilities of the psychiatrist managing an individual treatment are numerous and include the following: confirming that informed consent has occurred; ensuring that the patient has not eaten or drunk anything for the specified time interval; ensuring proper placement of stimulus electrodes and monitoring leads; choosing the electrical stimulus dose and parameter combination; delivering the electrical stimulus properly; determining that a seizure has in fact occurred and restimulating if not; stopping the seizure pharmacologically if needed; determining whether re-treatment is needed; assisting with recovery problems such as agitation or nausea; determining, along with the anesthetist, that the patient is sufficiently recovered after the treatment for discharge to the inpatient unit or to home; providing instructions to the patient/caregiver if an outpatient; providing any necessary information to the inpatient unit if an inpatient; and ensuring proper documentation. Decisions pertaining to managing the course of treatments as a whole, such as choosing electrode placement, monitoring therapeutic and adverse effect outcomes, and deciding on concomitant psychotropic usage, will be covered in Chapter 7.

As indicated, the first step is to confirm consent. Even if a patient has already signed an informed consent document, it is possible that there may be misgivings going into the electroconvulsive therapy (ECT) suite. If the patient declines treatment, that wish should be respected, unless legally obtained substituted consent has been undertaken. Also, there should be confirmation of nothing-by-mouth ("NPO") status. In patients who are unreliable in reporting this (e.g., patients with dementia or mute patients), separate confirmation should be obtained, because it is dangerous to undertake general anesthesia when the stomach is not empty.

The ECT Electrical Stimulus

ECT devices must deliver an electrical stimulus through two electrodes placed on the head. The original machines used electrical current straight from the wall socket of the buildings. These currents consisted of an undulating, bidirectional sine-wave form. The flow of electricity is bidirectional in the sense that a wave of electricity flows from one electrode into the brain and out through the other electrode, and then the next wave is identical except that it passes in the opposite direction. Thus, in the classic sine-wave ECT stimulus, there is a "to and fro" movement of electricity through the brain.

In the early 1940s, Vladimir Liberson, working at the Institute of Living in Hartford, Connecticut, realized that the amount of electricity delivered with the sine-wave stimuli was much greater than minimally needed to excite neurons. He reasoned that if a smaller amount of electricity could be used to induce seizures, the memory loss from ECT might be lessened. He developed a device that generated what he termed "brief stimulus therapy," whereby the municipal sine-wave stimulus emanating from the electrical socket in the building could be modified by the ECT device to deliver a stimulus consisting of a series of brief electrical pulses (Liberson 1948). He proved that clinically adequate seizures could be induced with this technique while causing much less memory impairment (Liberson 1948). Some decades later, a group at Duke University replicated the findings that this electrical stimulus technique, now termed "brief pulse, square wave" or simply "brief pulse" ECT, is preferable to sine-wave stimuli from a cognitive standpoint in ECT (Weiner et al. 1986). Sine-wave devices should no longer be used. In modern practice, brief pulse ECT is considered the standard of care. In between the brief pulses, there is no current. This contrasts with sine-wave stimuli, in which there is electricity flowing constantly. The brief pulse, square wave stimulus is also bidirectional—the flow of electricity in the pulses oscillates between the two electrodes on the head, with current making its way into the brain to excite neurons and causing a seizure.

There are four aspects of a brief pulse, square wave ECT stimulus that can be modified using modern ECT machines. These so-called stimulus parameters are frequency of pulses, current of each pulse, duration of each pulse, and duration of the pulse train. Total amount of electricity, or charge, of a brief pulse, square wave ECT stimulus can be calculated from these four parameters. Charge is quantified in units of electricity known as millicoulombs. The "dose" of electricity expressed in millicoulombs is analogous to a medication dose quantified in milligrams.

Frequency refers to the number of electrical pulses per second in the brief pulse, square wave stimulus. This is commonly communicated as cycles per second, where a cycle is a bidirectional pulse pair; thus, a frequency of 60 hertz (1 hertz, or Hz, is one cycle per second) reflects $60 \times 2 = 120$ pulses per second. Typical frequencies of ECT electrical stimuli are 40–100 Hz, or 80–200 pulses per second. On most modern ECT machines, frequency is typically expressed as units of Hz rather than pulses per second, even though the latter is more useful in calculating charge of an electrical stimulus (discussed below).

Current refers to the amount of electricity flowing per unit of time in each pulse and is commonly quantified in ECT in amperes (or amps) (1.0 amp = 1.0 millicoulomb per millisecond). During each pulse in the ECT stimulus, the current is constant. Typical currents in modern ECT devices are 0.8–0.9 amps. The reader is reminded that this current reflects amount of electrical flow per unit of time during each pulse—in between pulses, there is no current flow.

The next parameter is *pulse width*, which refers to the time duration of each pulse of electricity. Typical pulse widths in ECT stimuli are 0.25–2.00 milliseconds. Thus, if pulse width is 1.0 millisecond, and current is 0.9 amps, then the electrical charge of that pulse is 1.0 millisecond × 0.9 millicoulombs/millisecond = 0.9 millicoulombs. If the frequency of pulses is 60 Hz, or 120 pulses per second, then the charge rate of stimulation is 120 pulses/second × 0.9 millicoulombs/pulse = 108 millicoulombs per second of the pulse train. Please note that pulse train duration is the total time of all pulses plus inter-pulse intervals, and not just total duration of the accumulated pulses. Pulse widths less than 0.5 milliseconds are referred to as "ultrabrief," whereas those greater than or equal to 0.5 milliseconds are referred to as "brief" or "standard pulse width." This important variable will be discussed further in Chapter 7.

This *pulse train duration* is the final of the four stimulus parameters and refers to the total time the stimulus train is kept going. If the stimulus train of pulses just described is continued for 4 seconds, then the total charge for the electrical stimulus is 108 millicoulombs/second × 4 seconds = 432 millicoulombs. This latter figure is referred to by custom in the ECT field as the *stimulus dosage*.

The equation for calculating stimulus dosage in millicoulombs for an ECT electrical stimulus is as follows:

Charge (millicoulombs) = [pulse train duration in seconds] × [pulses per second (or frequency in Hz × 2)] × [pulse width (milliseconds)] × [current in amps (millicoulombs per millisecond)]

The reader can appreciate that the same stimulus dose can be achieved through different combinations of stimulus parameters. For example, a stimulus with 0.9 amps, 4-second duration, 100 Hz, and 0.5-millisecond pulse width has the same total charge as a stimulus with the same current and train duration but a frequency of 50 Hz and 1.0-millisecond pulse width. Clinical implications of different stimulus parameter combinations are discussed in Chapter 7. Suffice it to say here that the ECT practitioner in the suite needs to know which type of parameter combination has been selected and how to achieve it on the device being used. The latter is contained in the instructional manual of the ECT device, with which the ECT practitioner should be familiar.

Another aspect of the electrical stimulus that the psychiatrist needs to know about is *impedance*. When electricity passes through a circuit, as is the case with electrons passing through the ECT treatment electrodes and the patient's head and brain, the current can be expressed as a ratio of voltage to resistance (or impedance, which is roughly synonymous with resistance). The higher the resistance, then the higher the voltage must be in order to keep current constant. Modern ECT devices are termed "constant current," meaning that when electricity is being passed into the brain, the current is maintained at a constant level. Since impedance from patient to patient varies, the machine must be able to detect it and vary the voltage accordingly to maintain the constant current.

The amount of heat generated by the current is proportional to the voltage, which in turn is proportional to the resistance (impedance). If the resistance through the patient's head and brain is too high, then the voltage the machine must generate to achieve a constant current may cause too much heat, resulting in skin burns. Thus, before the actual electrical stimulus is passed through the patient's head and brain, there is an impedance check on the machine. During this impedance check, a very tiny, imperceptible amount of electricity is passed through the electrodes. The machine can instantaneously calculate the impedance, and if it is above the safe limit for that machine, then the ECT clinician must undertake measures to lower the resistance. This can be achieved by checking the contact of the electrodes with the scalp, making sure the hair is parted well, the scalp skin is cleaned, and there is plenty of conductive gel under the electrode, ensuring good contact between scalp and electrode. An assistant can use handles to push down on the treatment electrodes to further ensure good contact. Applying these measures will lower the impedance. If not, then checking to make sure the wires connected to the machine are still intact and functional is a good idea. The cables connected to the ECT machine carrying the electrical current may be damaged and need to be replaced. Thus, one must be sure that replacement cables are always available.

There are several commercially available ECT devices. These differ in terms of stimulus parameter combinations and electrical doses that the practitioner can choose. Thus, it is important for the ECT clinician to become thoroughly familiar with the device manufacturer's operations manual. Table 6–1 summarizes the steps needed in an individual ECT treatment.

TABLE 6–1. Steps in conducting an ECT treatment

1. Confirm correct identity of the patient.

2. Ensure placement of the intravenous line.

3. Connect pulse oximeter, ECG leads, and blood pressure cuff to anesthesia machine and ensure appropriate readings.

4. Apply stimulus electrodes.

5. Apply EEG electrodes and obtain baseline recording of a few seconds.

6. Apply ECG and EMG leads to ECT machine (optional).

7. Set stimulus dosage and stimulus parameter configuration.

8. Confirm induction of general anesthesia and muscular paralysis via communication from anesthesiologist.

9. Ensure stimulus electrodes have good contact with scalp via impedance check

10. Pretreatment pause: identify patient and procedure for all in attendance to hear.

11. Say "treat" and deliver the stimulus by pushing the button on the ECT machine.

12. Confirm occurrence versus nonoccurrence of seizure.

13. Confirm termination of seizure and induce pharmacologically if needed.

14. If no seizure occurs, increase electrical dosage and re-treat.

15. Follow patient through recovery and discharge to home if outpatient or to hospital service if inpatient.

Note.   ECG=electrocardiographic; EEG=electroencephalographic; EMG = electromyographic.

Treatment Electrode Placement

The ECT clinician must ensure that the two stimulus electrodes are placed in the proper location. Typically, the choice of electrode placement has been made by the time the patient arrives at the ECT suite for a treatment. This choice may have been made by a different clinician or perhaps by the ECT clinician if that practitioner is also the patient's primary treating clinician. Discussion of how to choose electrode placement for a course of ECT will be undertaken in Chapter 7. In this chapter, the focus is on how to place the electrodes. In some ECT suites, the ECT psychiatrist will place the electrodes and conduct the impedance test to ensure adequate contact with the scalp. In other suites, a nurse or other staff member may undertake this task, but it is still the psychiatrist's duty to oversee that it is done properly.

There are three commonly utilized electrode placements in modern ECT practice. *Bilateral* refers to placing one electrode on each side of the head, whereas *unilateral* refers to placing both electrodes on one side of the head. There are variations on each of these. The original electrode placement was *bitemporal,* a form of bilateral whereby each electrode is placed in the temporal fossa, about 3 centimeters above the halfway point between the outer canthus of the eye and the tragus of the ear on each side. In the *bifrontal* placement, the electrodes are located on the forehead. The version of bifrontal used by Abrams and Taylor (1973) involved placing the electrodes quite close to each other, whereas that used in modern studies of bifrontal placement involves placing the medial edge of each electrode along a vertical line perpendicular from the outer canthus of the eye (Kellner et al. 2010). It is this latter version of bifrontal that is standard for use today. In modern ECT practice and research, bitemporal placement is far more commonly used than bifrontal. Both of these are examples of bilateral electrode placement.

There have been several unilateral placements described over the decades, but the standard one used in modern ECT is the *d'Elia placement,* named after the investigator who first described it (d'Elia and Widepalm 1974). In the unilateral d'Elia placement, one electrode is placed in the temporal fossa as in bitemporal placement, but the other one is located about 3 centimeters lateral to the vertex of the scalp. The two electrodes are placed on the same side of the head. Thus, one could administer left or right unilateral d'Elia electrode placement. However, in modern ECT research and clinical practice, only right unilateral placement is used. Henceforth in this book, the expression "unilateral electrode placement" refers to the d'Elia placement on the right side, unless otherwise indicated. The reason why the right side is stimulated is that in the majority of people, even those who are left-handed, the left side is dominant for language. Thus, the ECT clinician will avoid stimulating that side to minimize language-based memory impairment. Figure 6–1 displays bitemporal, right unilateral, and bifrontal placement positions. Additionally, the interested reader can easily find images on the internet demonstrating these electrode placements.

There are two types of electrodes in use: reusable metal electrodes and disposable self-adhesive electrodes. Metal electrodes, about an inch or two in diameter, are circular and either flat (for use in the temporal fossa for bitemporal or unilateral placement) or concave (to conform to the curve of the head in the vertex position for unilateral or the forehead in bifrontal). Metal electrodes are inserted into a handle, which in turn is inserted into the treatment cable that is connected to the ECT machine. Thus, a staff member holds the metal electrodes in place on the head while the ECT practitioner pushes the button on the machine which delivers the electrical stimulus. Alternatively, if bifrontal or bitemporal placement is used, there are rubber straps wrapped around the head that can hold the

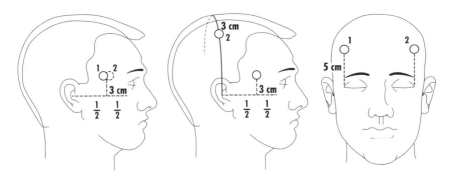

FIGURE 6–1. Bitemporal, right unilateral, and bifrontal electrode placement positions in ECT.

metal electrodes in place. After a patient is treated, the metal electrodes are cleaned thoroughly to be sterile for the next patient.

More commonly utilized in modern ECT practice are adhesive, disposable electrodes. These are available from the device manufacturers. The ECT clinician should be thoroughly familiar with the instructions for the device about how to use these electrodes. Typically, they are placed at the proper locations on the scalp and, like thick pieces of tape, adhere. However, the adherence is usually not stable enough to treat without having a staff member use handles to hold them in place. Once the treatment is finished for a particular patient, these adhesive electrodes are discarded.

Preparation of the electrode site is important, particularly for the vertex location in unilateral placement. This site may be densely filled with hair, which impedes electrical flow. Spacing apart the hair as much as possible for there to be good contact between electrode and scalp is essential. Cleaning of the electrode site can be accomplished with an alcohol wipe or, if need be, an abrasive scrub. Electrodes, whether metal or disposable, should be coated with a conductive gel to enhance good electrical contact. If the impedance check on the machine is acceptable, then the electrical stimulus can be delivered. If not, then one must undertake measures to ensure good contact, such as use of more conductive gel, firmer holding of the electrodes to the scalp, more vigorous scalp site preparation with an alcohol or abrasive scrub, and finally, inspection of the stimulus cables to ensure they are not broken or damaged.

EEG, ECG, and EMG Monitoring Technique

The other type of electrodes to be connected to the patient are those for EEG (electroencephalographic), EMG (electromyographic), and ECG (electrocardiographic) channels. The EMG and ECG are strictly optional in practice. The EMG availability on some ECT devices allows for connection of two electrodes to a muscle body, usually the forearm or calf, which are in turn connected via cable to the ECT device. That limb is then cuffed before succinylcholine administration to isolate it from paralysis and ensure motor convulsive activity. During the seizure, the printout from the machine displays activity that correlates with motor movement in that limb. The electromyograph can be tested by hooking up the two relevant electrodes to a muscle mass distal to the cuffed limb and running the paper feed from the machine while tapping the electrodes to see if there is a signal. Another capability on some ECT devices is an optical motion sensor attached to a fingertip on the cuffed limb. The device senses motor movements, and the machine printout displays large oscillations that correlate with these movements. The reason why the electromyograph or an optical motion sensor is unnecessary is that observation of the motor movements in the cuffed limb is trivially easy. These "extras" offer no further information beyond visual inspection and are gimmicks and a bit of a hassle to connect. Also, convulsive movements may be appreciated elsewhere on the body, such as in the neck or facial muscles, thus rendering the EMG or optical motion sensor readings on the cuffed limb moot. Visual observation of the whole body for convulsive movements should be the standard of care in ECT practice.

Similarly, ECG connection to the ECT device is also unnecessary because the anesthesia machine already has an ECG readout. A separate one is redundant. The ECG electrodes of course can be connected if desired, and the relevant ECG signal should be evident when the paper feed from the ECT device is started.

EEG monitoring during ECT seizures is, on the other hand, standard of care in modern ECT practice. First, it is necessary to document that a seizure has occurred. Also, occasionally, the EEG seizure is prolonged, necessitating pharmacological termination. If an EEG is not used, such cases would not be detected and undiagnosed status epilepticus could result. An EEG channel on the device printout reflects voltage differences between two EEG leads, the latter consisting of a wire from the machine connected to a scalp electrode. Thus, two EEG leads result in one EEG channel. For each EEG channel, one EEG lead should be connected to one side of the forehead and the other to the ipsilateral mastoid process. This constitutes a fronto-mastoid EEG channel. Some advocate using bilateral EEG channels, one on each side of the forehead, but one EEG channel is quite sufficient and is used by the author in his practice. It is recommended that the EEG leads be placed in the left frontomastoid position to ensure a generalized seizure when right unilateral electrical stimulation is administered. The ictal pattern seen on the EEG printout from the machine during the seizure is reflective of activity in the left prefrontal lobe. In contrast, motor convulsive movements during the seizure are reflective of ictal activity in the contralateral motor strip (the precentral gyrus). Each EEG lead wire can be snapped into an adhesive EEG electrode pad placed on the head. These pads are commercially available from device manufacturers. In addition to the frontal and mastoid leads, there is a ground lead that can be placed over the right side of the forehead. This lead does not detect electrical signals from the brain and does not contribute to the pattern on the device EEG printout.

Once the EEG channel is connected, the paper feed should be started to determine that a readable signal is being attained. Modern ECT devices have the capability of manipulating the gain (e.g., in microvolts per centimeter) of the electrical signal from the monitoring electrodes so that a signal that appears too small or too large can be modified to be more easily readable. If the gain in microvolts per centimeter is set too high, then the deflections on the paper printout during the seizure will be too small for the practitioner to detect reliably; if the gain is too low, the deflections will be higher than what can be accommodated on the paper and also be unreadable. The author, in his practice, utilizes a gain of 200 microvolts per centimeter and finds EEG seizure activity easy to appreciate. The ECT clinician should become familiar with how to set gain on the ECT machine.

Stimulus and monitoring electrode placement should be undertaken in a timely manner, generally starting before anesthesia administration, so that when the anesthesiologist indicates that muscular paralysis is adequate, the ECT clinician is ready to deliver the electrical stimulus.

Electrical Stimulus Delivery

At the point when anesthesia has been delivered, muscular paralysis has been determined to be adequate (by the anesthetist), the impedance check has been passed, and the person delivering ventilation has confirmed placement of the bite block with the mouth firmly kept shut, the electrical stimulus can be delivered by pressing the button on the machine. The person pressing the button will announce the name of the patient and the fact that stimulus delivery is about to take place so that all other personnel can be prepared. The person delivering ventilations should maintain closing of the jaw, as the electrical stimulus causes direct contractions of the jaw muscles. Leaving the jaw open would cause a forceful contraction of an open mouth, putting oral structures at risk (e.g., tooth or dental appliance fracture or dislocation or laceration of lips, cheek, or tongue). After passage of the electrical stimulus and confirmation that a seizure has been induced, the ventilating person resumes ventilations. Before electrical stimulus delivery, the ECT clinician should say the name of the patient being treated as final confirmation of proper identity, indicate that ECT is being done, and say "treat" to alert all personnel that the stimulus will now be given. It cannot be overemphasized how important it is not to simply press the button on the machine without all personnel knowing it is about to be done, lest there be somebody who is trying to manipulate one of the treatment electrodes or the bite block as the stimulus is being delivered. The ECT clinician should of course be familiar with how to deliver the electrical stimulus on the ECT device being used, which is available in the operations manual.

Threshold Determination and Electrical Dosing

Much of the electrical current that passes from the treatment electrodes travels directly along the patient's scalp into the other electrode, as the skull acts as a large resistor to electrical current. This part of the total charge obviously is not therapeutic because it does not reach the brain. However, some of the total current does penetrate the skull and reach the brain, causing a seizure if enough neurons are excited to depolarization. The smallest electrical dose that can elicit a seizure is termed the *seizure threshold*. This varies from patient to patient and within patients over the course of treatments. Factors that increase seizure threshold include older age, male gender, bilateral (vs. unilateral) electrode placement, and use of higher pulse widths as opposed to ultrabrief pulse width (Sackeim et al. 2008). Also, seizure threshold tends to rise over a course of treatments, indicating that ECT has anticonvulsant activity (Sackeim et al. 1987b). Colenda and McCall (1996) showed, also, that larger head size, as reflected by nasion-inion distance, predicted higher seizure thresholds. However, the majority of interpatient and intrapatient variance in seizure threshold remains unexplained.

At the first treatment session in a series, the ECT practitioner must decide on electrical dosage. The maximum setting on the machine could be used, but for most patients that would be more than is needed and cause excessive cognitive side effects. The method of dose titration, first elaborated by Harold Sackeim and colleagues at Columbia University, has become standard practice in the ECT field (Sackeim et al. 1987b). In dose titration, a very low dose is first used. If no seizure ensues, then another stimulation with a higher dose is used. Successively higher doses are administered until the patient has a seizure. The dose resulting in a seizure is considered the seizure threshold for that patient and is used to calculate electrical doses at subsequent treatments. During a titration, there should be at least 20 seconds between stimulations to allow enough time for either a motor convulsion or EEG evidence of a seizure to occur. In the author's practice, if there is a one-sided (i.e., jacksonian) seizure, then whatever stimulus dose resulting in that seizure is taken as the threshold. However, in future treatments, if such a seizure type occurs again, the electrical dose is raised in order to obtain a generalized seizure.

There is no standard dose titration schedule for ECT practice—different practitioners use different dosages. If one wished to fine-tune the threshold very precisely, one would have to start with the smallest dose on the device and use small increments in the titration. However, that would lead to many stimulations being used for some patients, which is to be avoided. Generally, a titration schedule should probably not have more than five levels. Unilateral ultrabrief-pulse-width ECT is associated with very low seizure thresholds (Sackeim et al. 2008). Thus, for that technique, one can start with the lowest dose available on the ECT device and progressively double the dose until a seizure ensues. Most patients with this technique will have a seizure at the first one or two doses (corresponding to electrical charges typically of 25–50 millicoulombs). Dosage at subsequent treatments for right unilateral ultrabrief technique should be five to eight times initial threshold, based on current literature showing greater efficacy than with minimally suprathreshold dosing (reviewed in Rasmussen 2015b). It was shown long ago that for unilateral electrode placement, electrical doses should be at least five times initial threshold—lower doses, especially doses barely sufficient to cause a seizure, are less effective (Sackeim et al. 1987a). In the author's practice, for right unilateral electrode placement, treatments subsequent to the initial threshold-determining session are set at six times threshold. This is a commonly used dose in unilateral ECT (Kellner et al. 2010).

For bilateral placements, a higher initial setting should be used to determine initial seizure threshold. For example, whereas an initial setting for unilateral ultrabrief ECT might be 25 millicoulombs, the initial setting for bitemporal placement (which is coupled with pulse widths higher than ultrabrief) might be 50 or 75 millicoulombs. Successive doublings of the dose would then constitute the titration schedule. For subsequent treatments with bilateral placements (including either bitemporal or bifrontal), the literature supports doses of 1.5 times initial threshold (Kellner et al. 2010). As noted, bilateral placement is not coupled with ultrabrief pulse widths, because the latter technique is associated with unacceptably low efficacy (Sackeim et al. 2008). Thus, when bilateral placements are used, pulse width should be at least 1.0 millisecond. Further discussion of the literature on electrode placement and stimulus parameter combinations will be found in Chapter 7. If electrode placement is switched during a course of treatments (i.e., bilateral to unilateral or vice versa), a new titration with threshold determination should be undertaken in order to deliver the proper electrical dose with the new placement.

The seizure threshold titration approach for unilateral ECT was supported by findings from a study by McCall et al. (2000), in which all patients were treated with unilateral electrode placement at the first session with a threshold determination performed. At subsequent sessions, the patients were randomly assigned to receive either a fixed high electrical dose that was unrelated to initial threshold, or an electrical dose five times higher than initial threshold. The results showed that the degree to which subsequent doses exceeded threshold correlated directly not only with therapeutic efficacy but also with cognitive side effects. Measuring threshold and basing subsequent dosing on that value maximized efficacy but spared cognitive effects for a significant number of patients compared with if they had been given a fixed high electrical dose. The titration approach has also been supported for bilateral placements, with research showing that doses of 1.5 times threshold are sufficient for good efficacy, with occasional patients who are refractory to this dose benefiting from higher doses (Kellner et al. 2006, 2010; Sackeim et al. 1993). Thus, it is currently advisable to measure seizure threshold at the first session and base subsequent dosing on this value rather than administer fixed doses to all patients.

As can be appreciated from this discussion, there are several ways to determine seizure threshold in ECT, ranging from methods resulting in a seizure with only one or two stimulations in most cases and those resulting in numerous stimulations. There is no currently agreed-on "standard of care" regarding how to measure seizure threshold. The electrical doses recommended above by the author, in his practice, result in seizures with no more than four stimulations in a titration session in the vast majority of cases.

Because seizure threshold tends to rise over a course of treatments, occasionally a patient will not have a seizure at a setting of 1.5 times threshold bilateral at subsequent treatments. In this case, the dose can be doubled. For example, if the original threshold is 50 millicoulombs, then at the second treatment the dose would be 75 millicoulombs. If during the course of treatments the patient does not have a seizure with that dose, then the dose can be doubled to 150 millicoulombs. It is exceedingly rare for a unilaterally treated patient not to have a seizure at six times threshold. However, if the patient is not responding well after several treatments, the electrical dose might be raised to enhance efficacy. Occasionally electrode placement is switched during a course of treatments. Either a patient is not responding well to right unilateral placement or he or she has unacceptable cognitive side effects to bilateral, so the clinician switches. For the first treatment session at the new electrode placement, it is recommended that the electrical dose be retitrated and the patient be treated at subsequent treatments with 1.5 times threshold for bilateral or six times threshold for unilateral.

Discussion of strategies to deal with lack of response or side effects during a course of treatments, including switching electrode placements, will be discussed in more detail in Chapter 7.

Seizure Monitoring: Motor Convulsion

After the stimulus button is pressed and the electrical stimulus is delivered, the ECT clinician must be able to determine whether a seizure has occurred. During presentation of the electrical stimulus, there commonly is tonic contraction of extremities and contraction of the jaw. However, this does not necessarily reflect the occurrence of a seizure. Tonic-clonic activity must be sustained beyond stimulus presentation in order to declare the activity a seizure. Inspection of the skeletal musculature will reveal a tonic-clonic seizure if one is elicited. First, there is a sharp tonic contraction, followed by clonic jerks. Depending on the dose of succinylcholine, there may be convulsive activity of other parts of the body as well, including other limbs, the platysma, lips, and eyelids. For timing of the duration of the seizure, the beginning of the motor convulsion is taken as the end of the electrical stimulus, even if activity is not observable until some seconds later. The motor end point is taken as the end of convulsive movements wherever they occur, not just the cuffed limb. If the seizure threshold is just barely exceeded, it may take up to 20 seconds or so for the convulsive tonic-clonic movements to be seen. Motor convulsive movements should not be confused with late-onset succinylcholine-induced fasciculations, which typically occur in the calf muscles, or with abdominal aortic pulsations. Finally, postictally, some patients may shiver, another movement that should not be confused with convulsion.

A very clever method of confirming the induction of a seizure was developed by Max Hamilton, the researcher famous for the depression scale bearing his name. Hamilton applied a blood pressure cuff on either the forearm or calf muscle and inflated it well above systolic blood pressure before administration of the muscle relaxant, thus blocking off the action of the agent in the muscles of the "cuffed" limb and thereby preventing those muscles from being paralyzed. When the seizure is elicited, convulsive movements are visually inspected in the "cuffed" limb. This is helpful because the EEG does not always show definite seizure activity even when there is clear seizure activity from a motor standpoint. Cuffing a forearm (not the one with the intravenous access) rather than a calf more reliably demonstrates motor convulsive movements. Preferably, one would cuff a limb ipsilateral to a unilaterally placed electrode in order to confirm a generalized seizure in the brain. That is, when the right side is electrically stimulated, if one appreciates motor convulsive movements in a right limb (calf or arm), one can be assured that seizure activity has spread to the left hemisphere. Thus, if the intravenous line is placed in the right arm, then cuffing the right calf would confirm generalization of the seizure to the left hemisphere, as motor activity in the right leg is reflective of seizure activity in the left motor strip. It is assumed that if the right hemisphere is stimulated in unilateral placement, then if ictal activity occurs in the left hemisphere, there must also be activity in the right hemisphere. In other words, stimulating the right hemisphere would not cause ictal activity only in the left hemisphere.

Patients who have had a mastectomy may prefer that a blood pressure cuff not be used on the site ipsilateral to the surgery so as not to provoke lymphedema, and patients with a hemodialysis access should not be cuffed on the forearm that has had that surgery. One would also not cuff the calf in patients known to have had deep venous thromboses of the lower extremities or in those with ankle edema. If multiple attempts at intravenous access were performed on both forearms, one would hesitate to cuff, because that would cause the failed needle-stick sites to pop up with a hematoma. A final reason not to cuff is when the patient is known to have methicillin-resistant *Staphylococcus aureus* or vancomycin-resistant enterococcus, in an effort to prevent cross infections. Using the cuff technique, though helpful, is not mandatory. Usually, there is detectable motor convulsive activity in uncuffed limbs or in the platysma or facial muscles.

The timing of the cuff technique is important. The cuff should be inflated only after the patient is unconscious from anesthesia but before the succinylcholine is injected. Inflating the cuff before the patient is unconscious causes pain. Also, once the seizure is elicited, the cuff can be deflated without having to wait until the seizure is terminated. Prolonged cuffing of a limb can cause nerve damage.

Seizure Monitoring: EEG

Of all the skills required of an ECT clinician, interpreting the EEG can be the most daunting to the novice practitioner. Expert interpretation of multiple-lead, clinically obtained EEGs in a hospital neurophysiology lab requires specialized training. Fortunately, that kind of training is not necessary in ECT practice. Interpretation of ECT-related EEGs is much easier but is also somewhat crude in the sense that only a small section of cerebral cortex is sampled to determine the presence of a seizure. Furthermore, there are multiple types of seizures, all with their own characteristic EEG pattern (Marcuse et al. 2016). In ECT, it is the tonic-clonic seizure type that is induced.

The two main goals of ECT EEG seizure monitoring are to determine whether a seizure has occurred and, if so, to determine that the seizure has stopped. Excessively short or prolonged seizures require intervention (as discussed below). Although the ECT clinician will observe and record an EEG duration for the seizure, determining a *precise* end point of the EEG seizure is not critical for good practice. The busy ECT clinician will see EEGs in which the seizure is clearly over at some point but in which the ictal activity slowly and imprecisely transformed into non-ictal activity. Whether the end point is, say, exactly 40 or 41 seconds or a few seconds later is not important.

Before undertaking independent ECT clinical practice, novice practitioners should view ECT EEGs with the instruction and feedback of experienced clinicians. In so doing, they will learn to recognize common ictal patterns and to determine when the seizure is over. Figures 6–2 through 6–9 outline some common patterns seen in ECT. It is a good idea to sample a baseline EEG reading before anesthesia is induced in order to have something with which to compare the post-stimulus recording. There are no published, explicitly defined criteria in the ECT field for EEG end-point determination, so such determination tends to be rather impressionistic in practice. This chapter provides guidelines for getting started interpreting ECT EEGs.

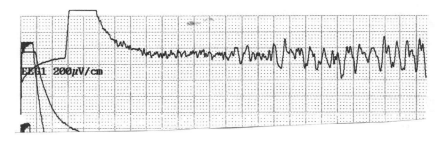

FIGURE 6–2.   **EEG showing early crescendo of increasing amplitude, termed *epileptic recruiting*.**

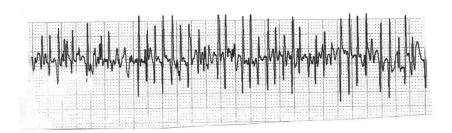

FIGURE 6–3.   **EEG showing hypersynchronous polyspikes indicative of ictal activity.**

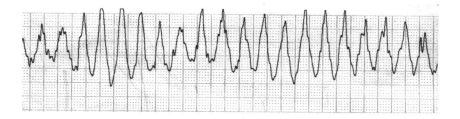

FIGURE 6–4.   **EEG showing large-amplitude, highly rhythmic slow waves indicative of ictal activity.**

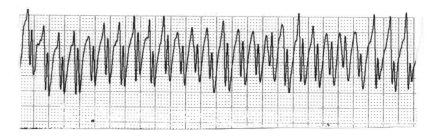

FIGURE 6–5.   **EEG showing mixed spike and slow wave activity, highly characteristic of ictal activity.**

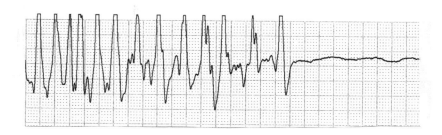

FIGURE 6–6.   **EEG showing seizure ending in an easily discernible flat line.**

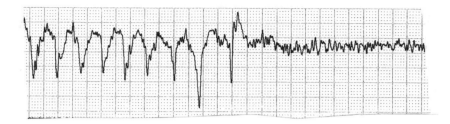

FIGURE 6–7. EEG showing seizure ending in low-amplitude, nonrhythmic activity.

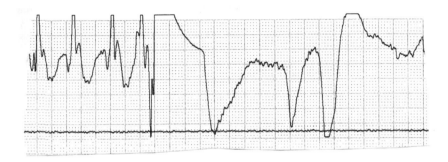

FIGURE 6–8. EEG showing ictal slow wave complexes followed by large motion artifact.

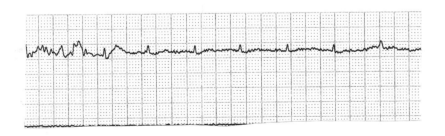

FIGURE 6–9. Electrocardiogram artifact.

The small deflections, which could be mistaken for ictal complexes, are synchronous with the anesthesia machine ECG rhythm strip and also with the pulse oximeter pulsation sounds and thus are QRS complexes.

Once the electrical stimulus has been delivered, the ECT device will stream out a printed EEG paper strip that ticks off the seconds elapsed since end of stimulus delivery. This allows for determining the duration of the ECT seizure in seconds. Additionally, the EEG recording itself, as well as any other channel being monitored, such as ECG or EMG, is displayed in real time.

The ECT practitioner must determine if the EEG signal constitutes ictal activity. The three main features of an EEG seizure are high amplitude, low frequency, and, most importantly, a highly regularly recurring or rhythmic pattern to the ictal complexes. The reader can peruse the figures and appreciate the various types of rhythmic activity. Ictal complexes are morphemes on the EEG that indicate seizure activity. With practice and supervision, the novice ECT practitioner can learn to recognize ictal complexes. As indicated, a key feature of ictal complexes is that they are regularly recurring, or rhythmic. It may take a few seconds—say, up to 20 or so—for the ictal complexes to be appreciated. Ictal complexes appear in one of three general forms: a) rhythmic spikes, b) rhythmic slow waves, or c) rhythmic combination spike and slow waves. The figures display examples of these. A given EEG may reveal one, two, or all three of these types of activity variably over the course of the seizure.

A second characteristic of ictal activity, as mentioned above, is low frequency. Generally, this refers to less than 8 Hz activity (recall that 1 Hz, or hertz, is one cycle per second). However, it is difficult to appreciate frequency of the ictal complexes in real time as the printout is streaming out of the machine. Furthermore, occasionally, especially in the case of continuous spike activity, the frequency of ictal complexes may be greater than 8 Hz. In Figures 6–3 to 6–5, the reader can appreciate the frequencies of the activity. The third characteristic of ictal activity is high amplitude, generally greater than 80 microvolts. However, the important point is that the amplitude of ictal activity is greater than that of the baseline activity, thus underscoring the value of obtaining preanesthesia baseline activity on the EEG strip.

In the author's experience, high amplitude and regularity of the ictal complexes are the most reliable and easily appreciated parameters in determining that the activity represents a seizure. The regularity or rhythmicity of the complexes may not be constant throughout the seizure, so the practitioner must be vigilant in inspecting the readout in real time to detect good rhythmicity. In contrast to frequency and amplitude of EEG complexes, which can easily be quantified in hertz or microvolts, respectively, there is no good way of quantifying regularity. Appreciating this crucial quality of seizure complexes on the EEG is something that requires practice and experience. Of note, occasionally there are highly rhythmic, slow-frequency but low-amplitude ictal complexes, which reflect seizure activity. The practitioner must be able to appreciate that there are no fixed rules on amplitude or frequency that determine whether the activity is ictal or non-ictal.

Generally, if the complexes are rhythmic (regular) in the face of either high amplitude or low frequency as defined above, then the practitioner can conclude they are ictal. Of course, other signs of seizure activity are quite helpful, such as motor convulsion, elevated heart rate, and piloerection.

Other authors have emphasized stages of the ECT EEG seizure (Krystal 2010; Weiner et al. 1991). These consist of pre-ictal, epileptic recruiting, polyspike, polyspike and slow wave, termination, and postictal phases. *Pre-ictal* refers to EEG activity, typically lasting only a few seconds, that is not ictal. This may be very small amplitude, nonrhythmic activity. Figure 6–2 demonstrates some pre-ictal activity briefly. *Epileptic recruiting* refers to ictal activity demonstrating progressively increasing amplitude. Figure 6–2 also features this. *Polyspike* ictal activity refers to deflections that are tall and narrow and have a spikelike morphology. Figure 6–3 demonstrates polyspike ictal activity. *Slow waves*, which indicate ictal activity as well, consist of large-amplitude, slow-frequency complexes and are nicely demonstrated in Figure 6–4. *Polyspike and slow wave* activity refers to a combination of spikes interspersed with slow waves and is featured in Figure 6–5. The *termination* phase of the seizure, according to Krystal (2010) and Weiner et al. (1991), refers to a stage of the seizure intermediate between the spikes and slow waves and the postictal phase and usually consists of progressively decreasing amplitude and rhythmicity of the complexes. The *postictal* phase, meaning that the seizure has ended, is most classically heralded by a flat line, as seen in Figure 6–6, but also occasionally by very small-amplitude, irregular, high-frequency activity such as seen in Figure 6–7. In the author's extensive experience delivering many thousands of ECT treatments, most EEGs do not display all these stages.

Visual inspection of the clonic movements of the cuffed limb and the EEG may reveal synchronization of each clonic jerk with one spike-wave complex on the EEG. The spike-wave complexes eventually give way to lower-amplitude activity that terminates in postictal suppression, which is a flat line. The point of maximal flattening is taken as the seizure end point, though the busy ECT clinician will see records where a definable end point is not apparent, though the activity eventually is noted to be non-ictal. Again, it is emphasized that the purpose at this stage of the EEG seizure is not so much to obsess about a precise end point but rather to be confident that the seizure is over, even though the ending of it may be a gradual process.

In general, an ECT electroencephalogram that demonstrates spikes, spike-and-wave complexes, or slow waves is considered ictal. Some electroencephalograms demonstrate all of these or only one or two. The termination of EEG activity in a flat line further confirms that a seizure in fact has occurred. Sometimes, there is activity that does not clearly seem ictal, but if it terminates in a clear flat line, then the practitioner can consider it as such. On the other hand, there are electroencephalograms that clearly show spikes, spikes and waves, or slow waves but do not terminate clearly in a flat line. These can be considered good evidence of a seizure as well, but the precise end point may not be apparent. If clearly ictal spikes or spike-and-wave complexes only slowly diminish in amplitude and regularity, Krystal (2010) and Weiner et al. (1991) recommend keeping the EEG streaming for some time to ascertain if a flat line appears, in which case seizure end point is taken as the point of flat-line appearance. However, if after many seconds of low-amplitude, low-regularity activity (and in the face of swallowing or diaphragmatic movements) it seems clear the patient is no longer having a seizure, the author recommends looking back at the point of maximal amplitude reduction as an estimate of seizure termination. This may be more easily appreciated by inspecting the EEG strip vertically rather than horizontally. In some cases, there is no discernible EEG activity at all, even in the face of clear motor convulsive activity. In such cases, the practitioner can indicate this on the patient record, making no attempt to record an EEG duration. The ECT clinician should remember that single, or even double, EEG channel monitoring during this procedure is a relatively crude representation of what is happening throughout the patient's cerebral cortex and as such should not obsess about EEG seizure end points. Evidence of termination of the seizure occasionally will have to be deduced from signs of patient awakening, such as swallowing movements of the thyroid cartilage or diaphragmatic respiratory effort, and obviously by the patient's resumption of consciousness. The heart rate can be of assistance when the cuffed limb and the electroencephalogram are not providing good data. A sharp rise in pulse rate after presentation of the electrical stimulus can be a good sign that a seizure has occurred, and then sharp reduction in heart rate is evidence the seizure has terminated. However, a caveat is that heart rate does not always sharply rise with the seizure, either because of a weak, poorly generalized seizure or because a beta-blocker was administered. Additionally, skin piloerection occurs during seizures and is another sign to use in determining that a seizure has occurred, albeit not a very reliable one.

Artifact on the electroencephalogram, which is typically characterized by very large undulations on the recording, should not be confused with ictal activity and may render end point determination difficult. Gently placing fingers on the frontal and mastoid EEG electrodes helps reduce artifacts on the record, as does having the ventilating person stop for a few seconds to reduce movement artifact. If ictal complexes terminate in a smooth, undulating pattern, the seizure is probably over, with some ventilation artifact, even though there may not be a flat line. A key feature of motion artifact is that it is nonrhythmic, in contrast to true ictal complexes. Figure 6–8 illustrates motion artifact on an ECT EEG recording.

Another type of artifact is that from the ECG. The EEG monitoring electrode positions, frontomastoid, are near enough to the heart that occasionally ECG activity is detected on the EEG. Such activity usually is discernible, if at all, after seizure termination, in which case there is a flat line interspersed with tiny QRS complexes, the frequency of which correlates tightly with pulse oximetry sounds. It is important not to mistake this for continuing seizure activity, lest one incorrectly diagnose a prolonged seizure and undertake pharmacological seizure termination efforts. Figure 6–9 illustrates postictal ECG artifact.

Most of the time, the motor seizure duration is shorter than the EEG duration by a few seconds, or at times both end points occur simultaneously. On rare occasions, there is clear continuation of motor convulsive movements after ictal cessation of the EEG, and rarer still, there are occasions of motor convulsion without EEG evidence of ictal complexes. Motor convulsive movements are reflective of ictal activity in the contralateral motor strip, while frontomastoid EEG ictal activity is reflective of seizure activity in the prefrontal cortex. Since it is likely that ictal activity in the prefrontal regions is related to therapeutic efficacy, vis-à-vis activity in the motor strip, the occurrence of this phenomenon may indicate the need for a more aggressive stimulation technique, such as increasing the electrical dose or switching from unilateral to bitemporal placement, if the patient is not showing improvement clinically.

It is standard of care in ECT practice for the ECT clinician to record in the patient's record the motor and EEG duration of the seizure. All modern ECT devices have a timer ticking off the seconds from end of stimulus that the clinician can use to determine motor end point. The EEG strips streaming out of the machine have the number of seconds recorded on them so that EEG duration can be determined. Modern ECT devices have automated EEG end point determination programs. However, the author has not found these helpful. When the EEG end point is unequivocal, the automated reading is not helpful because visual inspection easily pinpoints where the seizure ends. For those readings that are unclear, the automated end-point readings oftentimes do not seem accurate.

Management of Short or Prolonged Seizures

The importance of seizure length as a determinant of ECT efficacy has long been debated. For years, the "common wisdom" in the ECT field was that a certain total, cumulative seizure duration (calculated by adding the seizure lengths of the individual seizures) was needed, with the figure of approximately 200 cumulative seizure seconds being bandied about as necessary for an adequate course of treatments (Weiner et al. 1991). That notion was long ago discredited (Sackeim et al. 1987b). Modern ECT studies have usually considered 20–25 seconds of seizure activity a minimum for efficacy, and the methodologies have included provisions for restimulating the patient when a shorter seizure occurs (Kellner et al. 2006,

2010; Sackeim et al. 1987b, 1993, 2000, 2008). These studies have found that if seizures are at least 20–25 seconds, longer duration does not translate into better efficacy. What is not known is whether seizures less than 20 seconds are efficacious. Probably the most arbitrary custom that has developed in clinical ECT practice in the several decades of its existence is the "20-second rule" for adequate seizure duration.

The most important dictum is to assess clinical efficacy first and foremost over seizure length per se. If a patient is making the expected clinical progress with a course of ECT, then one need not undertake measures to prolong seizures. On the other hand, if early in a course of treatments seizures less than 20 seconds' EEG duration are occurring, then most practitioners will do something to make them longer. One common, highly recommended strategy is for the ventilating person to provide 2 minutes of vigorous hyperventilation after anesthesia induction, which has been shown to increase seizure duration (Bergsholm et al. 1984; Chater and Simpson 1988; Mayur et al. 2010; Pande et al. 1990). The mechanism of the seizure-lengthening effects of this maneuver is unknown but may involve reduction of blood carbon dioxide concentration, which is known to have proconvulsant effects. Alternatively, these effects may be due to the extra time allowing anticonvulsant barbiturate anesthesia to redistribute from the brain. "Hyperventilation" in this context has no precise definition in the ECT literature but typically involves ventilating the patient deeply and rapidly (say, every 2 seconds or so) for 2 minutes after anesthesia induction in order to prolong the seizure. This is a simple, safe maneuver if the ECT clinician desires longer seizures for a particular patient. It is important for the ECT clinician to discuss this with the anesthetist and ventilation person and record its use on the patient's chart for future reference.

Other seizure-prolonging strategies include use of nonbarbiturate anesthetics such as etomidate or ketamine and use of low-dose barbiturate supplemented with a high-potency opioid such as remifentanil or alfentanil (see Chapter 5 for a review of these agents). Intravenous caffeine administered a few minutes before anesthesia induction reliably prolongs seizures (Coffey et al. 1990) but fell out of favor after a preclinical study demonstrated that its use in electroconvulsive shock (ECS) in rodents was associated with brain damage (Enns et al. 1996). There is a theoretical advantage of using the benzodiazepine receptor–blocking agent flumazenil to prolong seizures in ECT patients in whom concomitant benzodiazepine administration is felt to be causing the seizure shortening (Krystal et al. 1998). However, this is not recommended because the duration of this drug is such that it can precipitate benzodiazepine withdrawal well after the ECT seizure is over. Strategies for reducing concomitant anticonvulsant medications will be discussed in Chapter 7. Doing so can result in longer seizures but obviously is not something immediately available on a particular day in the ECT suite. Increasing the electrical dosage does not reliably result in longer seizure durations; but it may result in more therapeutically effective seizures and thus is a reasonable strategy for poor clinical response during a course of treatments (see Chapter 7 for further discussion of efficacy-enhancing strategies during ECT). If no seizure at all is obtained, then higher electrical doses may result in a seizure.

A common question is whether to provide an immediate restimulation to a patient who has just had a short seizure. There is no scientific evidence that doing this speeds up efficacy, and it likely increases cognitive side effects. The author recommends only doing this with extremely short seizures—say, less than 10 seconds EEG duration. If this is done, then the electrical dose should be doubled. It must be pointed out, though, that increasing the electrical dose does not reliably increase seizure duration, though it may enhance the efficacy of the elicited seizure. If the ECT practitioner encounters a short seizure at a particular treatment session, the best strategy is to use hyperventilation and a non-anticonvulsant anesthetic regimen at the next session and to communicate to the primary psychiatric clinician that efforts be made to eliminate or at least minimize concomitant oral medications that may be inhibiting seizure expression.

The opposite of a short seizure, of course, is a prolonged seizure. It is reassuring from basic science research utilizing ECS in animals that many hours of continuous seizure activity are required before there is evidence of brain damage (Meldrum 1986). However, to be prudent, a seizure in ECT should be terminated if it is prolonged. The definition of "prolonged" may vary, but a conservative figure would be that if the seizure lasts 150–180 seconds, an effort should be made to stop it. There are various methods available. If the anesthetic agent used was a barbiturate or propofol, both of which are highly anticonvulsant, then simply giving a repeat dose works promptly in stopping the seizure. Etomidate, ketamine, alfentanil, remifentanil, or an inhalational anesthetic should not be used to attempt to stop a seizure. Rapid-acting intravenously administered benzodiazepines such as diazepam 5–10 mg or midazolam 1–2 mg also can quickly terminate a seizure. Lorazepam for this purpose is not recommended as a first-line agent because it has a longer onset of action. If methohexital, propofol, midazolam, or diazepam, after a couple of doses spread a minute apart or so, fails to stop the seizure, an urgent neurological consultation should be arranged, the same as if a medical inpatient suffers from status epilepticus. The neurological consultant may arrange for transfer of the patient to an intensive care unit. The author has only seen this as a necessary action once in almost three decades of busy ECT practice, however.

Occasionally a patient stops having a seizure in the ECT suite but has a recurrent seizure in the recovery room, a phenomenon known as a tardive seizure.

This type of seizure can be stopped in the same way that is used to stop a prolonged seizure. If a patient develops a spontaneous seizure between ECT treatments, a rare phenomenon, then a neurological evaluation should be undertaken before resuming further treatments, to assess for presence of brain disease that may be predisposing to the spontaneous seizure.

Determination of Seizure Adequacy

There are variable technical modifications in ECT practice, such as electrode placement, stimulus dosing, and treatment frequency. These will be discussed further in Chapter 7. Suffice it to mention here that a certain proportion of patients achieve remission with low-dose, right unilateral technique (about 20%–30% based on research), which causes minimal cognitive side effects (Sackeim et al. 1987a, 1993, 2000). It would be nice to know in advance which patients thus treated at the initial titration session will go on to achieve remission with low-dose stimuli and which ones will need either higher electrical doses with unilateral placement or the more intense bitemporal placement. In other words, ECT practitioners would benefit from information emanating from an individual treatment session that indicates whether the current technique ultimately will be sufficient or whether something more intense, such as a higher electrical dose or switch to bitemporal placement, will be necessary. Efforts to use biochemical blood analyses of postictal hormonal changes, though theoretically interesting in deducing biologic mechanisms of ECT action, have not proven sensitive, specific, cost-effective, or time efficient for clinical use (Abrams 2002, Chapter 11). EEG data, on the other hand, are immediately available in real time with each treatment and do not cost extra money. Researchers thus have focused efforts at discovering predictors of ultimate remission with EEG analyses.

The degree of postictal flattening of the EEG tracing, often referred to in the ECT field as *postictal suppression*, correlates with therapeutic efficacy (Mayur 2006). On some modern ECT devices, postictal suppression can be quantified. Figure 6–6 displays one extreme of postictal suppression, with prominent spikes and slow waves followed by a very well-demarcated flat line, indicating good postictal suppression. Other electroencephalograms show ictal activity that very slowly and gradually tapers off without a certain point being observable as the end of the seizure (i.e., poor postictal suppression). Modern research has confirmed that in general (at least for depressed patients), the more well-defined the postictal suppression, the better the therapeutic outcome (Mayur 2006). However, the predictive power of this marker has not achieved sufficient sensitivity or specificity to be used to guide clinical technique. Quite simply, there are enough patients whose electroencephalograms display excellent postictal suppression but whose symptoms do not remit and those whose electroencephalograms demonstrate poor postictal suppression but whose symptoms do remit that quantifying postictal suppression should not be used to guide technique, at least with modern methods of quantification.

Other of the so-called EEG indices have been described in addition to postictal suppression. For example, Minelli et al. (2016) showed that ictal wave amplitude and hemispheric brain wave synchronicity, which reflects the degree to which EEG recordings from the right and left hemispheres demonstrate synchronous activity during the seizure, correlate with good outcomes. Some modern ECT machines have automated printouts at the end of the EEG strip that quantify various of these indices (Rasmussen et al. 2007e). *Ictal regularity*, or rhythmicity, which refers to the degree to which the ictal complexes are repetitive and stereotyped on the EEG strip as opposed to chaotic and irregular, has also been shown to correlate with better efficacy (McCall et al. 1998). As is the case with postictal suppression, there are interesting correlations of some of these indices and clinical outcome (Kimball et al. 2009), but not enough to warrant their use in guiding technique in routine practice.

Though an attractive notion, the idea of using EEG indices to guide technique has yet to be tested in a manner that would allow for such indices to be confidently recommended for clinical practice. First of all, the correlations between the EEG indices and outcome are not firm enough to modify the technique based on them. Also, it has not been definitively demonstrated that modifying technique to higher electrical doses or switching from unilateral to bitemporal placement reliably enhances the EEG indices (Rasmussen et al. 2007e). As the literature stands now, the author's recommendation to the ECT clinician is not to rely on the EEG indices that are printed out at the end of the EEG strip on the modern machines. As far as determining whether a particular technique is "on the right track" toward good efficacy, the focus should be on careful daily clinical assessments of patient progress. The fancy-looking EEG indices that print out on modern ECT devices are appropriate at this stage of technological development for research purposes only.

Immediate Postictal Period

Once the seizure has stopped, the patient should be kept in the ECT suite until spontaneous respiration resumes without ventilatory support. Vital signs do not need to be back to baseline before transfer to the posttreatment recovery area. Heart rate may still be a bit fast and blood pressure may be elevated, because these parameters may take a few minutes or longer to return to baseline. Very high elevations in blood pressure or heart rate may prompt the anesthesiologist to administer medication such as the beta-blocker labetalol.

The patient will display gross movements of the body core and limbs as the succinylcholine wears off. If the awakening patient is aware of residual paralysis, there may be the sensation of not being able to breathe well, even if the pulse oximeter shows good oxygenation. This sensation of shallow breathing can be very anxiety provoking, and the heart rate may become highly tachycardic. One option to help the patient in this situation, which represents residual succinylcholine effect lasting beyond the wearing off of the anesthetic medication, is to give another dose of anesthetic, with the idea that by the time this second dose of anesthetic wears off, the patient's paralysis from succinylcholine will be completed and there will be a more comfortable awakening. Patients experiencing anxiety on awakening in the ECT suite will sometimes evince groaning sounds or even whisper "I can't breathe." Gentle reassurance from all the ECT staff will help the patient negotiate through this uncomfortable sensation. The author has noted this phenomenon to be particularly common in patients treated with right unilateral ultrabrief technique at the titration session (Rasmussen 2015c). The seizures thus induced are so light that unconsciousness normally caused by the seizure is short-lived, so there is commonly awareness of paralysis on awakening.

If a patient has consistently shown postictal agitation in the recovery room, then it would be appropriate in the ECT suite, after seizure termination, to administer a benzodiazepine, such as midazolam or diazepam, to prevent the behavioral restlessness in recovery. It is much easier to prevent that phenomenon before it occurs than to try and treat it once the patient is flailing about in the recovery area.

Occasionally, anesthetic medications cause shivering on awakening. It is important that the ECT clinician not mistake these shivering movements for recurrent seizure activity, to avoid requesting the anesthetist to give seizure-terminating medication.

Recovery Period

Once the patient is stable in the ECT suite, transfer to the recovery area can be undertaken. The recovery area may be a separate room altogether or a different section of the ECT suite room, depending on a particular hospital's setup. ECG, pulse oximetry, and blood pressure monitoring are standard. Post-anesthesia recovery rooms (PACUs, in common parlance) are under the supervision of the anesthetist, but the psychiatrist, of course, should be aware of the process and, in particular, can help out with behavioral disturbances that occur. Specific requirements for discharge from the PACU (and back to the inpatient unit if an inpatient or home if an outpatient) include blood pressure, heart rate, ECG rhythm, breathing, and pulse oximetry readings that are back to pretreatment baseline.

Common issues that occur in recovery that need attention include airway difficulty, tachycardia, and prolonged elevated blood pressure. For the latter two, labetalol is a good option. PACU personnel should be competent to assess adequacy of the airway and respiration and ask for help if needed and to provide basic ventilatory assistance, such as jaw lift, to aid patient breathing.

From a behavioral standpoint, the PACU period may be one of relative calm, or it may be characterized by flailing about. Some patients simply wish to lie on their side, and allowing them to do so alleviates restlessness. Others can be consoled and calmed down verbally, but if not, administration of an intravenous benzodiazepine such as midazolam 1–2 mg or diazepam 5–10 mg will calm them down. As discussed earlier, if this happens at the first treatment session, then a prudent strategy would be to administer the dose just after seizure termination at the subsequent sessions as a preventive strategy. Midazolam has the advantage of shorter duration of activity and may be suitable if needed serially during an ECT course, in which case blood levels will not accumulate. On the other hand, for patients whose postictal agitation is quite prolonged, diazepam would be preferable.

Some patients will complain of headaches or nausea while in the recovery area, and medications can be administered such as ondansetron for the former or ketorolac for the latter. Switching the anesthetic agent to one less likely to cause postictal nausea is another strategy. Gentle, ongoing reorientation by the PACU nurse will help reassure the disoriented patient, who may repeat the same questions over and over, such as "Where am I?" or "Did I get a treatment?"

If severe breathing problems or a disconcerting ECG rhythm occurs in the PACU, then consultation with the appropriate specialists will be necessary. Occasionally, transfer to a medical service is needed. Tardive seizures occurring in the PACU, a very rare phenomenon, can be terminated the same way as in the suite for a prolonged seizure, and if that is not successful, then an urgent neurological consultation is needed. Patients who normally have continuous positive airway pressure (CPAP) or bilevel positive airway pressure (BiPAP) prescribed should bring in their portable units for use in the PACU after ECT. Finally, fingerstick blood sugar monitoring repeated in the PACU for patients with diabetes may be helpful but is not mandatory, because research has shown very mild mean increases occur in blood sugar postictally during ECT (Rasmussen and Ryan 2005, 2006b).

Discharge from the PACU directly to the inpatient unit for inpatients will involve calling staff from that unit to transfer the patient back to the inpatient unit. Outpatients can be disconnected from the monitoring devices (electrocardiograph, blood pressure cuff, pulse oximetry) according to the same criteria as inpatients. ECT outpatients should only be discharged home in the presence of a responsible adult who will accompany them for at least 24 hours after the treatment.

Communication to Patient, Family, or Inpatient Staff

ECT patients forget many of the instructions or educational facts given to them, so ECT personnel, as well as other mental health staff, should be prepared for regular repetition and reinforcement of principles, especially those pertaining to outpatient care. Of high importance is communication with family members and others who will be involved in the patient's home care. Appointments for the next ECT visit, if there is one, should be given in writing with instructions about NPO status for the next treatment as well as not driving. Also, outpatients should be informed about which medications to take at home with a small amount of water prior to coming for the treatment (e.g., antihypertensive medications). These instructions should be provided to a responsible adult in addition to the patient, who likely will forget instructions. Phone numbers for whom to call with questions should be provided. Reinforcing at the time of discharge of outpatients to those accompanying them should include explaining what to expect from a memory standpoint; emphasizing that things will have to be repeated, especially the day of treatment and the next day; and so forth.

If there are any particular issues that will need attention for the next treatment, such as premedication with something for headaches, this should be communicated to the inpatient staff for inpatients and to family members for outpatients. In modern practice, we are swimming in a sea of regulatory requirements, and this includes documentation. Ideal would be computerized records where all aspects of the treatment, including technical parameters like electrode placement and stimulus parameters, motor and EEG seizure duration, and all anesthetic medications given, as well as vital sign data, are recorded.

Patients should be counseled to refrain from driving on the day of ECT treatments. It is not established whether there should be driving restrictions beyond that day. To be cautious the patient should not drive the day after ECT either. Beyond that, the anesthetic medication effects have worn off. The question then becomes, what effect does the seizure have on driving? There may be difficulty with directions as memory may be impaired. It is prudent for the patient not to do any driving during index ECT. This issue should be handled on a case-by-case basis, depending on how the individual patient responds to the treatments in terms of mental acuity and hand-eye coordination.

Beyond driving, the patient should be counseled about returning to work. This depends on the patient's job difficulty and how much recent recall is required. This issue will be discussed in more depth in Chapter 9.

Key Points

- The clinician conducting an ECT treatment must be aware of all aspects of the patient's care in the treatment room, including anesthetic technique, electrode placement, stimulus dosing and parameter configuration, stimulus delivery, how to ensure that a seizure occurs, and how to ensure that the seizure ends.

- Interpreting an ECT electroencephalographic pattern to discern seizure activity requires much practice.

- Determining that a seizure is too short or long necessitates appropriate action.

- The ECT clinician is responsible for ensuring proper stimulus electrode placement even if another practitioner, such as a nurse, is actually applying the electrodes.

7

ECT Technique, Part II: Managing the Course of Treatments

The initial acute series of electroconvulsive therapy (ECT) treatments is referred to as an *index course of treatments* by custom in the ECT field. The purpose of an index course of treatments, usually administered twice or thrice weekly, is to reduce psychopathology such as depression, mania, catatonia, or schizophrenic psychosis. In contrast, continuation or maintenance ECT treatments are given at spaced intervals after an index course and are designed to prevent relapse. That topic is discussed in Chapter 8.

Several issues must be broached before and during an index course of ECT treatments. These include managing concomitant psychotropic medications, making the choice of electrode placement and stimulus parameters, determining treatment frequency, monitoring therapeutic outcome, monitoring side effects and adverse events, monitoring and managing medical issues, and determining when to stop the course of treatments. These issues are covered in this chapter. Management after the index series of treatments is finished is covered in Chapter 8, and managing the treatment inside the ECT suite itself was covered in Chapter 6.

It is assumed that the ECT patient has a designated psychiatrist who is prescribing the treatments and following progress. This practitioner can be termed the "primary psychiatrist" and may be the same person who is conducting the treatments but often is not. Furthermore, in some clinical settings, the primary psychiatrist may change during the course of treatments. It is critical for these various personnel to communicate with one another and with other physicians involved in the patient's care during this time period in order to achieve consistency. The majority of ECT patients are being treated for depression, so much of this chapter pertains to management of depression during ECT. Mention will be made periodically of issues pertaining to patients with mania, schizophrenia, or catatonia. Table 7–1 summarizes common tasks of the psychiatrist who is managing a course of ECT treatments.

Managing Concomitant Psychotropic Medications During a Course of ECT

The majority of ECT patients have already been treated with multiple psychotropic agents during the index episode (Rasmussen et al. 2006a). The primary psychiatrist following the ECT patient needs to decide whether to taper and discontinue, continue, or add new medications during the course of treatments. In this section, each of the typical psychotropic classes is considered. Nonpsychotropic medications are considered in Chapter 4.

Antidepressants

Traditionally, it has been customary to taper off concomitant antidepressants during an ECT course. The rationale was that such medications presumably were ineffective and might contribute to ECT-related adverse events, such as cardiac risks, prolonged seizures, or memory impairment. While it is prudent to taper off any antidepressant agent that were ineffective prior to ECT, in spite of adequate dose and duration of therapy, one need not completely accomplish this before commencing with treatments. The tapering can proceed at a pace that is deemed comfortable for the patient. There is empirical support for the practice of tapering and discontinuing antidepressants during index ECT. Mayur et al. (2000) randomly allocated depressed ECT patients already taking antidepressants, mostly tricyclics, to continue receiving them during index ECT or to have them discontinued and receive placebo. The results indicated no difference in efficacy between the two groups. Similar findings were reported by O'Brien and Berrios (1993). The advantage to antidepressant discontinuation is that it prepares the patient for a new regimen.

This, of course, raises the issue of what to do with concomitant antidepressants that either have been partially effective or have just been started and have not been subjected to an adequate trial prior to ECT. It would be acceptable to continue such medication during the ECT course, and even to titrate up to therapeutic doses, in anticipation of continuation therapy post-ECT, even if mainte-

---

TABLE 7–1. Tasks of the psychiatrist managing a course of ECT treatments

---

1. Make patient selection (Chapter 2).

2. Obtain informed consent and provide patient education (Chapter 3).

3. Organize the pre-ECT medical workup (Chapter 4).

4. Choose electrode placement.

5. Choose stimulus dosage and configuration.

6. Choose treatment frequency.

7. Assess efficacy, cognition, other side effects, and medical stability throughout course of treatments.

8. Choose concomitant psychopharmacology.

9. Decide when to stop the acute course of treatments.

10. Plan post-ECT management strategy (i.e., pharmacotherapy and/or maintenance ECT).

---

nance ECT is anticipated. In the case of a partial response to an adequate course of an antidepressant prior to ECT, one could either taper off that medication in anticipation of starting something else or maintain it in the hope that it might confer some prophylactic potential in preventing relapse if ECT is successful. In Chapter 8 the strategy of adding lithium carbonate to an antidepressant medication for relapse prevention after the index ECT course is finished is discussed.

Assuming the index ECT patient is not taking an antidepressant medication or has been tapered off what was being prescribed before, the next issue to consider is whether to start a new agent concomitant with index ECT in the hopes that it might either enhance acute remission rates or at least provide extra prophylaxis against relapse after ECT. The theory is that by the time ECT is finished, the newly administered antidepressant will have had time to induce its neurobiological effects to enhance acute response or protect against depression recurrence. A multisite study, termed the OPT-ECT study, tested both these hypotheses (Sackeim et al. 2009). A group of depressed patients scheduled for ECT were randomly assigned to receive concomitant venlafaxine, nortriptyline, or placebo during index ECT. Those who achieved remission with index ECT and had been given either venlafaxine or nortriptyline were continued on that medication, with the addition of lithium carbonate. Those patients achieving remission with index ECT while having been given concomitant placebo pills were, on remission, randomly assigned to receive either venlafaxine/lithium or nortriptyline/lithium during the 6-month continuation phase. The results showed that both active medications enhanced acute remission rates vis-à-vis placebo. Both medications were well tolerated. This important study provides reliable evidence in favor of starting antidepressant medication along with index ECT, at least in patients with unipolar depression, to enhance initial remission rates. What is not known is whether the results are specific to nortriptyline and venlafaxine or would extend to medications from other antidepressant classes.

Other research groups have broached the strategy of starting antidepressant medication along with index ECT, albeit in studies with much less scientific rigor than that used in the Sackeim et al. (2009) study just mentioned (for review, see Rasmussen 2015b). Yildiz et al. (2010), in a small study, found no evidence that adding sertraline early in a course of ECT enhanced acute response rates versus starting it after the completion of the course of treatments. The study was probably not statistically powered enough to detect a benefit. Lauritzen et al. (1996) found that adding imipramine to index ECT was associated with higher acute response rates than adding paroxetine to ECT.

Nelson and Benjamin (1989), Muller (1961), and Seager and Bird (1962) all found that adding antidepressants, either tricyclics or monoamine oxidase inhibitors (MAOIs), to index ECT was associated with fewer treatments being needed. Baghai et al. (2006) retrospectively reviewed their experience treating several hundred depressed patients treated with ECT and concomitant antidepressants of various types and found no evidence of adverse effects of using the medications and even a suggestion of enhanced efficacy with this strategy.

Mention should be made of MAOIs. For some time in the anesthesiology literature, it was held as virtually immutable that general anesthesia could not be safely induced while a patient was taking an MAOI (Jenkins and Graves 1965). However, there is sufficient literature in the ECT field showing that such a combination can proceed safely (Dolenc et al. 2004b). It is acceptable practice to continue an MAOI in preparation for ECT if such medication has been partially effective and it is anticipated that the patient will continue taking it after ECT, or, if indicated, to start an MAOI concomitantly with index ECT.

In summary, the primary psychiatrist caring for the index ECT patient will need to have a strategy to deal with concomitant antidepressants. In general, those agents that were ineffective at adequate doses and durations for the index episode of depression should be tapered off. Medications that have just been started or have been partially effective may be continued, or the practitioner may taper them off, depending on choice of medication later on. It is recommended that the clinician choose an antidepressant, preferably nortriptyline or venlafaxine, to prescribe along with index ECT, although data on other antidepressant classes are lacking at this time. These recommendations pertain to the unipolar depressed patient. For bipolar depressed patients, the practitioner will probably decide to taper off previously used antidepressants and not start such medications along with ECT so as not to risk induction of a manic episode. A recent meta-analysis (Song et al. 2015) concluded that antidepressant medication should not be combined with index ECT. However, most of the studies were markedly inferior to the Sackeim et al. (2009) OPT-ECT study, which, as mentioned, did show that concomitant venlafaxine or nortriptyline enhanced acute efficacy. At this time, the ECT clinician can choose whether to add an antidepressant or not during acute ECT—either strategy is defensible.

Antipsychotics

It has become common practice to add antipsychotic medications to antidepressants in depressed patients. Thus, these are commonly encountered medications in patients referred for ECT. In the interest of medication simplicity, it is recommended these medications be tapered off if they have not been effective, but no delay in starting ECT is necessary to allow a thorough washout. This class of medication does not cause increased risks of medical complications during ECT, as reported in one large series of ECT patients treated concomitantly with antipsychotic medications (Nothdurfter et al. 2006).

For patients with bipolar depression, the clinician must assess whether currently prescribed antipsychotic medications have been helpful in the past in preventing manic states—if so, then they should be continued. In fact, a bipolar depressed patient may benefit from the addition of an antipsychotic medication during index ECT to prevent mania as a substitute for lithium or anticonvulsants, which may interact negatively with ECT (see next subsection). Manic patients almost always are co-treated with neuroleptics along with index ECT, because such patients tend to be quite behaviorally agitated.

Finally, schizophrenia patients are also co-treated with neuroleptics, and an older literature suggests a synergistic benefit between ECT and neuroleptics in this population (for review, see Chapter 2).

Anticonvulsants

Anticonvulsant medications are used for epilepsy, mood disorders, migraine headaches, fibromyalgia, and various chronic pain syndromes and are common in patients referred for ECT (Rubner et al. 2009). The most frequently encountered for syndromes other than epilepsy are valproate, lamotrigine, pregabalin, gabapentin, topiramate, oxcarbazepine, and carbamazepine. It is immediately obvious that the ECT clinician would rather not have to induce a seizure in a patient taking anticonvulsant medication, but the decision to taper off such medication cannot be taken lightly. However, the majority of ECT patients co-treated with anticonvulsants can obtain therapeutic seizures with ECT without having to reduce their anticonvulsant medications (Lunde et al. 2006; Rubner et al. 2009; Sienaert and Peuskens 2007). A recent study divided ECT patients with mania into those treated with concomitant valproate versus placebo and found no difference in antimanic efficacy of ECT or seizure duration (Haghighi et al. 2013; Jahangard et al. 2012). Lamotrigine has also been combined with ECT without apparent ill effect on seizure duration (Penland and Ostroff 2006; Sienaert et al. 2011). Zarate et al. (1997), in a very small series, found that co-treatment with ECT and either valproate or carbamazepine did diminish seizures but did not apparently reduce efficacy. Thus, a first strategy is to have anticonvulsant-treated patients continue taking the medication while commencing ECT.

Cautious downward tapering may be needed if excessively short seizures occur during ECT or if no seizures can be induced. In epileptic patients, this should only be undertaken in consultation with a neurologist to ensure it is done safely. For mood disorder patients taking anticonvulsants, it is also a conundrum with ECT: one might wish to taper off the medications so as to ensure maximally therapeutic seizures, but that might lead to a manic episode if the medication had been used to prevent mania. As with the epileptic population, one can commence ECT without having tapered off the anticonvulsant if it is determined that the latter was helpful as a mood episode prophylactic. However, if poor or no seizures are induced, then cautious tapering down can be tried. As noted above, antipsychotic medications provide good antimanic activity, and such a medication can be used instead of the anticonvulsant to provide protection against precipitation of a manic episode if the anticonvulsant is tapered off. Some ECT practitioners may insist on not worrying about treatment-emergent mania, on the theory that continued ECT treatments will treat the mania as well. However, an ECT-consenting depressed patient may turn into an ECT-refusing manic patient. The consequences of mania can be so severe that one must do all possible pharmacologically in the patient with a history of mania to prevent that from happening when ECT is used for depression by using the strategies outlined above. As for patients given anticonvulsant medications for various pain syndromes (e.g., migraine, fibromyalgia), since these are less risky conditions than epilepsy or mania, it is advisable to taper these medications off during ECT to obtain maximally therapeutic seizures and because in many of these patients, effective treatment of depression also leads to benefits in the pain complaints and may obviate the need for the medications.

Lithium

The question of whether lithium can be combined with ECT safely has received a surprisingly large amount of attention in the ECT literature for several decades

(Mukherjee 1993). There have been case reports, case series, and case-control series reporting excessive confusion, delirium, and prolonged or spontaneous seizures when lithium was combined with ECT (Ahmed and Stein 1987; Alexander et al. 1988; Conway and Nelson 2001; DePaulo et al. 1982; el-Mallakh 1988; Hagen 1976; Hoenig and Chaulk 1977; Jephcott and Kerry 1974; Lebovitz 1976; Mandel et al. 1980; Penney et al. 1990; Ray 1975; Remick 1978; Sartorius et al. 2005; Schou 1991; Small and Milstein 1990; Small et al. 1980; Stewart 2000; Weiner et al. 1980). Other case series failed to confirm this (Dolenc and Rasmussen 2005; Jha et al. 1996; Kukopulos et al. 1988; Martin and Kramer 1982; Thirthalli et al. 2011; Volpe and Tavares 2012; Volpe et al. 2003). Some papers have incidentally mentioned concomitant ECT and lithium without mentioning safety (Gagné et al. 2000; Hartigan 1963; Krishna et al. 1978; Sackeim et al. 1991). There are some individual cases of safe combination of lithium and ECT (Bright-Long and Fink 1993; DeQuardo and Tandon 1988; Gupta et al. 1998; Kramer 1999; Lippmann and Tao 1993; Mayur et al. 1999; Pearlman 1988). Vlissides et al. (1979) showed that ECT treatments did not cause an acute rise in lithium blood levels. Whether or not the combination is safe or is to be avoided in all cases has been the subject of persistent and intense interest in the ECT literature (see Adityanjee 1989; DeQuardo and Tandon 1989; El-Mallakh 1987, 1988; Lippmann and El-Mallakh 1994; National Institutes of Health 1985; Rudorfer et al. 1987a, 1987b; Schou 1991).

It is a possibility that in some patients, lithium may exacerbate posttreatment agitation or confusion temporarily. Of course, if the ECT patient is taking lithium and it has been determined that the latter has not been of help either in the current episode or for prophylaxis, then the medication should be tapered off in anticipation of ECT. However, a complete washout is probably not necessary before starting treatments. If lithium has been effective in treating the manic phase of bipolar disorder, and the patient is being treated with ECT for depression, then continuing the lithium during treatments can be recommended, with holding of doses 24 hours prior to each treatment. Alternatively, if excessive cognitive issues appear, lithium can be tapered off and replaced with an antipsychotic medication during ECT to prevent mania.

In the bipolar patient in whom lithium has been effective in preventing manic episodes, this medication should not be stopped without replacing it with another antimanic agent during ECT lest the clinician precipitate a manic episode. Some may argue that if mania does occur during index ECT, the treatments can be continued to treat the mania. However, the manic patient may not be willing to cooperate with ECT, and mania is a dangerous condition. Thus, there should be some medication prescribed to prevent mania in the bipolar depressed patient receiving ECT.

If lithium is not a current medication for the ECT patient but the plan is to start it to prevent mood episode recurrence after ECT, then the clinician should wait until the end of the ECT course to start the lithium, even if an antidepressant medication is started concomitantly with ECT. The question of whether starting lithium concomitantly with index ECT enhances acute remission or lowers continuation phase relapses has not been studied, but a randomized trial would be quite welcome. The use of lithium for post-ECT relapse prevention in unipolar and bipolar patients is discussed more thoroughly in Chapter 8.

Benzodiazepines

As is the case with the anticonvulsant medications, benzodiazepines might be expected to have an inhibitory effect on seizure expression or duration in ECT. One study indicated that such medications might interfere with ECT efficacy (Pettinati et al. 1990). However, another study indicated that lorazepam at dosages of up to 3 mg/day does not interfere with the antidepressant efficacy of ECT (Sackeim et al. 1987a). A prudent conclusion would be that short-acting, moderately dosed regimens of benzodiazepine medication can help the acutely distressed or agitated patient during ECT, with the expectation that as the course of treatments progresses and the patient improves, the usage would lessen substantially or even disappear. The patient who is already taking long-acting benzodiazepines before starting ECT presents a dilemma, but in general, a withdrawal state would confuse the picture clinically and make improvement from ECT difficult to discern. Thus, one must not insist on benzodiazepine withdrawal regimens in order to perform ECT, but the possibility of a slow taper should at least be considered on a case-by-case basis. Many catatonic patients have already been treated with lorazepam, usually in high doses, by the time ECT is commenced, with either no or partial improvement. The clinician should taper off this medication as ECT is started. In the case of a catatonically mute and stuporous patient in whom lorazepam clears the catatonia but reveals an underlying mood disorder to be treated with ECT, the lorazepam tapering can be done a bit more slowly so as not to lose the anti-catatonic benefits early in the ECT course.

Miscellaneous Psychotropic Agents

Many hypnotic agents are used to help patients with sleep, including those medications specifically designed for such use (e.g., zaleplon, zolpidem, eszopiclone, melatonin and its analogues), as well as benzodiazepines and sedating antidepressants/antipsychotics (e.g., trazodone, quetiapine). As far as ECT issues are concerned, the clinician should not be averse to a patient being given any of these medications if needed but would again try to avoid long-acting benzodiazepines.

Stimulant medications such as methylphenidate or amphetamine are commonly used for attention-deficit disorders or as antidepressant augmentation strategies. While there is no evidence for increased risk of cardiac adverse events with such drugs, it would seem prudent to withhold them during an index ECT course, especially if they have not been helpful for the current depressive episode. Thyroid preparations have come into some popularity as well for antidepressant augmentation and should be tapered off if ineffective. Of course, if such medication is given for a thyroid disease, then by all means it should be continued during ECT.

Nootropics are a class of medication used to attempt to enhance cognitive function in dementia patients. The most commonly utilized are cholinesterase inhibitors such as donepezil or the N-methyl-D-aspartate receptor–blocking agent memantine. There is some evidence that donepezil (Prakash et al. 2006) or memantine (Abbasinazari et al. 2015; Alizadeh et al. 2015) may lessen the cognitive effects of ECT, findings much in need of replication in larger samples before such strategies can be used in routine practice. However, these studies do document that use of such agents in ECT is safe. Thus, in dementia patients, these agents may be continued during ECT if the patient or family feels they have been helpful for cognitive function.

Electrode Placement, Stimulus Dosage, Stimulus Configuration, and Treatment Frequency

Historical Perspective on ECT Technique

During the first few decades of ECT usage, electrode placement was almost always bitemporal, with sine-wave machines used and with no strategy for quantifying electrical dosage. In the 1960s and 1970s predominantly, there was a flurry of "unilateral versus bilateral" ECT studies, about half of which showed therapeutic equality and half showing superiority of bitemporal (Pettinati et al. 1986). Most of these studies utilized the now-outmoded sine-wave electrical stimulus, and those that did not had no specification of electrical dosage. A landmark study in the history of ECT was published by Sackeim et al. (1987a) from Columbia University: for the first time, unilateral and bilateral (bitemporal) ECT were compared using a brief-pulse, square wave stimulus, the dosage of which was quantified with a seizure threshold–determining titration. Throughout the course of treatments, barely suprathreshold dosing was maintained, and bitemporal placement produced superior results. This study set the modern standard for ECT technique, which includes not only choice of electrode placement but also quantification of the electrical charge and specification of dosage in relation to seizure threshold. In addition to electrode placement and stimulus dosing, studies have examined the effects of different stimulus parameter configurations (standard pulse width versus ultrabrief pulse width) as well as treatment frequencies (usually twice vs. thrice weekly schedules). Henceforth in this discussion of ECT technique, only studies specifying information on all four of these aspects of ECT technique will be considered.

Before commencing with an index series of ECT treatments, the psychiatrist must decide on electrode placement, stimulus dosage, stimulus configuration, and treatment frequency. Additionally, as the treatment course progresses, outcome needs to be monitored, and if the patient either does not make expected therapeutic progress or experiences undue cognitive side effects, one or more of these technical parameters may need to be changed. Thus, index ECT patients must be followed carefully throughout their course of treatments.

The reader can appreciate the complexity of these choices. There are three electrode placements in modern ECT practice (bitemporal, bifrontal, and right unilateral), different stimulus dosing paradigms (i.e., low, moderate, and high dose, to be simplistic), and standard pulse width versus ultrabrief pulse width. Additionally, treatment frequency is generally twice versus thrice weekly. This amounts to $3 \times 3 \times 2 \times 2 = 36$ different combinations for the practitioner to choose from! A randomized study comparing all these options has not been conducted, nor will one ever be. Further, there has never been a study in which any three of these four variables have been systematically manipulated. In fact, there are only four studies in the era of modern ECT technique in which two technical variables have been manipulated (Janakiramaiah et al. 1998; Sackeim et al. 1993, 2000, 2008). In all the other studies reviewed below, only one variable (electrode placement, stimulus dose, stimulus configuration, or treatment frequency) was manipulated. Thus, it is impossible to describe the "one true" type of ECT technique for depressed patients, but review of the dozens of well-conducted studies that do exist leads to some confident recommendations for current practice. We will henceforth consider pertinent topics related to electrode placement, stimulus configuration, stimulus dosing, and treatment frequency, providing recommendations along the way. For most of the rest of this section, the discussion pertains to depressed patients treated with ECT. Manic, catatonic, and schizophrenic patients will be considered at the end of the section. Proceeding forth, the author will review the ECT technical literature, pointing out lessons that have been learned and suggesting a proposed algorithm to guide clinical practice. This discussion will focus mostly on therapeutic efficacy with relatively brief mention of cognitive outcomes. The latter topic will be discussed in more detail later in this chapter, as well as in Chapter 9, which is devoted to the effects of ECT on cognition.

Electrode Placement

Bifrontal Placement for Depression

Let us consider bifrontal electrode placement, first described by Golla et al. (1940). The theory behind its use was that stimulating the frontal brain regions presumably involved in the mechanisms of major depression might result in sparing of the temporal regions involved in memory consolidation (Inglis 1969). Initial open trials (Abrams and Fink 1972; Abrams and Taylor 1973) using a close spacing of the electrodes on the forehead (so-called anterior bifrontal placement) resulted in some skin burning and no apparent benefit for efficacy, so the technique was abandoned for some years until resurrected by Lawson et al. (1990) and Letemendia et al. (1993), who found an apparent therapeutic and cognitive benefit for the modern wider-spaced bifrontal versus right unilateral or bitemporal placement. However, subsequently, there have been numerous randomized comparisons of bifrontal placement in depressed patients with either right unilateral (Bjølseth et al. 2015; Eschweiler et al. 2007; Heikman et al. 2002; Sienaert et al. 2009b, 2010) or bitemporal (Amiri et al. 2009; Bailine et al. 2000), or both (Kellner et al. 2010; Ranjkesh et al. 2005), with no benefits seen for bifrontal in terms of efficacy or cognition. A meta-analysis of these studies concluded there was no benefit to bifrontal placement for depression (Dunne and McLoughlin 2012). The most extensive study (Kellner et al. 2010), in fact, found that delayed recall and retrograde memory were worse for bifrontal than for bitemporal placement. Thus, at this time, it is the author's opinion that there is no advantage to using bifrontal placement for depressed patients. The author has abandoned this placement in his practice.

Ultrabrief-Pulse-Width Bitemporal Placement

Next, let us consider the perplexing case of ultrabrief-pulse-width bilateral placement for ECT technique. *Ultrabrief pulse widths* are those less than 0.5 milliseconds, while pulse widths greater than or equal to 0.5 milliseconds are termed *standard pulse width*. In a randomized comparison of standard versus ultrabrief-pulse-width as well as bitemporal versus right unilateral lead placement (thus, four groups), Sackeim et al. (2008) unexpectedly found very low remission rates in the ultrabrief pulse width bitemporal group. In fact, patients in this group fared worse than patients in any of the other three groups, all of whom had good remission rates. Poring through the ECT literature uncovers a few other similar findings. Cronholm and Ottosson (1963b), in a study in which the term "ultrabrief" pulse was coined, similarly found low efficacy in the ultrabrief pulse bitemporal group. Robin and de Tissera (1982) also found low efficacy in a group treated with what is now termed ultrabrief pulse stimuli with bilateral placement. More recently, Niemantsverdriet et al. (2011) and Sienaert et al. (2009b) also found low remission rates with bitemporal and bifrontal ultrabrief techniques, respectively. It is not known why bilateral placement, usually considered the gold standard for efficacy in ECT, would have compromised efficacy when combined with ultrabrief pulses, but at this time, such a technique is not recommended for routine ECT practice. If bilateral placement is used, it should be combined with a standard pulse width—preferably at least 1.0 millisecond.

Is There a Reason to Use Bitemporal Placement for Depression?

The landmark studies of Lancaster et al. (1958) and Thenon (1956) established that unilateral placements were feasible for ECT practice and could lead to lesser memory side effects. The debate over unilateral versus bilateral raged on for much of the 1960s through the 1980s. In modern ECT research, there are plenty of studies showing that some form of unilateral ECT equals bitemporal for efficacy (Kellner et al. 2010; McCall et al. 2002; Ranjkesh et al. 2005; Sackeim et al. 1993, 2000, 2008, 2009; Sienaert et al. 2009b). However, as should be abundantly clear by now to the reader, there is much more to ECT technique than simply "unilateral versus bilateral." The modern studies showing unilateral equal to bitemporal or bifrontal have, as discussed earlier, used electrical doses several times initial threshold. Most of these studies have also demonstrated less severe cognitive side effects with the unilateral placement. Thus, the question arises, is there a place in modern ECT practice for bitemporal placement (standard pulse width) for depression? A caution is that the depressed patients enrolled in these studies were all sufficiently cognitively intact enough to process the consent form for complex studies. What about depressed patients who are too ill from psychotic ideations, ruminations, or pseudodementia to participate in such studies? Would unilateral ECT have the same efficacy in these patients? The answer is not known. Furthermore, as discussed later, nonresponders to initial treatment technique in multiple Columbia University Consortium studies were crossed over to high-dose bitemporal technique with excellent subsequent remission rates.

A prudent clinical recommendation is that for depressed patients with illness severity like that represented in modern ECT studies, unilateral placement is an acceptable option. There is no basis for the mind-set that unilateral ECT should not be used in modern practice, an attitude held by some practitioners for many years. For patients who are too ill to participate in the complex cognitive task of processing a randomized study, the author will be more likely to use bitemporal placement with standard pulse width. On the other hand, if a depressed patient is considered to be like the types of patients enrolled in modern clinical trials, then right unilateral ultrabrief technique will be used to begin an index course, with stimulus dosing at six times threshold. Additionally, if a patient thus treated does not progress sufficiently after, say, six to eight treatments, the next technique will be standard-pulse-width bitemporal placement. Table 7–2 summarizes factors weighing in favor of bitemporal versus unilateral electrode placement in depressed patients.

Stimulus Dosage:
Stimulus Dose-Response Studies

Electrical dose refers to the amount of electricity in units of charge that is delivered to the patient during a treatment. Note that this is different from the issue of *stimulus parameter configuration*, which refers to choices about the four stimulus parameters of pulse width, pulse frequency, pulse current, and stimulus train duration (see Chapter 6). On modern ECT machines, the clinician must choose an electrical dose in addition to parameter combinations. Different parameter combinations can be used to achieve the same electrical dose, so these two variables are not identical. As described in Chapter 6, at the first session, a titration is performed to determine seizure threshold. At subsequent treatments, dose must again be chosen based on the initial threshold. Studies have shown that the higher the electrical dose relative to initial threshold, the greater the clinical efficacy but also the higher the cognitive side effects.

The earlier-cited study of Sackeim et al. (1987b) at Columbia University established electrical dosing as a variable just as important as electrode placement. The Columbia University Consortium studies established that for unilateral placement to be effective, electrical doses several times initial threshold need to be used. Studies in which low, just barely suprathreshold, dosing was utilized for unilateral placement found around 20%–30% remission rates (Sackeim et al. 1987a, 1993, 2000), which are low by ECT standards. Studies in which higher doses were used have shown greater efficacy (Sackeim et al. 1993, 2000, 2008, 2009). This dose-response relationship has been confirmed by McCall et al. (2000, 2002) in two studies using a variety of dosing schemes. The standard that has emerged for unilateral electrode placement, whether ultrabrief or standard pulse width, is five to eight times threshold, with the modal dose in modern studies being six times threshold. Indeed, the latter is what the author uses in his practice. It should be noted that in one very small study, it was found that there was no difference in efficacy among 4, 7, and 10 times threshold dosing for unilateral ultrabrief technique (Quante et al. 2011). However, with only about 10 patients per treatment group, the study was quite statistically underpowered to detect a difference.

TABLE 7–2. Choice of electrode placement for depressed ECT patients

---

Factors favoring bitemporal placement

1. Psychotic or catatonic features

2. Intense suicidal drive

3. Profound functional impairment

4. Lack of patient concern about memory side effects

5. Previous good outcome with bitemporal placement

Factors favoring unilateral placement

1. Concern expressed by patient over memory side effects

2. Situations in which memory side effects may be particularly bothersome (e.g., students enrolled in school, professionals needing good recall of recent events)

3. Previous poor tolerance of bitemporal placement

4. Start of an acute course of treatments on an outpatient basis

5. Presence of a baseline cognitive disorder separate from depression-related cognitive dysfunction (e.g., dementia, Parkinson's disease)

For bitemporal placement, there is also a dose-response relationship, but the efficacy rates among dosage levels are not as dramatically different as with unilateral placement. Sackeim et al. (1987a) found that low-dose bitemporal (meaning an electrical dose barely suprathreshold throughout the treatment course) technique was associated with an approximately two-thirds remission rate, which was twice that for low-dose unilateral treatment. In a follow-up study, Sackeim et al. (1993) randomly assigned patients to receive low-dose versus 2.5 times threshold dosing and unilateral versus bitemporal placement (thus, four groups). In the bitemporal groups, efficacy was slightly greater in the higher-dose than in the lower-dose group. This is the only study in which depressed patients have been randomly assigned prospectively to low versus substantially higher doses for bitemporal placement. Thirthalli et al. (2009a) randomly assigned depressed patients to barely suprathreshold (1.0 times threshold) versus 1.5 times threshold dosing with bitemporal placement and found no efficacy difference, but most ECT practitioners would consider 1.5 times threshold not substantially greater than 1.0 times threshold. In two other Columbia University Consortium studies, in which bitemporal 2.5 times threshold was used (Sackeim et al. 2000, 2008), remission rates were about as high as with the 2.5 times threshold bitemporal group in the earlier study (Sackeim et al. 1993). Furthermore, in several of these studies, patients who did not respond to the initial randomized technique were given high-dose (i.e., 2.5 times threshold) bitemporal with excellent response rates (Sackeim et al. 1993, 2000, 2008, 2009). Taken together, these data strongly indicate that for bitemporal placement, higher electrical doses can be associated with higher efficacy, albeit with more cognitive side effects. As the field stands now, it is customary that if a depressed patient is treated with bitemporal placement, dosing subsequent to the initial threshold should be 1.0–2.0 times threshold, with the possibility of raising the dose higher if no response is achieved. The reader is reminded that all these data refer to standard-pulse-width bitemporal technique. Ultrabrief pulse widths (i.e., less than 0.5 milliseconds) should not be utilized for bitemporal placement.

Stimulus Parameter Configuration: Ultrabrief or Standard Pulse Width for Unilateral Electrode Placement?

Ultrabrief-pulse-width right unilateral technique has gained much popularity of late in the ECT field because of its relative lack of cognitive side effects (Sackeim et al. 2008). The ultrabrief pulses allow for less total electricity to be used to induce seizures, which is probably the basis for the lesser cognitive effects (Abrams 2002). One recent large-scale, multisite study utilized right unilateral ultrabrief, six times threshold thrice weekly, with elderly depressed patients and found an approximately two-thirds remission rate (Kellner et al. 2016a). Several randomized studies have compared right unilateral ultrabrief pulse width with right unilateral standard pulse width and either found equal efficacy (Loo et al. 2014; Sackeim et al. 2008) or slightly better efficacy or faster time to response, with standard pulse (Loo et al. 2007, 2008, 2011, 2012b, 2013; Spaans et al. 2013a). A meta-analysis and a literature review concluded that at that time, the evidence showed slightly better efficacy for right unilateral standard pulse width than for ultrabrief pulse width (Spaans et al. 2013b; Tor et al. 2015). However, confounded in the meta-analysis is one influential study showing much greater efficacy for standard-pulse-width unilateral in which treatments were administered twice weekly (Spaans et al. 2013b). The other studies used thrice-weekly treatment schedules. Moreover, using an ultra-high electrical dose of eight times threshold unilateral ultrabrief pulse width versus five times threshold standard pulse width, Loo et al. (2014) found equal efficacy but better cognitive profiles for the ultrabrief group. Thus, it is overly simplistic to ask "Is right unilateral ultrabrief equal to right unilateral standard pulse width?" without specifying treatment frequency or electrical dosing scheme. Perhaps at higher doses and more frequent treatment schedules, ultrabrief technique approaches standard pulse width for therapeutic outcomes.

At this time, the decision on whether to utilize standard-pulse-width or ultra-brief-pulse-width stimuli for unilateral placement is not settled in the literature. However, right unilateral ultrabrief pulse width has gained much popularity in clinical use because of its low cognitive side effect profile and is considered an acceptable alternative. If this technique is utilized, it should be administered thrice weekly so as not to compromise efficacy—cognitive side effects are so low that a twice-weekly schedule is not needed. Also, a stimulus dose of at least six times, and up to eight times, threshold should be used for right unilateral ultrabrief ECT. The ECT clinician, on the other hand, may choose to utilize standard pulse width for right unilateral placement until further data are available on this issue. In the author's current practice, unilaterally treated patients are given ultrabrief pulses at six times threshold.

It should be noted that pulse width is not the only ECT stimulus parameter of interest. There is research investigating the relative influence of pulse frequency (e.g., Roepke et al. 2011) and current strength (e.g., Peterchev et al. 2015) on efficacy and cognitive effects of ECT. However, the database for these parameters is in a preliminary state, so recommendations for current practice cannot be made at this time.

Treatment Frequency

The fourth ECT technical variable is treatment frequency. In most ECT studies, treatments are delivered thrice weekly. However, in some ECT services, twice-weekly schedules are also used, especially when there is a desire to minimize cognitive side effects. Several research efforts have shed light on optimizing treatment frequency. The fundamental issue at hand is balancing efficacy with cognitive side effects: more frequent treatments lead to more rapid efficacy but also to more cognitive side effects.

Abrams (1967) first broached the treatment-frequency issue by delivering unilateral treatments to schizophrenia patients daily (i.e., five times a week), comparing neuropsychological test performance to that of earlier patient cohorts treated thrice weekly and finding no essential difference. Strömgren (1975; Strömgren et al. 1976) compared unilaterally treated patients given treatments four versus two times a week and found the four-times-a-week schedule to be well tolerated cognitively and associated with faster time to remission. Also, Rasmussen et al. (2016) followed a cohort of depressed patients given right unilateral ultrabrief ECT, six times threshold dosing, treated five times a week, and found excellent cognitive tolerability of this aggressive schedule. None of these studies were randomized.

There have been several studies in which patients were randomly assigned to receive thrice- versus twice-weekly treatments, with most of these studies using bitemporal placement (Gangadhar et al. 1993; Lerer et al. 1995; Shapira et al. 1998; Vieweg and Shawcross 1998) but one using unilateral placement (McAllister et al. 1987). All showed equal efficacy for twice-weekly frequency, with a general trend in a meta-analysis showing fewer treatments needed in twice weekly but a longer time to remission with that modality as well (Charlson et al. 2012). Two studies comparing once-weekly versus thrice-weekly ECT, both with bitemporal electrode placement, found significantly lower improvement in depression with the once-weekly schedule (Janakiramaiah et al. 1998; Kellner et al. 1992). One interestingly designed study randomly assigned a small number of depressed patients to receive 2 weeks of thrice-weekly treatments or one real treatment followed by five sham (i.e., placebo) treatments and found equal efficacy (Jagadeesh et al. 1992). This intriguing finding goes against many decades of ECT practice and must be replicated in larger samples to be taken seriously.

Two recent well-designed ECT studies involved treatment with twice-weekly schedules. Spaans et al. (2013b) randomly assigned depressed patients to eight times threshold unilateral treatments given either with ultrabrief or standard pulse widths and found markedly lower efficacy in the ultrabrief group. This is the only data set currently published in which right unilateral ultrabrief ECT was given twice weekly, so the low efficacy should encourage caution in using this treatment frequency for that modality. Semkovska et al. (2016) randomly assigned depressed patients to receive either twice-weekly right unilateral high-dose standard pulse width or bitemporal moderate-dose standard pulse width, also at a twice-weekly frequency, and found no therapeutic differences but some cognitive advantage to unilateral. This study adds to the extensive literature documenting that unilateral ECT, if administered properly, can equal bitemporal ECT for efficacy.

The summary of the treatment-frequency literature is that twice-weekly treatments can yield results equivalent to those of thrice-weekly treatments, with fewer total treatments but at a somewhat slower pace and perhaps with some cognitive advantage. It is acceptable to treat ECT patients at a twice-weekly rate. However, as noted earlier, at this time the twice-weekly frequency cannot be recommended if the unilateral ultrabrief technique is used. For unilateral ECT, the clinician should treat twice weekly only if standard pulse width is used (i.e., at least 1.0 millisecond). If bitemporal electrode placement for depressed patients is chosen, either as the beginning strategy or as a crossover from ineffective unilateral placement, then the twice-weekly frequency is a viable choice and is probably underutilized. In the Semkovska et al. (2016) trial utilizing twice-weekly bitemporal placement, there was very little retrograde amnesia.

A Proposed Algorithm for
Initial ECT Technique in Depressed Patients

As indicated earlier in this section, there is no extant study in the ECT literature in which depressed patients were randomly assigned to all possible combinations of electrode placement, stimulus dosing scheme, stimulus parameter configuration, and treatment frequency. However, it can be confidently concluded that there is no need to deliver bifrontal placement and that ultrabrief pulse width with bitemporal placement should not be used. The author, in his own ECT practice, decides on initial ECT technique in depressed patients by judging whether the patient is well enough to participate in the types of randomized trials that have been published. If the answer (and admittedly this is a subjective judgment call) is yes, then right unilateral ultrabrief, six times initial threshold, thrice-weekly treatment is planned. If the answer is no—that is, the patient seems to be too ill to be able to process the complex cognitive demands of a clinical study—then bitemporal standard pulse width, 1.5 times initial threshold, is chosen, with treatment frequency being generally thrice weekly or twice weekly if cognitive concerns exist. If the patient has a history of good prior response to a particular technique, then that technique is used for the current episode. For example, if a patient has a history of poor response to unilateral ultrabrief with subsequent good response after crossover to bitemporal, then for a new episode, bitemporal is used from the beginning.

Modifying Technique as
the Treatment Course Progresses

During an index course of ECT treatments, the psychiatrist must monitor the patient daily for therapeutic efficacy, side effects (most prominently, cognitive side effects), and medical stability (e.g., assessing for evidence of cardiac decompensation in a patient with congestive heart failure). Medical monitoring was discussed in Chapter 4.

If the patient does not seem to be responding well in terms of depressive symptoms, or if there seem to be excessive cognitive effects, then measures need to be taken to address these concerns. Efficacy-enhancing alternatives include increasing electrical dose, switching from ultrabrief to standard pulse width, switching from unilateral to bitemporal placement, and increasing treatment frequency. There is usually a direct relationship between enhancing efficacy and the effect on cognitive side effects. Thus, alternatives to lessen cognitive side effects are the opposite of those to enhance efficacy. Striking this balance is one of the main goals of the psychiatrist during an index series of treatments.

In terms of efficacy assessment, the typical course of treatments for a depressed patient is 6–12 total treatments, assuming technique does not have to be changed because of lack of response. In the latter instance, if a patient is switched from, say, unilateral ultrabrief to bitemporal standard pulse width, then the total number of treatments may be up to twice as much. Unfortunately, there is no science guiding when to declare the first chosen technique a failure. That is, if a patient is not responding, when does the clinician switch to something more aggressive? After five treatments, eight treatments, or more? The appropriate study would be to randomly assign nonresponders after a given number of treatments—say, five—to either continue with the initial technique or switch to something more aggressive, but such research has not been done. In the meantime, the clinician is advised to balance severity of psychopathology with patient concerns about cognitive side effects when deciding when to switch. For example, a more severely ill patient who is not showing cognitive side effects should be switched earlier in a treatment course than a less ill patient who is either showing some bothersome cognitive effects or expressing a lot of worry about such effects. The author, in his own practice, usually considers switching if six treatments do not result in substantial improvement in depression. If the initial technique was unilateral ultrabrief pulse width, then the next step is switching to bitemporal standard pulse width (thrice weekly). If the initial technique was bitemporal standard pulse width, then the next step would be to increase the electrical dosage (e.g., doubling it). The author does not increase treatment frequency for bitemporally treated depressed patients to more than three treatments per week, as such a strategy builds up much cognitive side effect load. Some clinicians, faced with ineffective unilateral ultrabrief technique, may avoid switching to bitemporal by either increasing the electrical dosage—say, from six times threshold to eight times threshold—or converting from ultrabrief pulse width to standard pulse width. Such strategies are relatively untested, however, and may only prolong an already longer than average total course of treatments.

Cognitive monitoring, discussed in more detail in a later section and in Chapter 9, usually does not reveal bothersome effects when a unilateral ultrabrief technique is used, even when it is used five days a week (Rasmussen et al. 2016). Thus, a clinician will not be faced with having to lessen treatment frequency or lower electrical dose in patients thus treated. On the other hand, if initial technique is bitemporal standard pulse width thrice weekly, the clinician may need to back off to twice-weekly treatments later in the course if the patient seems a bit disoriented to place or time. Since initial bitemporal dosing is usually not much above threshold (i.e., 1.5 times threshold), lowering the electrical dose is not likely to help cognition much and will only increase the risk that a seizure will not be attained. Additionally, as has been emphasized several times thus far, ultrabrief pulse width should not be used when placement is bitemporal. Thus, this leaves lowering treatment frequency and switching to unilateral as options to lessen cognitive effects. The author recommends the former versus the latter, because if bitemporal placement was chosen initially, the clinical severity is probably so high that unilateral placement is not likely to be effective.

A final note should be made of when to stop the index treatment course. For patients who are improving, the clinician should not discontinue treatments until a confident plateau of improvement has occurred after, say, two treatments. One of the most common mistakes the author has seen is for clinicians to stop ECT prematurely. The source of information about improvement emanates not only from the patient's subjective self-report but also from mental status examination and discussion with those familiar with the patient, such as nursing staff for inpatients and concerned family members. For depressed patients who are not improving with ECT, a course of 10 treatments is considered an adequate trial (Husain et al. 2004).

ECT Technique for Mania, Catatonia, and Schizophrenia

There is a paucity of technical ECT studies in mania, catatonia, and schizophrenia. The most substantial recommendation for this very ill population is to administer bitemporal standard pulse width technique at least thrice weekly. Unilateral placement, especially if combined with ultrabrief pulse width stimuli, is not recommended in such patients. While there are limited data suggesting equal or at least good efficacy for right unilateral standard pulse width versus bitemporal standard pulse width in mania (Black et al. 1986; Mukherjee et al. 1988; Schnur et al. 1992), or equal efficacy in brief versus ultrabrief pulse width unilateral in schizophrenia (Pisvejc et al. 1998), the vast weight of clinical experience favors bitemporal placement. For patients who are fulminantly ill, such as delirious manic patients, malignantly catatonic patients, or highly agitated schizophrenic patients, daily bitemporal treatments—say, for the first three days or so—can be utilized until initial improvement occurs, with a subsequent switch to thrice-weekly frequency.

There are some studies emanating from one group suggesting that bifrontal placement is more effective than bitemporal placement in schizophrenia (Phutane et al. 2013) and mania (Hiremani et al. 2008), but these data need to be replicated before a recommendation can be made not to use bitemporal, which has been the standard placement for such patients for many decades. Thirthalli et al. (2009a), representing the same group, compared barely suprathreshold versus 1.5 times threshold dosing with bitemporal placement in schizophrenia patients and patients with mania and found no difference, which is not surprising because these two dosing schemes are very close together. Chanpattana et al. (1999b) randomly assigned schizophrenia patients to twice- versus thrice-weekly treatment schedules and found a faster time to recovery with thrice weekly. The same group (Chanpattana et al. 2000) also randomly assigned schizophrenia patients to receive 1.0, 2.0, or 4.0 times threshold bitemporal dosing and found the 1.0 times threshold group to have longer times to recovery. Thus, in patients with schizophrenia (and probably manic and catatonic patients as well), higher electrical doses than minimally suprathreshold and at least thrice-weekly schedules are recommended.

Monitoring Therapeutic Efficacy

The psychiatrist must assess response to ECT in an ongoing manner to determine if changes in technique are needed and when to stop the treatments. A good outcome implies remission of symptoms and signs as ascertained by patient self-report as well as observation by mental health staff and family members. A poor outcome implies that the suffering is not relieved after a course of treatments. However, there are three other scenarios that also represent suboptimal outcomes in ECT. The first of these is rapid relapse after apparent good initial response to index treatments, making the course of treatments a seeming waste of time. The second is self-reported improvement without objective signs of such. Rasmussen and Lineberry (2007) concluded that such patients tend to have severe personality or somatoform disorders and, in essence, take some reinforcing value from being an ECT patient that is separate from any true benefit for psychopathology. Such reinforcing value may result from the intensive social interactions and caregiving from the ECT staff and the primary and secondary gain from being in the sick role, which ECT sustains. A final poor outcome scenario in ECT practice is the demonstration of objective benefit from observation of mental health staff and family but with bitter complaints from the patient that ECT-induced memory impairment overrides therapeutic gain. The ECT psychiatrist should be aware of these complex patient outcome scenarios and evaluate accordingly throughout the course of treatments.

Another challenge to assessing ECT outcomes is the reliance in modern ECT research on depression rating scales as the sole outcome measure. Modern ECT studies exclusively utilize standardized rating scales for depression such as the Hamilton Rating Scale for Depression (Hamilton 1960) or the Montgomery-Åsberg Depression Rating Scale (Montgomery and Åsberg 1979). These consist of structured questions, conducted usually by research coordinators who are otherwise blind to patient status, asked of the patients with no consideration of information from other sources, relying almost exclusively on subjective patient self-report. Remission or response rates are defined in terms of degree of reduction of scores on these scales acutely with ECT based on the structured interviews performed within a day or a few days after the last treatment. Information from family and other mental health staff and findings from mental status examination are virtually ignored in modern ECT as well as much of other psychiatric research. This causes a loss of depth of information gained. This is especially true in depressed ECT patients, who over the course of treatments may forget some of the details of their depressive symptoms and may misreport certain aspects of function, such as sleep, appetite, or participation in activities. For some of the most severely ill depressed patients, it is information from nursing staff and family members from which the most reliable confidence in improvement emanates. It is not uncommon that elderly highly psychomotorically retarded patients do not accurately report the severity of their depression, answering no to many of the questions on the rating scale when it is quite obvious to caretakers and family that they are still profoundly depressed. Also, after several bitemporal treatments, patients may forget details of questions such as "How long does it take you to fall asleep?" or "How much have you been participating in enjoyable activities?" Observations from nursing staff and family are critical in assessing functionally impaired depressed patients' responses in terms of sleep patterns and level of interest in activities.

One source of spuriously reported ECT improvement is that ECT may have a nonspecific numbing effect on emotionality and memory that may in fact be experienced positively by patients who are dealing with either intense memories of past traumas or the distress of having to deal with current conflictual circumstances, such as unhappy marriages or jobs (Rasmussen and Lineberry 2007). Chronically impaired borderline personality disorder or prolonged complex posttraumatic stress disorder patients seem to fit this profile. They may insist that ECT helps them, but objective review of their lives reveals no fundamental change. The main point here is that the ECT practitioner should be aware that with patients in whom the only outcome assessment for ECT is subjective self-report, there are multiple complex factors at play. The author uses the term "spurious improvement" when there is self-reported improvement but in fact no observable evidence of real improvement exists.

There have been attempts over the years to develop laboratory test results that aid the ECT clinician in determining when to stop a series of treatments. These have included various electroencephalographic findings as well as the dexamethasone suppression test (DST). While there have been studies demonstrating that certain electroencephalographic indices correlate with efficacy (discussed in Chapter 6), none have been shown to indicate when to stop a course of treatments. For example, it would be helpful if a certain electroencephalographic finding, such as degree of slowing, reliably informed the ECT clinician that treatments could be stopped, even if clinical improvement was not yet maximal. However, the electroencephalographic research field in ECT has not matured sufficiently to do that. Additionally, some research has been conducted on the DST as an indicator of an adequate course of ECT (Shorter and Fink 2010), but as with electroencephalographic research, reliability of the findings is not sufficient to guide clinical decision making.

The idea behind these putative biologic tests is that some accurate, valid, reliable biologic measure allows one to determine an end point separate from that based solely on subjective patient self-report. The reason this may be helpful is that if a critical biologic result is found, it may mean that even if a patient is not feeling better yet, he or she might start to improve over time even if no more treatments are administered. The hoped-for benefit thus would be sparing the patient from having to undergo excessive treatments. Alternatively, there may be a biologic test that would indicate that the patient is not improving, even if he or she may be reporting improvement, and that treatments need to continue. In that scenario, the putative test would prevent stopping a course of treatments prematurely and thus might help prevent relapses. As of yet, such data are not available for any biologic indicator in determining ECT course end point.

Depression

Most patients being treated with ECT have depression, so it is important for ECT practitioners to become familiar with all aspects of improvement in depressed patients. It is essential that the patient be regularly evaluated for therapeutic efficacy throughout the course of treatments. For inpatients, this will mean being seen at daily rounds. For outpatients, this may mean formal visits in the psychiatrist's office weekly or perhaps at the times of treatments if that is feasible. Over the course of treatments, the clinician will want to focus on the target symptoms identified at the beginning of treatment. These tend to include the description of mood, which may be sad in nonpsychotic patients or irritable with admixtures of anxiety and ruminative worrying. Psychotic patients may not show a mood problem that is separable from whatever psychotic ideations they have, or they may not have a mood problem separable from their ruminations. Thus, the daily rounds may focus on a psychotic ideation or a rumination, and when those disappear or no longer cause distress, the clinician will know that improvement is taking place. Nonpsychotic patients will tend to report directly on their mood, separate from a specific ideation that is troubling them. Their moods may be reported as admixtures of sadness, worry, and irritability. Nonpsychotically depressed patients tend to have some element of mood reactivity, in which case there is some fluctuation of mood depending on daily experiences with other patients, staff, or family members, so the ECT practitioner should be observant for stable trends in mood improvement during ECT and not rely on a temporary good mood. On a rating scale such as the Hamilton Rating Scale for Depression, responses to the item for depressed mood will typically show over a few treatments that the amount of time during the day spent feeling dysphoric is decreasing, hopefully to none but often to something greater than zero but substantially less than at baseline. Family members should be consulted as well for their impressions of the patient's mood. Oftentimes, they will report a brightening before the patient self-reports feeling better, or family members might report that in conversations, troubling ideations/ruminations are taking less predominance and the patient is talking more of usually interesting topics such as family matters and is not so self-absorbed.

Anhedonia lessens with ECT treatments. In the hospital, this may manifest as willingness to attend groups without having to be prompted and more attention to self-care such as maintaining hygiene and eating meals. For outpatients, this may manifest as increased participation in usual activities as opposed to staying home all the time. Sleep becomes less disrupted and suicidal ideations diminish. A more positive outlook on the future becomes apparent. There tends to be a sense of "return to normal self."

A common clinical dilemma concerns how many treatments to administer in a course of ECT. The need for as full a remission as possible must be balanced against building up cognitive side effects. In an early paper, Barton et al. (1973) randomly allocated patients who achieved remission with ECT to either stop ECT treatments at the point remission was achieved or receive two more treatments. There was no difference in outcomes beyond the course of treatments, lending support to the notion that when remission is achieved, treatments may be stopped. This may be difficult to detect in some patients because one may not be confident that a full remission has been achieved. In that situation, a couple more treatments without any more noticeable improvement probably indicates that maximal ECT-induced efficacy has been reached. Review of the ECT literature indicates that typical courses of treatment for depressed patients fall in the range of 6 to 12, though an occasional patient seems to achieve remission with fewer than 6 and some patients need a few more than 12, especially if electrode placement is switched to bitemporal after nonresponse to unilateral. Patients should not be told up front that there will be a certain number of treatments, because it is impossible in advance to know how many treatments a particular patient will need. In a recent report analyzing the speed of response to ECT (Husain et al. 2004), it was found that a course of approximately 8–10 treatments was necessary before the course of treatments was considered to be a failure.

One of the challenges of determining end point in a course of ECT treatments for the depressed patient is differentiating continued depression from cognitive impairment caused by the treatments. A patient who begins by being psychomotorically slowed because of depression may, after a number of treatments, have varying levels of disorientation and anterograde amnesia that may seem to exacerbate the psychomotor abnormalities. In such cases, holding off on a treatment or two may help to clear up the confusional state so that a more accurate assessment of the status of depressive symptoms may be undertaken. If the patient starts to look brighter and has more psychomotor activity, then the previous signs were probably the result of ECT-induced memory impairment. If, on the other hand, the patient seems to worsen after holding off on a treatment or two, then the depression is probably worsening, which is an indication to proceed with further ECT treatments, albeit at perhaps a slower pace (e.g., two treatments per week rather than three).

There are also issues relevant to outpatient ECT courses in depressed patients. If the ECT clinician is also the patient's primary psychiatrist, then visits can take place at the time of ECT treatments to assess progress and monitor for cognitive side effects. If, on the other hand, the ECT clinician is different from the primary psychiatrist, then the latter should schedule outpatient appointments at least weekly to assess progress, and there must be good communication between the two clinicians in order to concur on any changes in treatment technique, such as electrode placement, stimulus dose/parameters, or treatment frequency.

In modern practice, it has become common to assess outcome through standardized depression rating scales. The ironies of using such scales include asking patients who are undergoing a procedure known to impact recall to recall symptoms, obtaining patients' versions of symptoms when the illnesses in question impact insight, and attempting to interview highly sick patients who at times cannot meaningfully participate in conversation. As noted above, the Hamilton Rating Scale for Depression and the Montgomery-Åsberg Rating Scale are the most commonly used depression scales. Both of these scales are clinician-administered and involve asking the patient questions. Of note, in the original form of the Hamilton scale, Professor Hamilton clearly intended for each question to be answered not just through a patient's immediate response but also by inquiry of other personnel and serial mental status examination (Hamilton 1960). Various self-report rating scales are available as well. Most modern ECT studies show that typical ECT patient populations have scores in the severely depressed range on rating scales. As the course of treatments progresses, scores gradually decline until the criteria for remission (generally being defined as scores less than 10 on the Hamilton Rating Scale for Depression or Montgomery-Åsberg scale) are met. Of course, not all patients follow a predictable course of improvement. Some patients might show an early dramatic drop in scores followed by an increase, with erratic fluctuations thereafter. Such patients are probably showing a placebo effect combined with a highly reactive mood that may change in response to environmental events such as family visits or interactions with other patients on the unit. Also, as noted earlier, some patients, especially the highly psychomotorically retarded elderly, tend to underreport their symptoms, and some patients may not be able to remember depressive symptoms in detail after having received several bitemporal treatments. Thus, decisions to end a course of ECT treatments should not be based solely on a depression rating scale score, but should always include assessments based on mental status examination and observations from all mental health staff as well as concerned family members. Finally, it bears emphasizing that in treating depressed patients with ECT, the focus of outcome assessment is on the core depression signs and symptoms—features of psychiatric comorbidity, such as borderline personality disorder, posttraumatic stress disorder, or obsessive-compulsive disorder, as well as others, are not expected to improve with ECT unless they are secondary to the depressive episode. Along these latter lines, it is important to realize that depression may cause personality dysfunction that abates with ECT along with the core depressive features. One should not diagnose a separate personality disorder unless there is evidence of such disorder having been present since young adulthood and present in a variety of contexts and not just during an episode of depression. Furthermore, especially for chronically depressed patients, it is the primary depressive signs and symptoms that abate with an acute course of ECT, not the long-term secondary complications, such as personality dysfunction or disability status, which may take longer periods of time, as well as psychotherapy, to improve maximally.

Mania, Schizophrenia, and Catatonia

In contrast to the case with depression, which is not a homogeneous syndrome and in which a variety of subjective dynamics are in place, confounding outcome assessment, improvement in mania is not at all subtle or difficult to assess. ECT patients who are manic can reveal dramatic ECT responses. The patient who begins in four-point restraints, is receiving intramuscular sedatives or antipsychotics, and spends much of the day in seclusion oftentimes will become quiet, calm, and cooperative with an adequate course of ECT treatments. Rating scales can be used, but usually the improvement in these patients is easy to appreciate. The total number of treatments needed will probably exceed that for a typical depressed patient by about two to four treatments.

The typical schizophrenia patient receiving ECT treatment will probably need a few more treatments than the average depressed patient. The end points or target signs and symptoms to assess include thought disorganization, bizarre behavior, delusions, and hallucinations. In other words, it is the positive symptoms of schizophrenia that respond best to ECT. Prominent negative symptoms such as avolition and lack of emotional expression are much more resistant to ECT, as they are to psychotropic medications as well.

Determination of an ECT treatment end point for schizophrenia patients can be difficult. In the case of depressed patients and manic patients, complete remission of psychopathology is a realistic goal for most patients treated with ECT. However, with schizophrenia patients, complete remission is rare. Thus, the treating psychiatrist must decide when maximal efficacy has been reached. Ongoing liaison with those who are quite familiar with the patient, such as family members or caretakers at group homes and such, can be invaluable to establish confidence that the ECT course has rendered the patient at baseline.

During the course of treatments with catatonic patients, the assessing clinician may notice dramatic fluctuations in severity. It is important not to stop ECT treatments as soon as improvement is observed, for it is the rule rather than the exception that catatonic patients show short-lived periods of improvement during ECT that progressively become more long-lasting. The clinician should not stop the course of treatments until a stable, several-day improvement is seen. Also, as the catatonic features remit with ECT, there may be unmasking of an underlying psychopathological syndrome, such as mania, depression, or nonaffective psychosis, depending on what the patient's underlying psychiatric diagnosis is. For patients with medical, neurological, and toxic causes of catatonia, usually as the catatonia remits with ECT, there is no underlying syndrome that is unmasked.

If the initially mute, stuporous catatonic patient becomes manic as the ECT course proceeds, then a decision must be made whether to continue with ECT or treat the mania pharmacologically. If the patient is cooperative and agreeable to ECT, then it would be appropriate to continue with treatments. Otherwise, the manic syndrome can be treated pharmacologically. For the catatonic patient who shows classic depressive psychopathology as the catatonic signs remit with ECT, continuing the ECT course to treat the depression is recommended. For the schizophrenia patient in a catatonic episode, it is recommended that the patient be treated with ECT until his or her baseline psychopathological status is reached.

Dementia

When dementia patients are being treated for behavioral dyscontrol, the target outcome is a state of behavioral calm. Most commonly such patients reside in a nursing home and the nursing home staff are familiar with a baseline. When dementia patients and depressed patients are being treated with ECT, as the course of treatments proceeds, there may be difficulty differentiating between behavioral worsening and the cognitive impairment with ECT. For example, a patient with cognitive impairment that cannot be definitively attributed to dementia versus pseudodementia may show substantial improvement of cognitive functions during ECT as the depressive syndrome remits, assuming that the cognitive impairment was related to the depression. If there is truly an underlying neurodegenerative dementia syndrome along with the depression, then it may be difficult to know when the depression improves after a few treatments because of the extra cognitive impairment such patients demonstrate. After treatments are stopped, careful observation over the next few days may well reveal a patient much less depressed than at baseline, the improvement having been masked by cognitive impairment. It is suggested that the clinician begin with right unilateral ultrabrief technique in dementia patients being treated with ECT.

Cognitive Monitoring

The important topic of cognition in ECT will be reviewed in detail in Chapter 9. This section presents a brief discussion of recommendations for cognitive monitoring during an index course of treatments. The most substantial side effect of ECT is memory impairment. Such impairment takes three forms. The first is *posttreatment confusion*. This may be as mild as simply taking a few minutes to become oriented after a treatment or as severe as persistent confusion over several days. On average, however, the posttreatment confusion clears up within an hour or two following the end of the seizure. Factors associated with longer time to orientation include older age, higher number of treatments, treatments spaced closely together, bilateral electrode placement, higher stimulus dosage relative to threshold, and higher pulse width.

The second type of ECT-induced memory disturbance is *anterograde amnesia*, which refers to inability to recall newly learned information. During the course of ECT treatments, patients typically have an adequate ability to register and process information (assuming no baseline deficit in this regard), but there is impairment in the ability to recall this information at a delayed time interval. Typical examples of this include having conversations that are later on forgotten and watching a television program one evening and forgetting about it the next day. The third type of ECT-induced memory dysfunction is *retrograde amnesia*, which refers to inability to recall previously learned information as a result of ECT treatments. Examples of retrograde amnesia include forgetting vacations or special family events such as birthday parties or weddings.

There is a dearth of clinically relevant literature informing the ECT clinician what type of cognitive testing is feasible and helpful during a course of treatments (Rasmussen 2016). While much research has focused on detecting statistically significant differences between various ECT techniques in certain neuropsychological domains (reviewed in Chapter 9), translating these in-depth, time-consuming neuropsychological batteries into usable tests during ECT has not been accomplished (Rasmussen 2016). In the meantime, it is advisable at a minimum to ask patients and caregivers (which includes nursing staff as well as family members) their own opinions on how they perceive the patient's memory function. Questions should include areas such as ability to focus and concentrate, ability to recall recent information, and ability to recall more remote information. Serial assessments of orientation for person, place, and time are appropriate. While some ECT clinics may be able to conduct a more in-depth neuropsychological assessment, it is not clear how a particular patient's performance can be used to guide alterations in clinical technique, such as making decisions to switch electrode placements or reduce the frequency of treatments for those with seemingly excessive memory side effects. As a rule of thumb, when the ECT clinician takes into account the patient's and significant others' subjective assessments, as well as orientation, if there is a feeling that the patient is significantly bothered by cognitive side effects, then some type of reduction in intensity of treatment is worth considering, unless clinical severity contraindicates such an adjustment. Such reductions in intensity most frequently would be to switch from thrice- to twice-weekly treatments or bitemporal to unilateral electrode placement. Reduction in electrical dosage is probably not a good idea because it might compromise the ultimate efficacy of the treatments. Occasionally, the treatment course should be stopped outright until return of orientation to place and time. Such circumstances usually occur in elderly patients receiving thrice-weekly bitemporal treatments.

Monitoring Other Side Effects

The primary psychiatrist following the patient over a course of ECT treatments should be aware of active medical problems and maintain vigilance for any emergent worsening during ECT, such as exacerbation of congestive heart failure or chronic obstructive pulmonary disease. Additionally, there are specific symptomatic side effects that occur commonly, as discussed below.

Nausea/Vomiting

Posttreatment nausea/vomiting is common with ECT. The mechanism for this is obscure but may be related in part to the anesthetic medication as well as the neurological effects of the seizure (such as temporarily increased intracranial pressure). Usually, nausea/vomiting occurs within half an hour or so following the treatment and peaks within a couple of hours or so, and then wanes. If this occurs after the first treatment, then it would be appropriate to administer ondansetron 4 or 8 mg intravenously along with anesthesia for subsequent treatments. This is a very safe medication that is essentially free of adverse effects. Other, older options for post-ECT nausea/vomiting include prochlorperazine, metoclopramide, and promethazine. These drugs are associated with the usual risks of dopamine blockers, such as dystonic reactions. As far as anesthetic medications go, etomidate and high-potency opioids are associated with nausea more so than the others.

Headache

Headache is one of the most common post-ECT side effects. As with posttreatment nausea, it would be appropriate at subsequent treatments to pretreat with a headache medication such as acetaminophen or ibuprofen. Intravenous ketorolac is also commonly used at the time of treatments but should only be used for those patients experiencing headache after the first treatment and not in all patients at the time of first treatment (Rasmussen 2013). Opioid medications such as oxycodone or hydromorphone are not recommended as treatments for post-ECT headache. Post-ECT migraine headaches can be treated with whatever medication the patient normally takes for such headaches.

Myalgia (Muscle Ache)

Posttreatment myalgia (muscle ache) occurs in patients after the first treatment but in very few patients after subsequent treatments (Rasmussen et al. 2008d). The etiology of post-ECT myalgias is unknown—they do not correlate with degree of fasciculations with succinylcholine or with degree of motor movements during the convulsion. Probably this side effect is an "all or none" effect of the succinylcholine but is unrelated to dose of that agent. Thus, if a patient has post-ECT myalgias after the first treatment, there is no reason to increase or decrease the succinylcholine dose subsequently (on the theory of too much motor movement or too much fasciculation, respectively). Patients can be reassured that myalgias occur after the first treatment and then abate after subsequent treatments. One can always pretreat with the same medications used for headaches. The effect is analogous to the myalgias experienced after a first intensive exercise workout that abate after subsequent workouts.

Jaw Ache

Patients commonly have a jaw ache after the first treatment. Like myalgias, this abates after subsequent treatments.

Urinary Hesitancy

Some patients, especially elderly men, experience urinary hesitancy after ECT treatments. This is due to the anticholinergic agent that is used as pretreatment (glycopyrrolate or atropine). If this happens, such medications should be withheld for subsequent treatments.

Angialgia

Angialgia is pain on injection with the anesthetic agent and probably arises from irritation of nerve endings in the venous endothelium. It is common with etomidate, propofol, and methohexital and less so with ketamine, thiopental, and high-potency opioids such as remifentanil or alfentanil (Rasmussen and Ritter 2014a). Strategies to lessen angialgia, which may be quite bothersome to some patients, to the point of severe anticipatory anxiety regarding the treatments, include use of a large-caliber vein for intravenous access, injection of a small dose of lidocaine prior to anesthetic induction, use of low-dose anesthetic combined with high-potency opioid, and use of the inhalational anesthetic sevoflurane to induce anesthesia, with intravenous access started after the patient is asleep (Rasmussen and Ritter 2014a; Rasmussen et al. 2005).

Key Points

- Deciding on electrode placement, stimulus dosing, stimulus parameter configuration, and treatment frequency may be done by the ECT clinician or a separate psychiatrist.

- Generally, bitemporal placement has been viewed as the gold standard for efficacy but has been associated with greater memory side effects than unilateral placement.

- Higher electrical doses are associated with greater efficacy but also more cognitive side effects.

- Treatment frequency is usually thrice weekly, but twice weekly may be equally effective and cause less severe cognitive side effects.

- Treatments are stopped when the primary psychiatrist has determined that maximal efficacy has occurred.

8

Preventing Relapse After ECT: Maintenance ECT and Pharmacotherapy

The psychiatric syndromes most effectively treated with electroconvulsive therapy (ECT) tend to be chronic, recurrent, and medication refractory. Post-ECT relapse rates are high regardless of diagnosis. Thus, maintaining acute treatment benefits is difficult. Managing the patient after the index course of treatments is finished is a challenging aspect of ECT practice. This chapter focuses on relapse prevention strategies.

First, a bit of clarity in terminology is in order. *Remission* refers to a complete abatement of the symptoms and signs of an episode such as mania or depression. *Lack of remission* in research settings refers either to no improvement or to partial remission not meeting research criteria for full remission. Thus, when one is assessing the literature on ECT outcomes and relapse prevention, it is wise to keep in mind that just because a patient's condition may not have formally "remitted" with index treatment, there still may have been clinically significant improvement that from the patient's standpoint made the treatment worthwhile. The term *response* is often used in reference to a 50% reduction in episode severity without full remission. *Recovery* indicates remission sustained for at least 6 months. In modern psychiatric literature, there has emerged a distinction between *relapse* and *recurrence* after remission of an episode, with the former referring to reappearance of the syndrome within 6 months, and the latter referring to when the syndrome recurs later on. Presumably, relapse represents a return of the same episode of illness, whereas recurrence indicates a new episode. There is no doubt that the disorders treated with ECT undergo relapses and recurrences, and anybody experienced in following such patients knows the challenges of keeping the illness at bay. For the sake of simplicity, in this chapter the word *relapse* refers to reappearances of psychopathological syndromes regardless of whether they occur before or after the 6-month mark. The interested reader is referred to the article by Frank et al. (1991) for an explication of modern terminology regarding the phases of illness and recovery in psychopathological episodes.

After index ECT is completed, the expression *continuation therapy* refers to the first 6 months of management, whereas *maintenance therapy* refers to management thereafter. For the purposes of this chapter, however, to keep things simple, all post–index ECT management will be referred to as maintenance therapy. Thus, *maintenance ECT* (MECT) will refer to post-index ECT designed to prevent return of symptoms, regardless of whether it is within the first 6 months or thereafter. In similar fashion, the term *maintenance pharmacotherapy* (MPharm) will refer to use of psychotropic medication after index ECT regardless of duration.

Post-ECT Relapse: The Scope of the Problem

Depression

Soon after early clinicians discovered the remarkable benefits of ECT for depressive episodes, they also discovered the high relapse rates thereafter (Kalinowsky 1943). Deducing a general figure for "the" post-ECT relapse rate for depression is complicated by a variety of factors: the definition of relapse, the method of psychopathological assessment, the duration of the study period (i.e., the longer the post-ECT period of observation, the higher the cumulative relapse rates over time), and the types of treatments given during the observation period. For example, in one study with a very long observation period, van Beusekom et al. (2007) followed ECT remitters for 4–8 years and found that there was a 42.3% rate of relapses during this period after the first 6 months of post-ECT observation. In another follow-up study over a long period of time, O'Leary and Lee (1996) followed patients treated with index ECT for depression and found that 20% were rehospitalized within 6 months. Over the 7 years of follow-up, only 27% of the original cohort remained free of hospitalization for the entire time period. These long-term naturalistic follow-up studies indicate the high relapse/recurrence rate over time in depressed ECT patients.

Bourgon and Kellner (2000), in their review, pointed out that many patients do relapse in the months following successful index ECT treatment for depression. There have been several large case series documenting a rough overall average of 50% relapse rates in the first several months after the initial series, depending on maintenance management strategy (Jelovac et al. 2013). One must note that the situation is not necessarily as dire as this high-appearing figure suggests, for in some studies in which relapse was defined quantitatively, a full syndromal worsening back to pre-ECT severity was not required in order to qualify as a "relapse." For example, in the CORE studies (Kellner et al. 2006), a patient with a baseline Hamilton Rating Scale for Depression (Williams 2001) score of, say, in the 30s, which indicates a profoundly severe episode of depression, who experiences remission of symptoms, with a score of 8 or so, would be classified as a relapser during the maintenance phase of the study, with a rising of the score to a 16, which is still half the original score. Thus, the patient may be functioning much better than at pre-ECT baseline and may feel that ECT was "worth it" but still is not doing as well as in the immediate post–index treatment days. Further, the maintenance-phase relapse rates may be roughly similar between patients who were treated with ECT and those who were treated with medication during the initial treatment phase. Along these lines, Stoudemire et al. (1998) followed elderly depressed patients who had achieved remission with either medications or ECT and found an 18-month relapse rate of 28.6% in both groups.

Bidder et al. (1970), in an early follow-up series of ECT responders over 1 year, found that approximately 38% relapsed, while the rest of those for whom follow-up was available did not relapse. These relapse rates seem rather low by modern standards and probably reflect the more sensitive methods of determining relapse— that is, by structured rating scale scores—used today.

As another attempt at assessing post-ECT depressive relapse rates, it is instructive to cull together studies in which at least one group of freshly remitted ECT patients was selected to receive either no treatment at all or placebo pills. This contrasts with studies, covered later in this chapter, in which patients are treated either with MPharm or with MECT.

Studies with groups of patients followed after index ECT without treatment have been described (Coppen et al. 1981; Imlah et al. 1965; Kiloh et al. 1960a, 1960b; Lauritzen et al. 1996; Sackeim et al. 2001; Seager and Bird 1962; van den Broek et al. 2006; Yildiz et al. 2010). Definitions of relapse in these studies varied and included full return to pretreatment severity, hospitalization for another episode of depression, and a predetermined rise in depression rating scale scores. Durations of follow-up were generally in the 6- to 12-month range. Despite these differences among the studies, there is a remarkable unanimity among the findings: patients with freshly remitted depression who are followed post-ECT and receive no or placebo treatment have very high relapse rates in subsequent months, generally in the 70%–90% range. One of the most instructive of these reports is from Sackeim et al. (2001) of the Columbia University Consortium. In this study's post–

ECT remission placebo arm, 89% of the patients relapsed over 6 months. In the van den Broek et al. (2006) series, which represented another randomized controlled post-ECT trial, the relapse rate in the placebo group was 80% over 6 months. A clear conclusion from these studies is that active treatment post-ECT for depressed patients is the standard of care.

Sackeim et al. (2000), following depressed patients for a year naturalistically treated after acute remission induced with various types of ECT, found an overall relapse rate of 53% regardless of electrode placement or stimulus intensity used for index ECT. This seminal finding indicates that "an ECT remitter is an ECT remitter" in the sense that even though low-electrical-dose unilateral technique may yield much lower remission rates than those seen with bitemporal placement at any dose, for those patients who do experience remission, the chances of sustaining the remission during follow-up are the same. This clinically important and meaningful finding was replicated by the same research group in their study of different medication strategies after index ECT remission (Sackeim et al. 2001). Additionally, Verwijk et al. (2015), following depressed patients after remission with either right unilateral ultrabrief- or right unilateral standard-pulse-width technique, found equal post–index treatment relapse rates. Thus, it can be concluded, with some confidence, that method of initial index ECT technique, though it may influence acute remission rates, does not seem to affect post–index ECT relapse rates.

In an interesting post–index ECT follow-up series, Tew et al. (2007) followed patients initially enrolled in an ECT trial just described (Sackeim et al. 2001)—in which remitting patients were randomly allocated to receive follow-up placebo, nortriptyline, or the latter plus lithium—who completed ECT with remission but who refused participation in the follow-up phase and were thus treated naturalistically. In this group of patients, treated with medication, there was a 6-month relapse rate of 51%, compared with 89% for the study patients randomly assigned to receive placebo, 60% for those randomly assigned to receive nortriptyline, and 39% for those randomly assigned to receive nortriptyline plus lithium (Sackeim et al. 2001). The CORE methodology, similar to that of Sackeim et al. (2001) but with an MECT group as well as a nortriptyline/lithium group, found relapse rates at 6 months that were similar to those of the combined-medication group in the Sackeim et al. (2001) trial, providing yet more data (Kellner et al. 2006). These modern studies with very precise longitudinal follow-up assessments probably provide the best estimates of post-ECT relapse rates in depressed patients in the modern era.

It is clinically useful to ask whether there are any particular predictive features that are associated with higher versus lower post-ECT relapse rates so that post-ECT treatment can be planned accordingly. What might such predictors be? Clinical features that come to mind include the usual demographics, such as age, gender, episode duration, age at onset of first depressive episode, and total number of prior depressive episodes; characteristics of the current episode, such as psychosis, melancholia, or atypical features; strength of failed pre-ECT medication trials for the current depressive episode; degree of improvement with ECT (i.e., full vs. partial remission); and, of course, type of post-ECT maintenance treatment.

Probably the most consistent predictor of relapse during the post-ECT phase is presence of residual depressive symptoms with index ECT, which underscores the need to treat aggressively in the acute phase in order to achieve as strong a response as possible. Degree of residual depressive symptomatology at time of index ECT completion correlates with relapse proclivity during follow-up (Sackeim et al. 2001), a finding that underscores the need for the ECT clinician to ensure during the index phase of treatments that a full remission is achieved if possible before undertaking MECT or MPharm.

Nordenskjöld et al. (2011a) followed several hundred depressed patients naturalistically after successful index ECT for a mean of 564 days. The rate of rehospitalization was 32% at 1 year, and the suicide rate was 2%. Sackeim et al. (1990), following 58 patients after index ECT for depression, found a 50% relapse rate at 1 year, with relapse being defined by depression rating score elevations. Most of the relapses were in the first 16 weeks after index ECT. Pre-ECT medication resistance was associated with higher relapse rates. Verwijk et al. (2015) followed a cohort of index ECT responders with depression, comparing the longitudinal course of those treated with right unilateral ultrabrief pulse width and those treated with standard pulse width, and found no difference in relapse rates, which were 25% at 3 months and about 40% at 6 months. Longer initial depressive episode tended to predict higher post-ECT relapse rates. Martiny et al. (2015) randomly assigned patients whose depression remitted post-ECT to receive one of several medication regimens, discussed in more detail below, and found overall relapse rates to be 35% at 6 months based on depression rating scale scores. This figure is commensurate with findings from other modern post-ECT follow-up studies. Medda et al. (2013) found a 36.1% depressive relapse rate over 1 year after index ECT and also found that longer index depressive episode duration correlated with higher relapse potential. Prudic et al. (2013) found an overall 50% 6-month relapse rate post-ECT in depressed patients whose depression had remitted. Martínez-Amorós et al. (2012b) also found that longer index episodes and greater number of prior depressive episodes were associated with higher relapse potential, in a 2-year follow-up study after ECT.

Another feature that has emerged quite consistently as a predictor of high or early post-ECT relapse for depression is degree of pre-ECT medication resistance. That is, patients beginning ECT whose depression has been refractory to one or more aggressive antidepressant medication regimens, versus patients who either received ECT before any medications were tried or had medication trials that were suboptimal in dose of medication or duration of trial, have been shown to have higher or earlier post-ECT relapse rates (Prudic et al. 2004; Rasmussen et al. 2009b; Sackeim et al. 1993, 2000, 2001, 2008). In the Sackeim et al. (2000) series, baseline (i.e., pre-ECT) antidepressant medication resistance predicted higher postremission relapses in comparisons with patients whose symptoms had not been refractory to an adequate antidepressant trial before ECT. This finding was partially echoed in the CORE trial (Rasmussen et al. 2009b), in which baseline medication resistance predicted higher relapse rates in the first week following ECT remission. This underscores the need for aggressive maintenance therapy in such patients, whether MECT or MPharm. However, relapse rates are still quite high even in patients with non-medication-refractory depression, so all patients need aggressive preventive strategies.

Presence of a personality disorder has strongly and consistently emerged as a predictor of high post-index ECT relapse among depressed patients. Sareen et al. (2000) found that clinical diagnoses of personality disorders in depressed patients referred for ECT predicted not only lower acute ECT responses but also, in those who did respond, higher relapse rates over the following year. This confirms the clinical experience that patients with personality disorders, especially borderline personality disorder, do not fare as well with ECT either acutely or in follow-up as nonborderline patients (Rasmussen and Lineberry 2007). This was consistent with the results of a study by Zimmerman et al. (1986), who found that although depressed patients with personality disorders responded acutely to ECT as well as did those without such disorders, the former had much higher relapse and rehospitalization rates during follow-up. Also, Prudic et al. (2004) found that baseline presence of personality disorder was associated not only with lower acute remission from ECT but also with higher posttreatment relapse in those patients who did experience remission of their illness.

Several investigators have assessed post-ECT relapse rates in psychotic versus nonpsychotic depressed patients. In the O'Leary and Lee (1996) report cited earlier, delusions in the initial index episode of depression predicted higher follow-up relapse rates versus nonpsychotic depression. Flint and Rifat (1998) studied psychotically depressed patients after remission. Of the 17 ECT-treated patients, 15 achieved remission (demonstrating the well-known dramatic efficacy of ECT for psychotic depression), and of those, 14 remained well for 4 months of follow-up. After the 4-month period, there were seven recurrent episodes, most occurring after the more commonly defined "relapse" interval of 6 months.

Birkenhäger et al. (2004) followed psychotic and nonpsychotic depressed patients naturalistically after remission with ECT and found that the latter had higher 6- and 12-month relapse rates (21% and 73%, respectively) than did the former (12% and 53%, respectively). A subsequent report by the same group (Birkenhäger et al. 2005), involving a sample of maintenance ECT depressed patients, also revealed much lower relapse rates for those patients whose episodes were marked by psychosis than for those whose episodes were not. Of note, Grunhaus et al. (1990), in a small sample of 10 formerly depressed MECT patients, found that psychotic depressive patients seemed to do better in the follow-up phase than did nonpsychotic depressive patients. However, in the Prudic et al. (2004) follow-up of patients whose depression remitted after ECT, psychotic patients had higher relapse rates compared with nonpsychotic patients. Spiker et al. (1985) followed 37 psychotic depressive patients who had achieved remission with ECT, none of whom received MECT, and found a 50% 1-year relapse rate. Most patients had been treated with tricyclic antidepressants and many with antipsychotics as well. Clearly, delusional depressive patients are at high post-ECT relapse risk.

The CORE investigators (Fink et al. 2007) attempted to correlate melancholic features with post-ECT course and found essentially no predictive value, at least if melancholia is assessed in the manner used in that study, which was with a structured interview, the Structured Clinical Interview for DSM-IV (First et al. 1996), conducted by study coordinators. If melancholia is associated with a post-ECT course differential from nonmelancholic patients, then the method of diagnosing melancholia will have to be much more in-depth than use of structured questionnaires and will have to involve observation of patients. In this regard, the study by Hickie et al. (1990) showing clear predictive value of psychomotor abnormalities and ECT response provides a good lead for future studies of melancholia and ECT responsivity and posttreatment course.

Longer depressive episode duration is associated with higher post-ECT relapse rates (Prudic et al. 1990). Age and gender have generally not been associated with predictive value for post-ECT relapse (Bourgon and Kellner 2000; Kellner et al. 2006), although one trial did find that females had higher relapse rates post–index ECT compared with males (Sackeim et al. 2001). Attempts have been made to correlate biologic variables with post-ECT relapse but without success (for a review, see Bourgon and Kellner 2000). Dexamethasone testing probably has been studied the most, with a bit of a hint that return to escape from dexamethasone suppression during post-ECT follow-up may herald an incipient relapse, but this has not been a consistent finding (Bourgon and Kellner 2000).

Mania

There are fewer published series for post–index ECT relapse rates in manic patients than in depressed patients. Winokur and Kadrmas (1988) retrospectively reviewed extensive treatment and follow-up data from patients hospitalized at a state psychiatric facility in Iowa during the early 1940s. These authors compared data from manic patients treated with ECT with data from manic patients not treated with ECT during this time period. Of the 45 manic patients treated with ECT, 84% had more than one affective disorder episode during the approximately 5 years of follow-up, versus 61% for those not treated with ECT, a statistically significant difference. Those treated with ECT also had a 24% incidence of having at least six such episodes during the follow-up period, versus only a 9% incidence among those not treated with ECT. Focusing on manic recurrences, there was a 55% incidence of having more than one such episode during follow-up among the ECT-treated patients, versus 31% for patients in the non-ECT-treated sample. Thus, from this interesting data set, it appears that manic patients who are treated with ECT have more recurrences of illness over time than nontreated patients, a finding that could not be explained by the investigators. In a follow-up report of a more modern sample using similar methodology by the same group of investigators, Winokur et al. (1990) followed 23 manic patients treated with ECT and compared them with a matched group of 23 manic patients not treated with ECT and found no difference in number of episodes per year during follow-up, even though the ECT-treated patients had more hospitalizations per year during the follow-up period. In all these studies, there was no randomization to ECT versus medication for mania, so it is likely the manic patients treated with ECT had more severe illnesses, which may have accounted for the more highly recurrent longitudinal courses after ECT. Whether or not treatment with ECT somehow confers greater numbers of affective episodes over time is not settled, but these studies do indicate that manic patients whose illness is successfully remitted with index ECT courses are at high risk for affective disorder relapse over time and should be treated aggressively.

In another follow-up sample of manic patients acutely treated with ECT, Thomas and Reddy (1982) followed 10 such patients and found that 1 patient was readmitted in the first year and that by 5 years of follow-up, 8 of the 10 had had at least one hospitalization. Finally, Small et al. (1988a), in their randomized comparison of lithium and ECT for acute mania, found that among the ECT-treated patients, there was a 24% rehospitalization rate for manic episodes during 2 years of follow-up, which was comparable to the rate in the lithium-treated group. These data sets provide further evidence of the high relapse potential of manic patients treated with ECT.

Chronically manic patients who have successfully been treated with index ECT tend to have high relapse rates after ECT, with relapse occurring quickly. Thus, post-index ECT treatment needs to be very aggressive in this population. Medication refractoriness and psychopathological chronicity predispose to rapid post–index ECT relapse among manic patients. On the other hand, a patient with a history of long intervals without mania in between manic episodes probably would not have a high chance of rapid post-ECT relapse compared with a chronically manic patient treated with ECT.

Schizophrenia

Shortly after the dramatic antipsychotic effects of ECT were appreciated in the late 1930s, Moore (1943) pointed out the high relapse rates in otherwise successfully ECT-treated schizophrenia patients. In an early review of ECT for schizophrenia, as well as other disorders, Kalinowsky (1943) noted that if the initial series of treatments is too short, then early relapse is almost inevitable. He felt that courses of treatments consisting of 20 treatments or more resulted in much more stable, long-lasting improvement, and in a sample of 111 patients given at least 20 treatments, rehospitalization over the next several months to 2 years occurred in only 13. In a several-year follow-up study of schizophrenia patients treated with a variety of methods, May et al. (1976, 1981) found a trend for ECT treated patients to spend less time in the hospital over 2–5 years than a cohort of patients treated with psychotherapy, a treatment method probably not relevant to modern samples. In another data set, Palmer et al. (1951) found that about two-thirds of schizophrenia patients who acutely improved with ECT relapsed either while hospitalized before discharge or within 5 months of discharge. Smith et al. (1967) found that the combination of chlorpromazine and ECT in the hospital was associated with fewer relapses in the year of follow-up versus treatment with the drug alone.

Hustig and Onilov (2009) provide some good follow-up data on a cohort of 27 schizophrenia patients who achieved significant acute benefits from index ECT. Over the following year, just over one-third remained clinically stable while taking antipsychotic medications, while almost two-thirds relapsed into a fulminant psychosis and required retreatment with ECT. Some of the patients benefited from MECT. This case series demonstrates the high relapse potential of this chronically ill and difficult-to-treat population.

Chanpattana et al. (1999d), in the most systematic follow-up data set for patients with schizophrenia diagnosed according to modern DSM methods and assessed with structured interviews, found that 6-month post–index ECT relapse rates were 40% for patients receiving follow-up treatment with both MECT and neuroleptics, versus 93% for patients treated with either modality alone. Either way, clearly schizophrenia patients have high relapse rates post-ECT.

As mentioned in Chapter 2, ECT does not effect complete remission of psychopathology in schizophrenia patients, especially that pertaining to the negative signs of the illness, such as lack of motivation and blunted emotional expression, as it might in depressed or manic patients. There tend to be two general scenarios for post-ECT course in recently treated schizophrenia patients. If the patient's initial presentation was one of chronic psychopathological features, such as dis-organized behavior, agitation, deluded thinking, and hallucinations, that were highly medication refractory (thus leading to the indication for ECT), then rapid post-ECT relapse is almost guaranteed without aggressive preventive measures, such as MECT(to be discussed later in this chapter). On the other hand, if the patient's longitudinal course was characterized by chronic negative symptoms with acute, superimposed positive symptoms or catatonia prompting an acute course of ECT, there is a lesser likelihood of quick post-ECT relapse, because in this case ECT was given more for an acute episode of an illness rather than for a chronic set of signs and symptoms. It seems that ECT is not given as often for schizophrenia now as it was in the first couple of decades of ECT practice because of the emergence of antipsychotic medication.

Catatonia

As indicated in Chapter 2, catatonia tends to respond quite dramatically to ECT acutely. Longitudinal course after this is variable depending on the underlying psychopathological diagnosis. For example, if the catatonic episode is part of schizophrenia, then one can expect that with clearing of the catatonic signs with ECT, there will be a return to the patient's baseline functioning, often consisting of prominent negative signs such as lack of motivation or blunted emotional ex-pression. If the underlying diagnosis is bipolar disorder, as is most often the case, then manic symptoms and signs may be "uncovered" by the use of ECT for the catatonic presentation and will thus have to be addressed. If the catatonic presen-tation is part of a depressive episode, then one might expect full remission of both the catatonia and underlying depressive features with ECT, and the longitudinal course will be that seen in samples of depressed patients. Finally, if the catatonic features are part of an acute neurological disease, such as postviral encephalitis-induced catatonia or another of the "organic" catatonias (e.g., neuroleptic malig-nant syndrome [NMS]), then the clearing of this state with ECT will likely con-stitute a more-or-less cure with no recurrences. On the other hand, if the organic catatonia is caused by a chronic neurological, medical, or toxic condition, then there may be high relapse potential after successful index ECT.

Other Indications for ECT

There were some reports of mostly depressed Parkinson's disease patients who received index ECT in which the investigators noticed and quantified improve-ments in motor function that were followed over time. In some cases, without MECT, the sometimes dramatic reported improvements in motoric function were sustained over many months or even years, whereas in other cases there was rapid relapse. One follow-up report (Pridmore and Pollard 1996) of 14 Parkinson's patients receiving ECT just for the motor signs (i.e., no depression was present) found that after 30 months, about one-third of the patients had experienced no or little and short-lived (i.e., a couple of weeks or less) improvement with ECT, while about a third each had experienced modest or marked improvement that lasted from a few weeks to all the way through the 30-month follow-up period without any intervening MECT. One of course wonders whether, if MECT had been offered, especially to the early-relapsing patients, there might have been more sustained improvement. It is intriguing indeed that patients with such a chronic condition as Parkinson's disease would show acute benefits with ECT and then would have what seems to be essentially a permanent improvement even without MECT. One might be tempted to speculate that in such patients, ECT caused neurobiological changes that were longlasting.

Other neurological indications for ECT, which are considered non–standard of care and experimental (along with using it solely for the motor signs of parkinsonism) include NMS; agitation due to dementia; epilepsy; movement disorders such as tardive dyskinesia and dystonia; and acute delirious states associated with neurological illness and catatonic features. In the case of NMS, as indicated earlier, one would expect a course of treatments, if effective, not to necessitate specific maintenance treatment, unless for underlying psychopathology (but not for NMS, which will be unlikely to recur once remission with ECT has taken place). As for agitated dementia patients, if index ECT helps calm them down, aggressive MECT is needed to sustain the benefits. Otherwise, rapid relapse (e.g., within days to a week or two) is common. If ECT is used for psychopathology in epileptic patients, and if one incidentally notices a reduced frequency of spontaneous seizures with ECT, then there probably will not be a long-lasting anti-epileptic effect of index ECT.

Maintenance ECT

After an initial series of index ECT treatments is finished, the provision of further treatments for prophylactic purposes is termed *continuation* or *maintenance ECT*, depending on whether the time period is the first 6 months after index ECT (continuation) or beyond that point (maintenance). As discussed earlier in this chapter, for ease of communication herein, all ECT beyond the index series that is used to prevent return of symptoms or signs is termed *maintenance ECT*. In typical practice, MECT is usually conducted weekly for a few weeks and then tapered off from there with the goal of eventually spacing the treatments out as far as possible, usually with monthly being the target inter-treatment frequency goal. The frequency is highly individualized, though, as discussed in the subsections below.

Depression

Efficacy of MECT

There is an extensive literature covering the use of MECT following index ECT for depression. Several reviews provide exhaustive discussion of this literature (Bourgon and Kellner 2000; Brown et al. 2014; Martínez-Amorós et al. 2012a; Monroe 1991; Petrides 1998; Petrides et al. 2011; Rabheru 2012; Rabheru and Persad 1997; Trevino et al. 2010; van Schaik et al. 2012; Youssef and McCall 2014). Interestingly, all these reviews come to the confident conclusion that MECT for depression is efficacious at preventing return of symptoms. The literature includes naturalistic MECT case series as well as controlled trials.

Karliner and Wehrheim (1965), providing data from a group of patients with a variety of psychiatric diagnoses, reported that those who accepted MECT after index ECT had a 12% relapse rate over the multiyear follow period as compared with 79% for those patients not accepting of MECT. Of course, with lack of randomization, this difference may represent, in part, factors other than choice of post–index ECT management, such as initial-illness psychopathological features, but it is highly suggestive of a prophylactic effect of MECT.

In an early expostulation of the presumed benefits of MECT, Wolff (1957) described its use in a very large ($N=505$) population of patients at a state psychiatric facility and found that, in general, it seemed to reduce relapse and rehospitalization rates, though precise statistics are not presented. Bourne (1954) provided an early description of highly recurrently ill depressive patients who could only be stabilized for relatively long periods with MECT, which he termed "convulsion dependence." Moore (1943) reported that recurrent mood episodes in a large series of MECT patients seemed to be less frequent with MECT. In yet another early series on MECT, Geoghegan and Stevenson (1949; Stevenson and Geoghegan 1951) provided 5-year follow-up data on "manic depressive" patients who were initially treated with index ECT. As with the Karliner and Wehrheim series (1965), those accepting MECT had fewer long-term recurrences of illness than did those not agreeing to receive this modality.

In more modern times, numerous relatively small case series of apparently successful MECT have been described (Abraham et al. 2006; Clarke et al. 1989; Decina et al. 1987; Dubin et al. 1992; Fox 2001; Grunhaus et al. 1990; Jaffe et al. 1990; Kramer 1999; Wijkstra et al. 2000; Zisselman et al. 2007). Many such series provide data indicating reduced hospitalization or relapse rates in the follow-up period during MECT compared with during a similar period prior to use of ECT (Beale et al. 1996; Bonds et al. 1998; Gupta et al. 2008; Lim 2006; Minnai et al. 2011; Nordenskjöld et al. 2011b; O'Connor et al. 2010b; Odeberg et al. 2008; Rodriguez-Jimenez et al. 2015; Russell et al. 2003; Schwarz et al. 1995;

Shelef et al. 2015; Thienhaus et al. 1990; Thornton et al. 1990; Vanelle et al. 1994) or after MECT is discontinued (Huuhka et al. 2012). Thus, even though at first blush MECT may seem a financially costly and aggressive modality, these reports suggest that in highly recurrent, chronic, or medication-refractory cases, on balance it may yield better quality of life, with less total cost, than if not used.

Some studies provide comparative naturalistically derived data on post–index ECT follow-up with MECT plus MPharm versus MPharm alone and generally find that the combination results in fewer relapses and hospitalizations (Gagné et al. 2000; Martínez-Amorós et al. 2012a; Rapinesi et al. 2013; Serra et al. 2006; Swoboda et al. 2001; Williams et al. 2010, as reported in Brown et al. 2014; Vothknecht et al. 2003). There is one naturalistic follow-up study in which MECT without concomitant medications was compared with MPharm, with the finding that those patients who complied with MECT generally had fewer relapses (McDonald et al. 1998).

There are five post-index ECT randomized controlled trials in which one group received MECT with or without MPharm and another group received MPharm alone (Brakemeier et al. 2014; Kellner et al. 2006, 2016b; Navarro et al. 2008; Nordenskjöld et al. 2013). In the Kellner et al. (2006) study, MECT was compared with MPharm, the latter consisting of a combination of nortriptyline and lithium. The two groups had the same sustained remission rate over 6 months (46%). There were slightly more relapses in the MECT group but more dropouts in the MPharm group. Of note, patients in the MECT group were not treated with concomitant medications as had been the case in the nonrandomized MECT versus MPharm comparisons cited above. It is possible that in the CORE study (Kellner et al. 2006), if there had been augmentation of MECT with medications, sustained remission rates could have been higher.

Navarro et al. (2008) randomly assigned psychotically depressed patients whose illness remitted with index ECT to follow-up MECT plus nortriptyline versus nortriptyline alone and found 2-year relapse rates to be about 38% in the medication-only group versus about 8% in the combined-modality group, a difference that was highly significant despite the relatively small sample size of each group (about a dozen patients per group).

Nordenskjöld et al. (2013) randomly assigned patients who had recently achieved remission of their depression after ECT either to MPharm, consisting of their doctors' choice of medications, or to MPharm supplemented with MECT and found that the combined treatment group had fewer relapses. Brakemeier et al. (2014) randomly assigned depressed ECT patients after successful index ECT to receive medication alone, medication plus cognitive-behavioral therapy (CBT), or medication plus MECT and found equal sustained remission rates (slightly over 40%) in the medication-alone and medication-plus-MECT groups, but almost twice the sustained remission rate (about 77%) in the medication-plus-CBT group. Kellner et al. (2016b) randomly assigned remitted depressed patients after ECT to MPharm consisting of lithium carbonate plus venlafaxine versus this combination plus four weekly ECT treatments followed by "as needed" supplemental treatments for return of depressive symptoms thereafter. This method of using MECT was termed "STABLE," meaning "symptom-titrated, algorithm-based longitudinal ECT." The follow-up period was 6 months, at the end of which the combined-modality group had a mean four-point-lower Hamilton Rating Scale for Depression score. At all other time points, the difference between groups in such scores was less than that, indicating a marginal at best advantage for their schedule of MECT. Thus, when a clinician is prescribing MECT, it is advisable to use a more aggressive schedule of treatments than was used by Kellner et al. (2016b).

In summary, the weight of current evidence indicates that MECT does add efficacy beyond MPharm alone. Unanswered questions about MECT include whether there are predictors of who benefits the most from it and what the best schedule of treatments is.

Patient Selection for MECT

In recommending MECT for clinical practice, the same question can be posed: Why not give it to all patients who have successfully completed an index course of treatments? After all, it makes sense that if a person responds well to an index course of ECT and has a history of medication refractoriness, chronicity, or recurrence, continued treatment with a successful modality probably has the best chance of keeping the illness at bay. MECT is an acceptable treatment alternative for virtually all patients from a strictly psychopathological standpoint if index ECT was successful. However, some patients may not be willing to accept it. Reasons for this include living a prohibitive distance from the ECT service, the inconvenience of MECT treatments (i.e., transportation time and time away from work for the patient as well as caregivers, who need to take time out from their schedule to transport and monitor the patient at home), continued memory impairment with MECT, and other aspects of ECT the patient may dread, such as the needlesticks or fear of undergoing general anesthesia. Additionally, some psychiatrists may not offer it because of lack of knowledge about the prophylactic efficacy of MECT.

As far as expense goes, each MECT treatment will cost much more as opposed to the relatively low cost of most antidepressant medications. Clearly, the direct costs of MECT are greater than the direct costs of MPharm. However, as discussed earlier, MECT, if successful in preventing hospitalizations, can be cheaper than MPharm if in fact it is superior to the latter, and several series were strongly suggestive that at the very least MECT reduces longitudinal costs vis-à-vis the time period prior to institution of index ECT. Thus, the cost issue is more complex than at first blush.

There is no question that MECT is time intensive in comparison to MPharm, which consists of simply taking pills each day. MECT involves at the very least the patient taking a day off from whatever he or she normally would do (such as work or school), and usually more than just one day. There is the transportation to and from the treatment, a long distance for many patients. Added to this is the time it takes away from the person who is transporting the patient, for the patient cannot do his or her own driving, and monitoring the patient for the rest of the day and night (patients also should not be left alone at least the rest of the day after a treatment). Oftentimes, patients may need such supervision and assistance with driving for longer than merely 1 day. Indeed, probably the main barrier to MECT in many patients is that they either live too far away from an ECT suite or are unable to find proper transportation and monitoring.

The memory impairment from an index course of treatments is likely to leave the patient, in the first few days after the last such treatment, with some modicum of anterograde and retrograde amnesia, which, if treatments are ceased, will clear up within a few weeks in the case of the former and get to the point of not necessarily being bothersome for the latter. If MECT is performed, both types of memory impairment are likely to be more extensive (see Chapter 9 for further discussion of the cognitive effects of MECT). For patients who have to return to a job requiring ongoing memory for work-related issues, this can be annoying. Some patients thus prefer not to attempt MECT in order to let their memory clear up.

The American Psychiatric Association Committee on Electroconvulsive Therapy (2001) report emphasizes that patients should only be treated with MECT if there is a history of an ECT-responsive psychopathological state and if they can comply with the demands of safe outpatient treatments.

The next consideration in deciding whether to offer MECT, beyond whether the patient can access it and is willing to undergo it, is how much of an improvement was obtained with the index series. This can be a complex issue. On the one hand, if there has been essentially complete remission of the index episode, that would favor MECT unless the longitudinal course of illness consisted of rare, very discrete episodes of illness. However, MECT may also be indicated for patients who obtained partial response during index ECT, for such patients are at very high risk of relapse, especially if the longitudinal course was characterized by a highly chronic, long-standing illness refractory to multiple medication trials. In that case, whatever benefit was obtained with index ECT may be worth trying to sustain with aggressive MECT.

Other considerations include refractoriness to medication trials (i.e., the more medication-refractory the illness is, the more likely it is that the patient will be offered MECT) and longitudinal course of illness (i.e., a chronic course of psychopathology favors MECT vs. a course characterized by highly discrete, widely spaced illness episodes). Overall, higher illness burden over time tends to favor offering MECT.

High episode severity, especially if the patient was suicidal before ECT, would also weigh in favor of offering MECT. If the patient has a history of good response to index ECT followed by relatively rapid relapse while taking adequate MPharm, then that would be a strong indication for offering MECT. Perhaps the most important consideration of all is patient preference. The psychiatrist should broach with the patient and family the possibility of MECT, taking time to discuss how the treatments are scheduled and spaced, what type of time commitments are needed from patient and caregiver, and what types of memory issues are expected. Patients and families are able to take into account all these factors and offer their own view of MECT. If a patient expresses a strong desire for it, and the clinician is convinced the improvement with index ECT was real and not based on spurious beliefs, then it is appropriate to offer it. The bottom line is that there is no universally agreed-on indication for MECT; judgment on a case-by-case basis is the rule. In general, though, the trend in recent years in the ECT field has been to offer MECT more commonly than in previous eras (Kellner et al. 2016b).

The Conduct of MECT

Once the decision to proceed with MECT is made, the schedule of treatments, ECT technique, and duration of therapy must be planned. The importance of starting the first MECT treatment quickly cannot be overstated. Waiting longer than a week risks early relapse. Review of the extensive clinical literature earlier in this chapter revealed a remarkable near-unanimity in MECT scheduling: in the early weeks, treatments are spaced closely together, with a gradual tapering off over subsequent months. One must wonder why this is the case. There has been no empirical study comparing ongoing weekly (or some other relatively aggressive schedule) with the gradually tapering schedule. The situation is analogous to the old tradition in pharmacotherapy of depression to gradually lower the dose of antidepressant as one progresses onward from the acute remission phase. This practice was abandoned after research found that maintaining full doses of medications prevented relapses. The same principle may be at work with MECT. However, if one were to attempt to maintain ongoing weekly treatments, many patients simply would not be able to tolerate that schedule cognitively or from the standpoint of the logistics of the schedule. The results of the McDonald et al. (1998) trial comparing MECT with MPharm in elderly patients are instructive. One of the reasons for the superior findings in the MECT group (albeit a small group) was the aggressive schedule for MECT: after a few weekly treatments, patients were maintained on a biweekly schedule. This is in contrast to the tapering off of the MECT to monthly treatments that so many other groups have reported.

In general, most clinicians prescribe four weekly MECT treatments to start off. If the patient seems to be doing well, then tapering to biweekly treatments, generally aiming for four consecutive treatments at that schedule (thus, 2 months of biweekly treatments), is appropriate. If at this stage the patient continues to do well, one can taper to every 3–4 weeks. If along the way there seems to be a tendency for the symptoms/signs to return toward the end of the inter-treatment interval, then holding off on spacing them further is recommended, because full-relapse potential is much greater if the patient seems to be slipping. The final "steady state" frequency of treatments is highly individualized: some patients will need ongoing weekly treatments to maintain stability, whereas others can be tapered off the MECT to once every 4–6 weeks without a hint of relapse. Additionally, when a patient who is being treated at an interval of every 2–4 weeks experiences a return of symptoms, then one or two "booster" treatments spaced a couple days apart may allow a return back to the maintenance schedule.

In addition to treatment frequency, there is the question of electrode placement, stimulus dosing, and stimulus parameter combinations. Common sense would indicate to continue with whatever technique worked well for index treatments. Research on whether changes in technique are needed for MECT versus continuing with whatever was done during index ECT has not been done. The question, from a neurobiological perspective, is whether the biologic basis of the initial index ECT response is the same as the biologic basis of maintaining that response. If there is some type of separation of these phenomena, then one might speculate that if bitemporal placement is optimal for index ECT, then perhaps a switch to unilateral, and maybe even lower electrical doses, may be sufficient to sustain the benefit during MECT, at much lower cognitive cost. Conversely, if unilateral placement was successfully used for index ECT, some have speculated that a switch to bitemporal placement during MECT, in which the treatments are spaced out, may be necessary for sustained improvement. As indicated, this important area of research has been neglected.

A common clinical question arises during MECT regarding the possible significance of seizure duration. Is it important during MECT? Several case series have reported on trends in seizure length during courses of MECT (Di Pauli and Conca 2009; Jarvis et al. 1993; van Waarde et al. 2010b; Wild et al. 2004). One should not worry about apparent seizure shortening during MECT and should pay more attention to patients' clinical status. Commonly, as the inter-treatment interval is increased during MECT, with presumed lowering of seizure threshold to baseline, there is an increase in seizure duration.

It is necessary to decide, of course, when to terminate MECT. Considerations include chronicity of the index episode, with longer durations indicating longer courses of MECT. Generally, a year of MECT is the modal goal, though much variability around this occurs in routine practice. For example, if the clinician concludes that MECT is a failure, then stoppage at that point is indicated. When can one conclude failure? The answer is not always, when early relapse occurs— for a few twice- or thrice-weekly index treatments may reestablish euthymia such that a return to MECT will be worth doing. Because depressive illnesses are so variable and recurrent in many cases, the MECT course may be characterized by periods of relatively spaced treatments interspersed with periods of return to index treatments. If during MECT there seems to be frequent depressive worsening— that is, the patient just does not seem to be maintaining stability—and cognitive side effects have built up to an uncomfortable level, then perhaps stopping MECT is indicated. One must balance the severity of the index depression with current functioning during MECT and side effect and inconvenience burden when deciding whether to discontinue MECT. Most often, the patient and family will render an opinion as to whether they consider it worthwhile to continue with MECT.

In some cases of patients with highly recurrent illnesses who tolerate MECT without problems, one may continue MECT indefinitely beyond a year. There have even been a few patients who continue with very long-term high-frequency MECT, much as in the case series presented by Zisselman et al. (2007). Again, balancing chronicity and disability burden of the illness, previous medication refractoriness, and patient tolerance, the clinician can make rational decisions about MECT treatment frequency and duration on a case-by-case basis. The importance of listening to patients and their families register their opinions cannot be overstated.

A final issue pertinent to MECT for patients treated during the index episode for depression is whether the overall diagnosis is unipolar depression, bipolar depression, or depression occurring during schizophrenia or schizoaffective disorder. Generally, MECT is the same, in terms of indications and technique, for these patients. MPharm will differ among these groups, as bipolar patients will need something to prevent mania, and chronically psychotic schizophrenic or schizoaffective patients will need an antipsychotic. MPharm issues will be discussed in further detail in the section "Maintenance Pharmacotherapy After Index ECT" later in this chapter.

Mania

Relapse is a major problem for chronically manic patients. Chanpattana (2000) described a young chronically manic patient whose condition was stabilized with a combination of clozapine and index ECT; improvement was sustained for over a year with an aggressive schedule of MECT. Vaidya et al. (2003) described in detail 13 patients with medication-refractory bipolar disorder who were stabilized with index ECT and continued with a decreased rate of hospitalizations during MECT courses. Other case reports exist of patients with refractory bipolar disorder whose illness was stabilized with index ECT and MECT (Husain et al. 1993; Tsao et al. 2004). Nascimento et al. (2006) described a patient with highly recurrent manic episodes, refractory to medications, whose condition was stabilized with index ECT and was sustained for many months on follow-up with MECT along with neuroleptic medication. Vanelle et al. (1994) and Petrides et al. (1994) have also provided data supporting a prophylactic role of MECT in patients with bipolar disorders. There are no clinical trials comparing MECT with medications in patients treated with ECT for mania.

Manic patients treated successfully with a course of index ECT should be offered MECT if the mania had a chronic course, for in such a case, relapse potential is very high. On the other hand, if the manic episode was of relatively short duration, with a discrete change from a euthymic baseline, and the past history is one of a small number of other such discrete manic episodes with long intervals between each one, then MECT might not be necessary. If MECT is not offered in such a context, there should be careful ongoing post-ECT follow-up to ascertain signs of relapse so that ECT can be reinstated and then followed by MECT.

The schedule of treatments should be aggressive for MECT after index ECT for mania, starting with weekly treatments for at least a month and probably 6 weeks or so before cautiously prolonging the inter-treatment interval to 10 days for several treatments, then to 2 weeks. The patient should be followed very carefully for signs of manic relapse and treated promptly. Some patients with chronic mania may need indefinite weekly or biweekly treatments to sustain euthymia. This is obviously a challenge for compliance. Such patients typically reside in state psychiatric hospitals and are disabled by their illness, and their illness has been refractory to highly aggressive psychotropic regimens. Fortunately, this is a relatively rare scenario. More common is the bipolar patient with a relatively acute, discrete manic episode that is highly responsive to ECT, and most such patients can be managed effectively if they comply with MPharm.

Schizophrenia and Schizoaffective Disorder

Schizophrenia patients can present challenges similar to those presented by chronic manic patients. They often reside in state psychiatric hospitals or other highly structured living environments such as group homes and have been given numerous medications that were at best partially effective. Index courses of ECT can help reduce behavioral and thought disorganization as well as psychosis and render the patient more interpersonally appropriate.

Several groups have published data regarding MECT for schizophrenia patients who respond well to index ECT. For example, Moore (1943) published a large series of chronic psychotic patients who in general seemed to have sustained benefits with courses of MECT, though systematic psychopathological data are lacking. Kho et al. (2004) gave index ECT to 11 schizophrenia patients who had not responded to clozapine , and the combination resulted in a good response in 8 of these patients. Of these, 4 experienced a relapse of symptoms without MECT within 3–19 weeks, and of these 3 responded to repeat index ECT. Two of these 3 then did well with MECT. This report demonstrates the systematic, stepwise application of MECT only to those initial index ECT responders who then relapse during MPharm.

Stiebel (1995) described several schizophrenia or schizoaffective disorder patients who achieved remarkable behavioral stability with index treatments followed by MECT. Lévy-Rueff et al. (2008, 2010) described 19 schizophrenia patients successfully treated with index ECT. These patients were then treated with MECT for a mean of 43 weeks at 1- to 5-week inter-treatment intervals. All were given antipsychotic medications and a few other classes of psychotropics. The yearly hospitalization rate during MECT was 80% reduced compared with the year before institution of ECT, demonstrating a probable prophylactic effect of MECT. Sajatovic and Meltzer (1993) described nine schizophrenia patients who received index ECT, of whom five were considered good responders. To these patients, MECT was added at a mean rate of monthly; not surprisingly, considering this long inter-treatment interval (especially at the beginning of MECT), there were a lot of relapses in this cohort of patients. MECT was undoubtedly administered too infrequently. Lohr et al. (1994) described two cases of aggressively pharmacologically treated patients with chronic schizophrenia whose illnesses were highly refractory to the medication trials but for whom good initial index ECT results were achieved that were sustained out to 11 months with aggressively applied MECT.

Chanpattana and colleagues (Chanpattana 1997, 1998; Chanpattana et al. 1999a, 1999c, 1999d) have published data on the use of MECT for schizophrenia patients responding to index ECT. In a unique technical aspect of this group's use of MECT, during the index ECT process once remission was noted, the patients received three more treatments in a week, followed by a treatment a week later; those who sustained the improvement were then transitioned to MECT, whereas those not sustaining the initial improvement received more thrice-weekly treatments. Only when patients received at least 20 treatments without remission criteria being met did the investigators consider the patients to have not responded to the index ECT, echoing Kalinowsky's (1943) view from half a century earlier that it takes that many treatments for stable remissions in schizophrenia patients. This strategy, in these authors' hands, resulted in good sustained improvements for their patients during the MECT phase of treatment. Demonstrating the need for long-term MECT in many schizophrenia patients, Sutor and Rasmussen (2009) reported on the use of multiyear MECT for several patients with schizophrenia whose condition would not remain stable if MECT were tapered down in frequency. This, of course, underscores the often chronic, unremitting nature of schizophrenia.

Some excellent controlled, systematic data were provided in the report by Chanpattana et al. (1999a) from Thailand. In these studies, schizophrenia patients whose illness had been stabilized with the combination of flupenthixol (an antipsychotic medication similar to fluphenazine) and index bitemporal placement ECT were randomly allocated to receive, for 6 months thereafter, MECT alone, flupenthixol alone, or the combination of these two modalities. The combination-therapy group clearly had better 6-month outcomes: 40% relapse rates versus 93% relapse rates in the groups of patients receiving either MPharm or MECT as sole treatment. This is reflected in clinical experience with the population of schizophrenia patients, indicating that highly aggressive continuation and maintenance regimens are needed.

For schizophrenia patients, ECT can make the difference between residing chronically and in a behaviorally disorganized and agitated manner at a state hospital versus living peaceably in a community resource such as a group home, and MECT can sustain such gains. Thus, for essentially all schizophrenia/schizoaffective disorder patients treated with index ECT and who demonstrate good improvement, MECT is recommended. As with manic patients, the schedule for such treatments will often need to be weekly or biweekly for prolonged periods. For the schizophrenia or schizoaffective disorder patient for whom ECT was prescribed for a highly discrete, acute exacerbation of illness (as opposed to chronic symptoms/signs), MECT may not be necessary if compliance with aggressive ongoing MPharm can be assured. Some patients, as described by Sutor and Rasmussen (2009), may need essentially indefinite MECT to function in the community. In this setting, the cognitive disturbance induced by such aggressive ECT schedules must be balanced against the therapeutic efficacy.

Catatonia

Suzuki et al. (2004) reported on 11 catatonic schizophrenia patients older than 45 years who responded well to index ECT. While the patients were being followed receiving neuroleptic medication but no MECT, there were seven relapses in 6 months. In another report from the same group, Suzuki et al. (2006) described a cohort of 14 catatonic schizophrenia patients, of whom 13 responded well to index ECT. Eight of these 13 experienced a relapse within a year while taking neuroleptic medication alone. A second index ECT course for these 8 patients resulted in good improvement in 7, of whom 3 relapsed during subsequent MECT. The 3 patients who experienced relapse during MECT were given a third index ECT course followed by a more intensive schedule of MECT and did well during the follow-up period. This report on a very systematically described and treated cohort details how relapse-prone patients with catatonic schizophrenia can be and the need, in some of these patients, for highly intensive (i.e., weekly) ongoing MECT schedules.

Most catatonic patients have an underlying psychiatric disorder such as schizophrenia, schizoaffective disorder, bipolar disorder, or unipolar depression or have catatonia due to a medical/neurological condition or substance. Whether to offer MECT for catatonic patients who have been successfully treated with index ECT depends on the underlying condition. If, for example, index ECT unmasks a manic episode, then that should be treated either with continued ECT or with antimanic pharmacotherapy as described above for manic patients. If a chronic schizophrenia patient had relatively stable functioning, with a superimposed acute catatonic episode treated with index ECT, then MECT is probably not needed. If the catatonia is part of a deep, psychotic depression, then the criteria described above for depressed patients should be considered. Medical/neurological/substance-induced catatonic episodes successfully treated with index ECT usually do not require MECT if the aggravating medical condition has been treated. Some patients have periodic isolated catatonia, in which case MECT should be offered if the longitudinal course is characterized by prolonged or highly recurrent episodes.

Other Indications for ECT

As indicated in Chapter 2, there are other, mostly neurological conditions that are occasionally treated with ECT. The use of ECT for these conditions should be considered experimental. These include ECT for the agitation of dementia (separate from depression), the motor signs of Parkinson's disease (again separate from depression or mania), epilepsy, NMS, some acute deliria, and other movement disorders such as dystonia or tardive dyskinesia.

Regarding patients with dementia, mostly involving Alzheimer's or Lewy body disease, agitation or screaming can be common. MECT can sustain gains from successful index ECT for such patients. Typically, the patient resides at a nursing home and has been aggressive toward others or screams relentlessly. Index ECT may calm the patient down. Starting with weekly MECT for the first few weeks—say, 4–6 weeks—is prudent, with a cautious increase of the inter-treatment interval from that point, going to every 2 weeks and ultimately to monthly if possible. Some such patients need to be treated, as is the case with schizophrenia patients or chronic manic patients, every week or two in an ongoing manner in order to sustain the initial benefits, given that agitation in dementia tends to be a chronic issue. Over time, as the dementing process progresses, the patient's agitation and screaming may be replaced by apathy and behavioral withdrawal such that MECT no longer becomes necessary. Thus, dementia patients receiving MECT need periodic reviews. MECT can be quite helpful in sustaining gains with index ECT for agitated dementia patients. There are several case reports and small series attesting to this utility (Rasmussen et al. 2003; Sutor and Rasmussen 2008; Wu et al. 2010).

Parkinson's disease motor signs may respond well to ECT, as reviewed in Chapter 2. In depressed Parkinson's patients, one must be on the lookout for excessive confusion and emerging dyskinesias. Close collaboration with the patient's neurologist or primary care physician can help determine optimal dosing in the patient's dopaminergic regimen along with the MECT. There is a smattering of case report literature on the apparently successful relapse prevention of the motoric signs of Parkinson's disease after index ECT gains utilizing MECT (Aarsland et al. 1997; Balke and Varma 2007; Fall and Granérus 1999; Höflich et al. 1995; Holcomb et al. 1983; Wengel et al. 1998; Zervas and Fink 1991). Because ECT is only rarely used for Parkinson's patients strictly for the motoric signs, confident recommendations are difficult to provide, but common sense would indicate that with a chronic degenerative condition such as this, MECT would be advisable if an index course of treatments is substantially beneficial. The clinician would have to titrate inter-treatment frequency carefully with regular assessments of motor function, as always balancing the desire for sustaining initial gains with probable cognitive effects of aggressive MECT schedules. Patient and family input regarding striking this balance is critical for success. If, on the other hand, the index ECT and MECT are given primarily for depression in a Parkinson's patient, then the issues relevant to the depression would be given primary consideration in determining whether and how often to administer MECT, with the motor signs being a secondary consideration unless the latter respond better than the depression does.

The anticonvulsant effect of ECT is one of the most fascinating neurobiological findings in the ECT field. However, it is extremely rare to find a patient who needs ECT in modern times for epilepsy itself. Some reports of suppression of spontaneous seizures exist, but MECT is not practical in these cases.

Index ECT can be lifesaving for neuroleptic malignant syndrome, as discussed in Chapter 2. However, MECT would not be necessary for the NMS signs themselves, because they constitute an acute and not a chronic condition. Rather, the need for MECT in ECT-treated NMS patients would be determined by the underlying psychopathology and the desire not to treat with ongoing neuroleptics for safety. For example, if a schizophrenia patient developed NMS that was eventually treated with ECT, with good resolution of the NMS as well as psychopathological features, it would be logical to continue with MECT. If the ECT was administered for a relatively acute condition, such as a psychotic depression, and that condition has now resolved, then MECT may not be necessary, as neuroleptic medications would not otherwise be needed for continuation therapy.

Finally, ECT is occasionally used for acute neurological delirious states (Rasmussen et al. 2008b), such as viral encephalitides, that defy other management. MECT would not be needed in these acute conditions. The rarity of use of ECT in other movement disorders, such as dystonia or tardive dyskinesia, precludes any evidence basis in the literature, but because these conditions are chronic, if such a patient did respond acutely to index ECT, one would expect MECT to be needed to sustain the gains.

Maintenance Pharmacotherapy After Index ECT

Depression

Literature Review

There have been a few controlled, systematic studies testing various post–index ECT MPharm strategies. Lauritzen et al. (1996) randomly assigned patients whose depression had remitted after index ECT to treatment with placebo, paroxetine, or imipramine and found 6-month relapse rates of 65%, 10%, and 30%, respectively. What stands out in this study is the remarkably low relapse rate with the selective serotonin reuptake inhibitor (SSRI) paroxetine. This rate is so low, quite frankly, that it is hard to believe it is not a spurious finding. van den Broek et al. (2006) compared placebo with imipramine post-ECT and found that the 6-month relapse rate for placebo was 80%, while that for imipramine was only 18%, a figure so low that it was only "bested" by paroxetine in the Lauritzen et al. study.

In another controlled MPharm study, Yildiz et al. (2010) randomly assigned patients whose depression remitted with ECT to receive sertraline early during index ECT, sertraline started after index ECT was finished, or placebo. Though the follow-up phase was relatively short (18 weeks), relapse rates were 12.5% for the "early sertraline" group, 28% for the "late sertraline" group, and 67% for the placebo group. These findings suggest that adding an antidepressant early in the course of treatments helps prevent relapses better than starting it after ECT is finished.

Grunhaus et al. (2001) randomly assigned patients whose depression remitted with ECT to treatment with fluoxetine plus placebo versus fluoxetine plus melatonin, the latter on the theory that helping with sleep may prevent depressive relapses. However, the two groups had similar relapse rates at 3 months' time (28.5%). In the Navarro et al. (2008) MECT trial alluded to earlier, the nortriptyline-alone group had an approximately 38% relapse rate over 2 years of follow-up, an outcome that actually compares quite favorably to outcomes of other medication-only groups in the other controlled trials and is quite superior to outcomes in the Sackeim et al. (2001) nortriptyline-only group, which had a 60% 6-month relapse rate. Martiny et al. (2015) randomly assigned patients whose depression had remitted with ECT to 6 months of one of three doses of escitalopram (10 mg, 20 mg, or 30 mg) or 100 mg of nortriptyline, finding a combined 50% relapse rate in the escitalopram groups taken as a whole versus 20% in the nortriptyline group. Thus, there are four studies in which at least one MPharm group's treatment consisted solely of a SSRI (Grunhaus et al. 2001; Lauritzen et al. 1996; Martiny et al. 2015; Yildiz et al. 2010), with generally favorable sustained remission rates.

There has been a surprisingly large amount of attention to the potential utility of lithium in preventing relapses after successful index ECT in depressed patients. In a relatively early study from the Columbia University Consortium (Sackeim et al. 1993), in which patients were randomly assigned to index ECT with unilateral or bitemporal electrode placement at low and high stimulus doses, naturalistic (i.e., nonrandomized) follow-up treatment with tricyclic/lithium combination therapy was associated with lower relapse rates than for nonlithium regimens. In another study from the same group, Sackeim et al. (2000) randomly assigned depressed patients to one of four different methods of ECT (three different electrical doses with unilateral electrode placement and one electrical dose with bitemporal electrode placement) and followed the patients naturalistically. Those patients who had been treated by their psychiatrist with a combination of lithium and a tricyclic antidepressant had lower relapse rates than patients not treated with this combination. One problem with the lithium/tricyclic combination is tolerability—in the McDonald et al. (1998) and Kellner et al. (2006) studies, this combination was associated with more "drop outs" than was MECT. Several other case series found a protective effect when lithium was added to antidepressants (Atiku et al. 2015; Nordenskjöld et al. 2011a, 2013; Rehor et al. 2009). Perry and Tsuang (1979) randomly assigned post-ECT patients to receive a tricyclic antidepressant versus lithium monotherapy and found equal relapse rates, indicating that lithium as sole medication therapy may be effective, a finding echoed by Coppen et al. (1981) in a study comparing lithium with placebo post-ECT.

Testing the hypothesis of a protective effect of post–index ECT lithium/tricyclic combination therapy in a randomized trial, Sackeim et al. (2001) randomly assigned a similar group of ECT remitters to treatment with placebo, nortripty-line, or the combination of nortriptyline and lithium and found 6-month relapse rates of 89%, 60%, and 39%, respectively. Whereas the placebo relapse rates were roughly comparable to those of the Lauritzen et al. (1996) study, the rates with a tricyclic alone (nortriptyline) were double those with another tricyclic (imipramine) from the latter study, which utilized similar criteria for discerning a depressive re-lapse. In contrast, in a later ECT trial from this group (Sackeim et al. 2008), pa-tients given a combination of a tricyclic antidepressant and lithium fared no better during follow-up than patients treated with other medications. Kellner et al. (2006) found the 6-month relapse rate in a lithium/nortriptyline-treated group to be 31.6%. Prudic et al. (2013), following patients treated with either lithium combined with nortriptyline or lithium combined with venlafaxine, found relapse rates of approximately 50% over 6 months in both groups.

Shapira et al. (1995) followed 24 patients whose illness was successfully re-mitted with index ECT and treated them with MPharm consisting of lithium car-bonate in isolation; these authors found that 65% of the patients sustained the remission for 6 months, suggesting that this medication alone may provide suffi-cient prophylaxis for most patients. Coppen et al. (1981) followed 38 patients after ECT-induced remission for depression, randomly assigning 18 to receive lithium and 20 to receive placebo for a year. There were more relapses and more time spent depressed in the placebo group than in the lithium-treated group, two of whom required repeat ECT courses over the year of follow-up. In a further anal-ysis of these data, Abou-Saleh (1987) determined that the prophylactic effect of lithium was predominantly seen in the second 6-month period after ECT.

The potential prophylactic effect of lithium after index ECT has been men-tioned in a case report in which a patient experienced relapse after ECT while be-ing given single-agent antidepressant pharmacotherapy and then after a second course of ECT stayed well when lithium was added (Okamoto et al. 2005). Jaffe et al. (1991) also mentioned the use of lithium in MECT failures in a very small case series. More recently, Kellner et al. (2016b) added lithium to all patients' regimens after successful index ECT for depression, and in the group receiving MPharm alone (lithium plus venlafaxine), the 6-month relapse rate was 20.3%, which is quite low by historical standards.

Recommendations for Practice

As indicated earlier, virtually all post-ECT patients will be treated with some form of MPharm, even if MECT is also used. The choice of MPharm is partially guided by the literature and practitioner preference. The best data available indicate that a combination of an antidepressant (nortriptyline and venlafaxine have been most systematically studied) plus lithium carbonate provides better protection than single-agent antidepressant pharmacotherapy (Sackeim et al. 2001). What is not clear is whether lithium alone would provide as much protection as when combined with an antidepressant. It is a shame that in the landmark Sackeim et al. (2001) study, in which index ECT responders were randomly allocated to receive placebo, nortriptyline, or nortriptyline plus lithium, there was no group treated with lithium alone. There are some hints from other studies of a benefit of post-ECT lithium monotherapy. The Coppen et al. (1981) and Shapira et al. (1995) studies described above suggest lithium monotherapy may suffice, which is good news for bipolar depressed patients in whom the practitioner wishes to avoid use of an antidepressant. It is a good idea to start lithium after ECT is completed. There has been disagreement in the literature regarding whether lithium is safe to combine with index ECT, a topic discussed in detail in Chapter 7, but it is prudent to avoid the combination when it is not necessary. Recently, Kellner et al. (2016b) have shown that using lithium in combination with MECT is safe. In that study, the dose of lithium was withheld the day before each ECT treatment.

In the absence of better data on the use of lithium in isolation after ECT for depressed patients, it is wise to combine it with an antidepressant (at least in those patients with unipolar depression). Tricyclic compounds and venlafaxine have the best databases of usage in this setting (Sackeim et al. 2001, 2009), but if a patient cannot safely tolerate those or his or her illness has clearly been refractory to those in the past, using some other antidepressant is recommended. Unstudied options include use of lamotrigine for relapse prevention. Several second-generation antipsychotics have now been U.S. Food and Drug Administration–approved as antidepressant augmentation agents, and one wonders whether one or more of them may also have prophylactic efficacy against relapse of depression post–index ECT. Given the high post-ECT relapse rates, it is advisable to consider aggressive strategies, especially in patients with a history of highly relapsing/recurring bouts of depression. Many such patients are not willing to undergo MECT, are not in a position to tolerate its cognitive side effects, or do not have MECT available, so practitioners should be prepared to try multiple medication strategies.

Virtually all MECT patients are also receiving MPharm (Russell et al. 2003). Mostly this is not a complicated issue. However, if anticonvulsant medications (e.g., valproic acid, lamotrigine, carbamazepine) are used, seizure induction may be difficult, and it may be necessary to hold off on the medication a day or two prior to each treatment (see Chapter 4). Another conundrum is whether to combine lithium carbonate with MECT. Both strategies are effective, and in the interest of relapse prevention, one would want to combine them. However, with concerns about excessive cognitive side effects with this combination, some practitioners may advocate holding off on lithium a day or two prior to treatments. Reassuring are findings from the PRIDE (Prolonging Remission in Depressed Elderly) study, in which MECT was combined with lithium, which was held a day or two before each ECT treatment (Kellner et al. 2016b). This combination was well tolerated.

A question arises whether to treat psychotically depressed patients whose illness remitted with ECT with an MPharm regimen that includes an antipsychotic. One trial randomly allocated such patients to nortriptyline plus placebo versus nortriptyline plus the first-generation antipsychotic perphenazine and found no difference in outcomes over the next 6 months (25% relapse rate in both groups), a result that argued against using neuroleptics (Meyers et al. 2001). Thus, when treating psychotically depressed patients, who most often are elderly and especially prone to medication side effects, with index ECT, one should discontinue antipsychotics if they have already been prescribed and maintain the patients after ECT with combination lithium/antidepressant without an antipsychotic medication if MPharm is chosen. Also, one should be certain that the diagnosis really is psychotic depression and not a more sinister ongoing psychotic disorder like schizoaffective disorder, in which case antipsychotic medication should be continued to prevent psychotic relapse.

Patients treated with ECT for bipolar depression should be managed pharmacologically after index ECT in accordance with practice guidelines for bipolar disorder, generally using medications such as lithium, carbamazepine, lamotrigine, valproic acid, or second-generation antipsychotics either as monotherapy or in various types of combinations. In particular, avoidance of antidepressant medications is a goal of such therapy. The two goals of MPharm for bipolar patients are to prevent mania and to prevent depression.

Mania

For the manic patient whose illness has just remitted with ECT, it is mandatory that some type of medication strategy be instituted. This probably also is the case even in those patients receiving MECT, given the very high relapse potential of these patients. Choice of medication should follow usual guidelines and practitioner preferences for treatment of bipolar patients. A dilemma, discussed in Chapter 5, is whether to use antimanic medications during index ECT. It is wise to use atypical antipsychotics, which help potentiate antimanic responses to ECT and prevent relapses. One would hold off starting an anticonvulsant or lithium until after the last index ECT treatment is finished.

Schizophrenia and Schizoaffective Disorder

As is the case with manic patients given ECT, all schizophrenia patients will be given concomitant antipsychotics, even clozapine if needed. An exception would be the patient treated with ECT for NMS. In that setting, pharmacology experts have provided a variety of opinions on whether to rechallenge the now-recovered NMS patient with an antipsychotic medication. In the initial weeks after index ECT in that scenario, MECT should be used aggressively to prevent relapse.

Catatonia

MPharm for patients with catatonia depends on the underlying psychopathology. If ECT uncovers a manic episode, then pharmacology will be prescribed accordingly. If it is schizophrenia/schizoaffective disorder, then a neuroleptic should be used. If a unipolar depressive episode is apparent, then in like manner a lithium/antidepressant combination should be considered. If the catatonia was due to a medical/neurologic/toxic cause the active phase of which is remitted, then there may be no need for any pharmacotherapy after successful ECT.

Other Indications for ECT

The database for post-ECT MPharm for parkinsonism is nonexistent. Common sense would indicate that the "usual" MPharm for depression should be instituted if MECT is not done. Regarding the pharmacotherapy for the motor manifestations of parkinsonism, there may be a lesser need for dopaminergic agent dosing if such signs improved with index ECT, but this matter should be decided by a neurologist. Abrupt reductions in or discontinuation of dopaminergic agents in Parkinson's disease patients has been associated with precipitation of a syndrome identical to NMS.

If a dementia patient was treated with ECT for behavioral agitation and there was substantial improvement, and MECT either is unavailable or is refused by the family, then MPharm could consist of the various pharmacotherapy strategies employed and advocated by geriatric psychiatry expert consensus publications. The use of antipsychotic agents in particular has been controversial, because the efficacy of such medications has been questioned for dementia-related agitation, and these agents have been associated with higher mortality rates in prospective trials. The use of SSRIs has some support as a possibly safer alternative for agitation in dementia. However, in the post–index ECT situation, the patient presumably was treated with ECT in the first place because such medication strategies did not work, so one wonders if better efficacy is to be found in prophylaxis after successful ECT. No data currently are to be found in the literature supporting any particular MPharm strategy in this setting.

Since ECT use expressly for tardive dyskinesia, dystonia, or epilepsy is so rare, recommendations for post-ECT MPharm would be purely speculative, and besides, one would expect such decisions to be made by the attending neurologist. Post-ECT MPharm for NMS would be guided by the underlying psychopathology, such as schizophrenia, mania, or some other state in which a neuroleptic was used. One would not expect anticonvulsant medications or lithium used as mood stabilizers or antidepressants to be a problem, though as mentioned earlier, use of antipsychotics is controversial. At least in the first few months after ECT-induced NMS remission, if the patient ordinarily would require a neuroleptic, one would try as best as possible to arrange MECT for psychopathological relapse prevention.

Post-ECT Psychotherapy

Most psychiatrists endorse psychotherapy and encourage their patients to receive it. However, many patients do not have access to anything but very limited psychotherapy services, because of geographic distance from practitioners, limited time due to busy personal schedules, or lack of insurance coverage. In addition, many patients simply do not wish to attend psychotherapy. It has been one of the challenges of the psychiatric profession to try and separate those depressed patients who need "biologic" treatment from those who need "psychosocial" treatment. The logical flaw of this simplistic thinking is that psychotherapy, when conducted properly, undoubtedly has neurobiological effects as patients improve, and ECT or medications can have profound effects on the way a patient perceives life circumstances (e.g., witness the dramatic reduction in psychosis with ECT). Thus, the boundary between so-called biologic and psychosocial treatments is artificial.

In the case of patients receiving index ECT, attempts at ongoing psychotherapy might be considered futile given the anterograde amnesia. However, there is not any research specifically looking into the question of whether index ECT patients might benefit from some form of psychotherapy, perhaps with the sessions given on nontreatment days. In the post–index ECT continuation/maintenance phase, with a patient whose depression has recently gone into remission, common sense would indicate that the time is ideal for the patient to commit to psychotherapy to deal with dysfunctional cognitions—say, in CBT—or interpersonal dysfunctions with interpersonal therapy. Fenton et al. (2006) offered CBT to several patients whose depression had remitted who also were receiving MECT. They found that the patients seemed to recall and benefit from the therapeutic principles. However, this was simply an uncontrolled case series. Brakemeier et al. (2014) did randomly assign patients whose depression had remitted after index ECT to receive medication alone, medication plus CBT, or medication plus MECT and found the lowest relapse rates over a year clearly to be in the psychotherapy add-on group. The field would greatly benefit from more controlled trial data on post–index ECT psychotherapy in which one post–index ECT group receives formal psychotherapy, with assessments of the degree to which patients recall the therapeutic principles to be included in the outcome assessments. Patients whose lives tend to be complicated by psychosocial disruptions and stresses in particular probably benefit the most from maintenance psychotherapy.

Maintenance Treatment for Patients Who Do Not Respond to ECT

As a follow-up to the question at the beginning of this chapter regarding what to do with the index ECT responder, the next question might be: For the patient who has *not* responded to a course of index ECT—now what? This highly important topic is almost completely neglected in the ECT literature. So much attention has been placed on how to sustain hard-won improvement with index treatments that the field has ignored what to do with nonresponders (or ultrarapid relapsers). Thus, there is no scientifically based or even naturalistic case series–based advice to the reader. Probably the most important thing to do is communicate to the patient the attitude that one will not give up hope. The reason this is so important is that most ECT nonresponders are patients who had fairly aggressive medication trials and psychotherapy attempts prior to ECT. Such patients may be prone to hopelessness and suicidal ideations in the face of still feeling poorly and not having responded to what they often perceive as their last hope, ECT. These patients should be followed very carefully. Attempts should be made to review prior medication trials thoroughly for dose and duration adequacy and to pick a medication that was not used adequately before. Using combination strategies that have an empirical basis in the literature, such as lithium augmentation of an antidepressant, is advisable (Jaffe et al. 1991). Perhaps even more than the robust ECT responders, the nonresponders may be the best candidates for intensive ongoing psychotherapy, given their frail emotional state and treatment refractoriness. The literature desperately needs attention for this neglected population.

Key Points

- Post-ECT relapse rates are high.

- Aggressive post–acute ECT treatment with pharmacotherapy and/or continuation ECT is necessary to prevent relapse risk.

- Continuation pharmacotherapy in unipolar depressed patients should include lithium along with an antidepressant agent.

- Continuation ECT is administered at progressively more spaced intervals over the 6 months after acute ECT is finished.

9

Cognitive Effects of ECT

Shortly after the introduction of electroconvulsive therapy (ECT), clinicians noticed that memory dysfunction was associated with the treatments. The importance of memory dysfunction as a side effect of ECT, with all its ramifications, simply cannot be overstated. Memory problems are the main side effect of ECT. If ECT did not cause amnesia at all, it would be used more frequently in routine practice. Imagine that a patient could be given a course of treatments, and even followed with maintenance ECT (MECT), without forgetting any aspect of his or her life or knowledge base or having any problem learning new information. What would be the downside of ECT then? Other than financial expense and a few relatively minor discomforts, such as headaches, nausea, and so forth, there would be practically none. Patients could return to work the next day without forgetting anything of their job and return to family life similarly without having forgotten vacations, interpersonal experiences, and the like.

Those who either oppose or are disconcerted by ECT because of amnesia accuse the psychiatric profession of essentially ignoring this issue (Donahue 2000). This accusation is patently incorrect. In fact, of all interventions in the medical field in the last century, and this includes surgical procedures, medical devices, medications, and invasive diagnostic methods, probably none has had a side effect so thoroughly studied and discussed among its practitioners as amnesia with ECT. Allusions to memory side effects of ECT occurred shortly after its introduction in 1938 (Janis 1950). Clinical ECT trials have been funded in large measure to assess methods of lessening ECT-induced amnesia. Reports on attempts to elaborate and reduce such a side effect have emanated from countries in all inhabited continents. Further, there have been U.S. government–sponsored conferences dedicated to hearing all opinions on ECT (McDonald et al. 2016; National

Institutes of Health 1985). These facts dispel any notion that psychiatry as a profession has ignored memory dysfunction. However, despite these attempts to reduce ECT-induced amnesia, it has not been eliminated and remains a critical issue to deal with all the way from initial planning stages during patient selection, through the consent process, to the conduct of the treatments and into post-treatment management. In sum, memory problems are virtually inseparable as an issue to be dealt with in ECT practice from other technical issues. Thus, a chapter devoted to discussion of the various relevant issues is in order as part of an effort to teach ECT practice. Herein will be discussed the various aspects of human memory affected by ECT and how to assess and manage such side effects.

Before a review of the specific neuropsychological effects of ECT is undertaken, it is important to point out that the illnesses treated with ECT are known to cause cognitive problems. For example, major depression is associated with problems in focusing and concentrating, which can interfere with memory and are in fact part of the diagnostic criteria for a major depressive episode in DSM-5 (American Psychiatric Association 2013). Additionally, research has shown that depression is associated with impairments in autobiographical memory recall (see discussion of studies on retrograde amnesia later in this chapter). Typically, depressed patients about to undergo ECT treatment have difficulty processing information and staying on task; they are prone to becoming negativistic while performing cognitive tasks and have low energy and poor self-esteem. All these factors contribute to reductions in work or school performance, and indeed, many ECT patients have already either dropped out of school or taken a leave of absence (or permanent disability) from work. The most prominent cause of this is the cognitive problems associated with depression.

Patients with schizophrenia and mania are also treated with ECT. The bulk of the neurocognitive studies on ECT pertain to depressed patients, so the data are limited with this population. However, manic patients (and catatonic ones as well) typically cannot undergo neuropsychological evaluation because of lack of cooperation. Research into the cognitive impairments in patients with schizophrenia and bipolar disorder is active and ongoing.

It is also appropriate to point out that ECT can dramatically help certain aspects of neuropsychological functioning. Learning, or registration, can be improved with a course of ECT treatments. Psychopathologically ill patients in the throes of an acute episode of illness often have a hard time focusing and concentrating. This difficulty is manifested by impaired performance on neuropsychological tasks requiring sustained attention, freedom from distraction, or divided attention. With improvement of the psychopathology, patients can focus better and show improved performance on such tests. It is likely the improvement in this aspect of cognitive function that is most noticeable to patients who improve with ECT and probably is driving the subjective reports of improved memory performance with ECT shown in some studies (as discussed later in this chapter). Thus, as part of the consent process, patients can be rightly told that it is quite possible they may feel mentally sharper and more "tuned in" to their environment (e.g., conversations, work duties) with a course of ECT treatments.

In this chapter, the effects of ECT on memory will be divided into postictal disorientation, anterograde amnesia, retrograde amnesia, and impairment of subjective memory function. Other sections will cover the nonmemory cognitive effects of ECT, cognition in patients undergoing MECT, and recommendations for clinical practice monitoring of cognition.

Postictal Disorientation

For the purposes of patient education and research on the cognitive aspects of ECT, acute disorientation following each treatment has been treated as qualitatively distinct from anterograde and retrograde amnesias. In fact, all three of these issues are probably continuous aspects of the brain's memory system. That is, from the point at which a relatively specific memory is formed, there are changes over time in the likelihood of recall that may be conceptualized as acute disorientation, anterograde amnesia, or retrograde amnesia depending on how much time has elapsed from incident to testing and whatever kinds of interventions have taken place in between.

Postictal orientation is a relatively straightforward cognitive function to quantify. After the seizure terminates, the anesthetic medication effect wears off and the patient starts breathing. Reaction to verbal stimuli initially consists of turning the head in the direction of the patient's name being called out, perhaps with eye opening. Eventually, the patient can answer questions about orientation to place or time; this typically occurs after a few minutes or so, though the time it takes to become oriented is highly variable depending on the ECT technique. In ECT research, postictal orientation has been measured in two ways. One way is to have a staff member stand at the patient's side in the post-anesthesia recovery area and continually ask orientation questions such as "What is your name?" or "What is the location of this facility?" and so forth. When a predetermined proportion of the questions are answered correctly, the patient is said to have reached "oriented" status, and the time to reach this state is recorded. Thus, time to orientation can be compared among different ECT techniques, such as electrode placement or stimulus parameter variations.

The other method of assessing postictal orientation is to assess degree of orientation at a fixed time period after the seizure stops. For example, a 10-question orientation questionnaire has been used that is administered at 20 minutes postseizure (Kellner et al. 2010). This method has successfully differentiated degree of orientation among different ECT groups (Kellner et al. 2010). The advantage of this method over the time-to-orientation method is that a dedicated staff member doing nothing but paying attention to that patient is not needed. One can easily have ECT recovery nurses perform the battery of questions at 20 minutes without impairing their ability to monitor other patients.

Sobin et al. (1995) and Martin et al. (2013) found that longer time to orientation correlated with greater retrograde amnesia after cessation of treatments. Theoretically, this may be useful in clinical practice. Presumably, if a particular patient takes a very long time to become oriented after a treatment, then ECT technique can be altered to lessen the delay, such as switching from bilateral to unilateral electrode placement, changing from thrice- to twice-weekly frequency, lowering the electrical dosage, or shortening the pulse width. Whether this strategy actually works and enhances clinical outcomes in terms of memory without compromising efficacy is yet to be tested. Also, in the Kellner et al. (2010) study, postictal orientation did not correlate with retrograde amnesia.

The Columbia University Consortium has found that time to orientation is longer for bitemporal electrode placement as well as for longer pulse widths (Sackeim et al. 1993, 2000, 2008). In another report of electrode placement and ECT outcome, however, there was no benefit to right unilateral placement for postictal orientation compared with bitemporal or bifrontal placements (Kellner et al. 2010). In that study, degree of orientation was assessed at 20 minutes postseizure, with the score on a 10-item orientation questionnaire used as a way to quantify orientation.

More factors than ECT electrode placement or electrical stimulus impact postictal orientation, such as neurological illness, concomitant medications, or type of anesthetic medication and dosage utilized. Furthermore, in the studies cited above, there was a lot of variability in postictal orientation times, so one piece of data in a single patient may not be too helpful in planning future technique. Thus, postictal orientation speed may not necessarily provide much useful clinical information in routine ECT practice.

Anterograde Amnesia

Anterograde amnesia refers to the inability to recall newly learned information at a later time point. For example, if a patient receiving ECT watches a television show one evening and then the next day cannot recall it, that would be an example of anterograde amnesia. Anterograde amnesia is fairly easily assessed and quantified with standardized materials, if it is assumed, of course, that one has trained personnel available to perform them with patients. This usually requires a special research grant, as most typical personnel (e.g., doctors and nurses) are too busy with other tasks to administer these tests. The paradigm for anterograde amnesia testing in ECT research consists of three steps: presentation of information, assessment of immediate recall (registration), and assessment of recall at a delayed interval, the latter being anywhere typically from half an hour to 24 hours (Squire and Miller 1974). The crux of the issue is to test how much of the material that was registered is recalled at the delay interval. The presented information consists of either verbal or nonverbal material. The former can be simple word lists, in which case a list of words is provided one or more times. Another common verbal stimulus is called *paired associate learning*, in which case a series of pairs of words is provided and testing is performed by providing the first word of each pair to see if the patient can recall the word it was paired with. Finally, the verbal stimulus can be in the form of information, such as a story told to the patient, to test how many elements of the story can be recalled. As far as nonverbal stimulus materials go, a commonly used test is the Rey-Osterrieth Complex Figure Test (Lu et al. 2003), which is a complex geometric figure the patient must first copy and then try to recall later on. The advantage of this test is that it is very commonly used in neuropsychology and has well-established norms available for comparison. Other nonverbal stimulus materials include pictures of faces to be recalled later on.

In anterograde amnesia testing, after the delay interval transpires, testing can consist of *free recall*, in which case the patient is asked to recall the stimulus materials without any prompting or cues, or *recognition*, in which case cues are provided (e.g., multiple-choice questions in which the correct answer must be picked from a set of choices). Generally, patients perform better with cued recognition tasks than with free-recall tasks.

The assessment of anterograde amnesia is much more standardized than that for retrograde amnesia, especially regarding autobiographical memory. The challenge in routine care is finding personnel who have the time and training to administer stimulus materials such as word lists, paired associates, or geometric figures; establish immediate recall; and then retest after a delay interval. Furthermore, the literature provides no formal guidance on what to do with the information obtained (Rasmussen 2016). Asking patients on rounds about events of the day before is easy—if they have forgotten, then establishment of significant anterograde amnesia has occurred. Simple reassurance that this will clear up after ECT is finished may be all that is needed. If the forgetting of recent events seems disconcerting or profound, then alteration of technique can be considered.

In contrast to retrograde amnesia, anterograde amnesia is much easier for the researcher or clinician to test and quantify. Rather than guessing at what autobiographical data, public events, and knowledge a patient may have forgotten after ECT, with anterograde amnesia testing, the researcher can provide information to be recalled and then test for recall of that information later with a high degree of specificity. The ability to register new information, as manifested by essentially immediate recall of such information, is a reflection more of focus and concentration than of other memory functions and correlates with severity of depression. In other words, depressed patients tend to have poor focus and cannot learn as much information for immediate recall. On the other hand, the ability to recall newly learned information after a delay interval is normal with depressive patients and is impaired by ECT. Rather unequivocally, long-term testing has shown that there is no permanent effect of a course of ECT on anterograde memory function (Semkovska and McLoughlin 2010; Semkovska et al. 2011; Verwijk et al. 2014), with anterograde memory difficulties induced by ECT usually clearing within a few days of the last treatment. Many studies in these two reviews included in-depth assessments of anterograde amnesia and invariably found them to be temporary, although in the acute post-ECT period there is measurable deficit compared with baseline that tends to be greater with bitemporal electrode placement and less with ultrabrief pulse width. Nonverbal material is forgotten to a greater extent than verbal for right unilateral ECT (Squire and Slater 1978). In one study of unilateral, bitemporal, and bifrontal placement, bifrontal fared the best in terms of anterograde memory function (Lawson et al. 1990), but this difference was not replicated by Kellner et al. (2010), who found no cognitive advantage to bifrontal placement.

From the standpoint of clinical care and patient education, it is appropriate to broach the subject of anterograde amnesia with patients when they are in the first week or two after the course of treatments (in addition to during the consent process, of course). Typically, at this stage, patients are feeling better from a depression standpoint and are eager to get back to typical life activities but might not be aware that they are not able to hold onto new information such as that related to work duties. Thus, a convalescent period for a week or so after ECT is completed is appropriate to let the anterograde amnesia clear up before the patient goes back to work. This period can be individualized on a case-by-case basis depending on how severe the anterograde amnesia is and what type of activities are required. For example, if a patient has a job requiring procedural memory—that is, a repetitive task highly learned—then that would not be as hard to go back to after ECT as a job requiring learning and retaining new information, such as teaching.

Retrograde Amnesia

The topic of retrograde amnesia is the most important of all the memory-related issues in ECT practice. Most patients are not bothered by postictal disorientation or even temporary anterograde amnesia. It is loss of memories for events and knowledge that leads to the most complaints from ECT patients. Before we review the literature on this, it is instructive to provide a brief overview of different types of memory for past events. Memory types are generally divided into declarative and procedural, or explicit versus implicit, respectively. *Declarative*, or *explicit*, *memory* refers to events or information that can be "declared," so to speak, in an explicit way. Declarative memory is subdivided into episodic and semantic. *Episodic memory* refers to events experienced by the person, such as a vacation or social situations. The *semantic* type of declarative memory refers to knowledge about the world, such as answering history questions or questions about recent public events, or to information about the person that is not referable to a specific episode in his or her life (e.g., knowing one's date of birth or favorite restaurant to visit). Memory can also be divided into personal and impersonal. Personal memories are autobiographical and can be either episodic or semantic. Impersonal memories are all semantic (e.g., knowledge about public events or cultural information). Generally, people are more bothered by loss of personal than impersonal memories.

Procedural, or *implicit*, *memory* refers to a variety of types of memory in which the person has recalled a skill or association of a stimulus with a response; these cannot be explicitly described in an informational manner. One type of procedural memory is learned skills such as how to dress or drive a car. Other types include associative learning, such as classical or operant conditioning. Examples of *classical conditioning* include pairing a previously neutral stimulus with an unconditioned stimulus until the latter brings about the conditioned response. *Operant conditioning* refers to the shaping of behavior via pairing it with consequential positive or negative reinforcers. Nonassociative types of procedural memory include *habituation*, in which a stimulus initially brings about a response but fails to do so after repetition, and *sensitization*, in which a stimulus initially does not bring about a response but does so after repetition. In ECT research on retrograde amnesia, declarative memory has been studied most intensely.

There has been much research using various memory inventories or questionnaires. Sorely needed is to translate the research instruments to clinically useful tools, and this has not been done. Also needed are normative data on published questionnaires for clinicians to compare to their own patients' data in order to make informed decisions about what to do with an individual patient who is showing a given score on a given memory scale; again, this has largely not been done, so it is premature to recommend any specific autobiographical or personal/impersonal memory questionnaire at this time for routine clinical use.

Retrograde amnesia is the most difficult, but probably most important, of the various types of memory for ECT research. The three steps of stimulus presentation, immediate recall, and delayed recall are fundamentally the same as in testing for anterograde amnesia, but the first two steps are uncontrolled and nonstandardized. In other words, recall is being tested for the memories people have for their lives. These are unique to each person. For an investigator to assess recall of a person's memories, it must be known what those memories are at baseline. Investigators have used a variety of techniques to try and standardize research of autobiographical memories and knowledge. Of note, retrograde amnesia was detected shortly after the introduction of ECT in 1938. Flescher (1941) performed a crude examination of recall with ECT, the results of which are uninformative, but this report does demonstrate that in contrast to those who accuse psychiatry of ignoring the issue of retrograde amnesia with ECT, this in fact has been studied intensively for many decades.

The first in-depth data collection on retrograde amnesia in ECT was carried out by Janis (1950), who asked patients a detailed set of questions about recall of recent and remote life events before and then again after ECT. This has been the most common method of autobiographical memory assessment in ECT research and will be reviewed below. Typical questions in this paradigm include "What is the name of your first school?" and "What is the name of the last restaurant you visited?" As one can imagine, there are many such questions about all phases of life, from childhood up until the last few weeks. The disadvantage is that experiences are not shared by all people (e.g., not everybody goes to restaurants or went to school). Additionally, the accuracy of recall even before ECT may be questionable.

Another technique of retrograde amnesia assessment is to test the patient's recall of impersonal material, such as public events, famous people, or knowledge of television shows. The advantage of this technique is that tests can be constructed that have right and wrong answers (e.g., asking which of the following was a real television show with four choices provided). The disadvantage, as before, is that some people do not follow public events or watch television much.

The final method of retrograde memory testing used in ECT research consists of presenting material to patients prior to commencing treatments and then testing recall or recognition at a later time. The advantage of such testing is that information is standard across patients, but the disadvantage is that it only assesses for recently learned information—that is, information presented within a day or so of the first treatment. It is life memories going back farther periods of time that are more precious to people. That is, most patients are not bothered by forgetting word lists learned the morning of the first ECT treatment, which is a typical task in this form of retrograde amnesia testing paradigm.

Despite these difficulties, several investigative groups over the decades have studied retrograde amnesia and have reported some interesting findings, to be discussed below. The problem with this type of testing is translating this time-consuming and nonstandardized type of testing into methods that are clinically useful.

It is likely that we forget much of our lives. Can very many people recall what they were doing exactly 1 year ago to the day? Probably most people cannot, unless something really significant happened that day (e.g., marriage, childbirth, death of a loved one). More precisely, it can be said, if one doesn't recall that day, that time as a cue is not causing one to remember. Perhaps if somebody mentions a conversation that occurred that day, then that may be enough of a cue to give one the feeling of truly remembering that event. Thus, in day-to-day life, when confronted with so-called forgetting of a personal event, perhaps the memory of that event still exists in the brain; it is just that one has not encountered the right cue to allow recall. It is likely that the recent memories that get forgotten with ECT are probably not gone from the brain, but rather, that the available cues to allow recall have been lessened. Patients who have had ECT may recall a forgotten memory if the right cue is presented, such as by a family member who was present at the time of the event in question. Thus, if a patient seems distressed that an event occurred that others are talking about which the patient cannot recall, then exploration of as many details as possible might lead to recall.

An exercise for the reader: try and recall as many of your life events of the 1-month period preceding the reading of this passage. You probably can recall many events (e.g., going to a movie or a restaurant, conversations with people, small trips around where you live). Now try and recall the same 1-month period (i.e., same time of year) 2 years ago, or 3 years or more. You probably cannot recall any events unless something really noteworthy happened in your life (e.g., marriage, birth of child, death of loved one, new job, purchase of a house). Yet, most do not complain about this or do not seem bothered by it. However, if you happened to have ECT and at the time perceived a loss of (then recent) events, you may carry with you in your ongoing conscious view of yourself that you "have a blank" for that period, even though almost everybody has a similar "blank." In large part, ECT causes forgetting of recent events that ultimately will be forgotten anyway, but because it causes that forgetting relatively soon after the events occur, amnesia sensitivity sets in. ECT patients, sensitized by some forgetting of recent events, may focus in an exaggerated manner on any aspect of their entire life they cannot immediately recall and inappropriately blame the "forgetting" on ECT. This phenomenon will be discussed in greater detail later in this chapter.

There are a few other interesting points to be noted about life memories and retrograde amnesia. When a patient suffers a traumatic brain injury, recent memories tend to be forgotten while older memories remain intact, a phenomenon known as *Ribot's law*. The same is true in ECT retrograde amnesia—that is, recent memories, say, memories of the last 6 months, tend to be forgotten more than more remote memories (Squire et al. 1975b). This is useful information to provide patients during the pretreatment ECT education and consent phase. Often, patients have been so miserable and depressed lately that the prospect of forgetting recent events may not be frightening to them.

Memories that have been forgotten can be relearned even if not re-remembered. That is, if one forgets a vacation, a third party can recite the facts of the vacation so that they are now known, but one still may not remember them. In other words, one now *knows* what happened without *remembering*. This essentially means that information that formerly was recalled as part of episodic memory now is recalled as part of semantic memory.

With the passage of time, most memories fade. Thus, in an ECT study, if psychiatrically healthy control volunteers or non-ECT psychiatric control patients are followed over time, it will be found that many of the recent memories forgotten by the ECT group will eventually be forgotten by the non-ECT control group. Few studies have gone out beyond 6 months for recall. It is likely that if an ECT group and non-ECT control group are followed far beyond that time—say, 1 or 2 years—the memories of the 6-month time period prior to initial testing will be quite similar.

Squire and Slater (1975) studied recognition of television shows and famous racehorses in control patients and amply demonstrated what is intuitively obvious: recall for recent events is much better than for remote events. However, with conditions causing retrograde amnesia, such as ECT or temporal lobectomy, remote recall is much more resistant to alteration than recent recall (or at least, over time the number of cues that lead to recall is reduced). Probably over time, memories are processed either at the cellular level or at the system level in the brain (e.g., transfer from the hippocampus to the cortex), and those that remain are resistant to insult.

Because the forgetting of personal and impersonal memories is bothersome, literature on this important topic will be reviewed. The first type of methodology to be discussed is the presentation of standardized material to patients prior to ECT with testing of recall at a later time. Lancaster et al. (1958), in a landmark study comparing bilateral and unilateral electrode placement, presented patients with a sentence just prior to an ECT treatment and then tested recall a few minutes after the treatment. Although statistics are not presented, nor is quantification of degree of recall, it is mentioned that most of the unilaterally treated patients could recall the sentence, whereas almost none of the bilaterally treated patients could recall it. A systematic series of studies with this methodology was conducted by a group of Swedish investigators in the late 1950s and early 1960s, headed by Borje Cronholm and Jan-Otto Ottosson. In their paradigm, the information presented consisted of three tests: word pairs, figures, and story-type information. They would assess immediate and 6-hour delayed recall the day before ECT to get a baseline and then retest using different versions of the stimulus materials the day of the first ECT treatment whereby stimulus presentation occurred shortly before the treatment and recall was 6 hours after the treatment. In one such study (Ottosson 1960), there were four groups: high-electrical-dose bilateral, usual-dose bilateral, usual-dose bilateral with lidocaine added as a seizure-shortening maneuver, and anesthesia only. Results showed that high-electrical-dose bilateral ECT treatment caused greater forgetting of the material than did usual-dose bilateral technique, which in turn was associated with greater forgetting than usual dose modified with lidocaine (all of which caused greater forgetting than simple anesthesia without a seizure induced). The investigators concluded that both electrical dose and seizure length contributed to the cognitive impairment of ECT. In another of these investigators' studies utilizing this methodology (Cronholm and Ottosson 1961), the treatments consisted of the ECT stimulus as usual versus the ECT stimulus along with what was called a "countershock" (an extra electrical stimulus presented after the one that induced the seizure). There had been a theory that use of "countershock" may actually lessen ECT-induced memory impairment. The results showed that there was no such effect and that in fact the countershock may have only worsened the memory impairment of ECT. Finally, Cronholm and Ottosson (1963a, 1963b), in an early study of ultrabrief-pulse-width technique (in fact, these investigators coined the expression "ultrabrief"), compared forgetting using the same three tests described above at the same time points in three groups: ECT as usual (a modified sine-wave stimulus), a 0.1-millisecond ultrabrief pulse stimulus, and the modified sine-wave stimulus with lidocaine to shorten seizure length. Those patients treated with the ultrabrief stimulus had less forgetting of the material presented just prior to treatments than did patients in the other two groups, who had about the same level of forgetting. This was the first scientific demonstration of lower retrograde amnesia with ultrabrief electrical pulses.

Daniel et al. (1982, 1983) have also studied retrograde amnesia for stimulus materials presented just prior to treatments. In two small trials comparing unilateral versus bilateral and sine-wave versus brief-pulse ECT (thus, four treatment groups), stimulus materials consisting of either verbal or nonverbal material were presented just prior to treatments 5 or 6 in a series, and then retesting occurred 24 hours after the treatment. In both trials, there were clear main effects for both electrode placement and stimulus waveform (bilaterally and sine-wave-treated patients recalled less). More recently, O'Connor et al. (2008) used this method and found that recognition of faces and names taught just before ECT was better than free recall. Recall of stories taught just before ECT, tested after the course of treatments was finished, did not change. Interestingly, there was no difference between patients given only unilateral versus those started on unilateral and switched to bilateral placement, though the sample sizes were quite small (11 in each group).

The Columbia University Consortium has presented similarly collected memory testing (i.e., recall for materials presented just prior to a treatment) in addition to other cognitive data. Their results in several well-controlled trials have been quite consistent: bitemporally treated patients recall less of this material than unilaterally treated patients, and ultrabrief pulse width (0.3 milliseconds vs. 1.5 milliseconds) is associated with more recall (Sackeim et al. 1986, 1993, 2000, 2008). In summary, the literature on retrograde amnesia for standardized materials presented just prior to treatment clearly indicates that patients treated with an interspersed ECT treatment often forget substantial amounts of this material and that bilateral electrode placement and longer stimulus pulse widths are associated with greater forgetting. However, most patients are not bothered by forgetting this type of material, namely, incidental information that occurs close to the course of treatments. It is the forgetting of other types of memories—namely, personal life events as well as knowledge about the world—that may be bothersome, and it is this literature that is now reviewed.

Janis (1950) first attempted a systematic study of the effects of ECT on autobiographical memory. He developed a method that has been used by numerous investigative groups in the decades since that time—namely, the questioning about personal memories such as vacations, schools attended, addresses, and relationships. Like some other investigators since, he did not actually publish the list of questions he used, making precise replication impossible. Nonetheless, in a sample of mostly schizophrenia patients, he recorded baseline memories before ECT as well as in non-ECT control patients. The ECT patients were given bilateral sinewave electrical stimuli, with a mean of 17 treatments, which is an aggressive course of treatments. Follow-up testing with the same questions was repeated 4 weeks after termination of ECT and again 2–3 months after ECT. In the non-ECT control group, testing was repeated at roughly similar time points. In the non-ECT group, repeat testing showed the patients giving essentially the same answers as at baseline. The ECT-treated patients clearly had forgotten some of the events they provided at baseline, but importantly, they recalled more than they forgot. Thus, there was no evidence, despite aggressive treatment, of a "blank period" in memory being induced by ECT. Ribot's law was followed, in that recent events were more likely to be forgotten than more remote events. Finally, at the 2- to 3-month follow-up interview, much (though not all) that had been forgotten at the 4-week time point was recalled. Interestingly, a review of essentially all the retrograde amnesia literature that has followed in the decades since the Janis (1950) report confirms these essential findings: acute reductions in memory for life events and knowledge acutely after ECT, but no "blanking out" of memory (rather, memory loss is spotty); measurable improvement on follow-up some months later; and Ribot's law being followed. The only thing that has been added since Janis's study is looking at the differential effect of various ECT technical modifications on the degree of acute forgetting.

Stieper et al. (1951) studied 12 schizophrenia patients receiving ECT (mean number of treatments was 15) and 12 non-ECT-treated schizophrenia patients. Patients were administered a 40-item personal memory questionnaire (20 items of recent events and 20 of remote events) before ECT and 3 weeks after ECT, and at similar time points for the non-ECT control patients. The ECT-treated patients had a reduction in identical answers and more "I don't know" answers than the controls, though there was no clear temporal gradient. The small sample sizes undoubtedly lowered the sensitivity of the study.

Strain et al. (1968) and Bidder et al. (1970) reported on a group of 46 unilateral and a group of 50 bitemporal electrode placement patients treated with ECT who were administered a "personal data sheet" consisting of 50 questions about autobiographical events. Over the course of treatments, the interview questions were repeated. At 36 hours after the last treatment, there were reductions in answers consistent with baseline, a bit more so in the bitemporal patients and more so for recent events versus remote events. Ten days after the last treatment, there was no difference in scores between unilateral and bitemporal patients; scores in both groups had improved since the 36-hour post–last testing, but in neither group were the scores back to pre-ECT baseline levels. Weeks et al. (1980), utilizing 28 items from the battery used by Strain et al. (1968), studied 15 right unilateral and 36 bitemporal ECT patients along with non-ECT depressed and nondepressed normal control patients (the latter at time intervals similar to those used with the ECT patients). Testing sessions were conducted at baseline, 1 week after the last ECT treatment, 3 months afterward, and 6 months afterward. At 3 and 6 months, there was no difference in the autobiographical memory performance among all the groups. However, at 3 months, the ECT patients were less able to recognize recent (vs. remote) famous faces than the non-ECT-treated patients. This study employed not only unilateral and bilateral electrode placement ECT groups but also two control groups of non-ECT-treated subjects: depressed and nondepressed. This was an influential study in providing evidence that ECT does not seem to cause a permanent loss of personal memories.

The study of retrograde amnesia caused by ECT was greatly enhanced by a series of studies led by Professor Larry Squire and colleagues in the 1970s and 1980s. In their first study (Squire 1974), 20 depressed patients treated with bitemporal sine-wave stimulation were compared with 20 control volunteers. The memory test consisted of 50 multiple-choice questions about public events covering the three previous decades. ECT patients were tested about an hour after either treatment number 1 or 5, and their scores were compared with those of the control volunteers. Patients had lower scores for all decades, especially after treatment number 5. In this data set, there was no evidence of a temporal gradient in memory—that is, of forgetting recent events more so than remote events. In the next study from this group (Squire 1975), the test subjects were the same as those in the above-referenced study, only data from testing 24 hours after the first or fifth treatment were presented, with the results being the same at the 1-day mark versus 1 hour after the treatments. Squire et al. (1975a) administered multiple-choice tests covering television shows from previous decades to bilaterally sine-wave-treated ECT patients at baseline before treatment and then 1 hour after ECT treatment number 5 and then again 1–2 weeks after the last treatment. The investigators found that scores dropped at the 1-hour post–treatment number 5 from baseline only for recent shows but returned to pre-ECT levels by 2 weeks post-treatment. This provided evidence of the temporal gradient of forgetting. Squire and Chace (1975) studied patients given right unilateral sine-wave ECT, patients given bitemporal sine-wave ECT, and non-ECT control patients. Testing was for television show recall at baseline and 6–9 months after ECT. At the final testing session, there were no differences among the three groups in test scores. However, a subset of bitemporally treated patients were tested 1 hour after treatment number 5 and were found to have lower scores than at baseline. Squire et al. (1976) studied 20 patients given bitemporal sine-wave ECT and 30 control volunteers. Testing was for memory of television shows of recent decades and was performed at baseline, 1 hour after the fifth treatment, and 12 days after the last treatment. A temporal gradient of forgetting, mostly of recent shows, was demonstrated. Of note, the 12-day post–ECT session was probably too early to allow full return of memory. Squire and Cohen (1979) assessed bitemporal sine-wave-treated ECT patients for recall of as many facts as they could pertaining to television shows from different eras. Time of testing was at baseline prior to the first ECT treatment and 1 hour after the fifth treatment. The number of facts recalled per show went down, but only for relatively recent shows, once again confirming the temporal gradient of ECT-induced retrograde amnesia.

Squire et al. (1981) assessed patients treated with bilateral, sine-wave ECT using a battery of questions regarding public events, television shows, and personal events conducted at baseline, after ECT treatment number 5, and at 1 week and 7 months post-treatment. All of the impersonal memories seemed to be recovered by 7 months. For personal events, all except for memory of very recent events were recovered by 7 months. The only decrement in memory detected at 7 months was recall for personal events, especially those in the days preceding commencement of ECT. Thus, the temporal gradient (Ribot's law) was confirmed in this study. In summary, these studies conducted by Larry Squire and colleagues, utilizing the creative tests of recall of television shows as well as personal information, reveal that by several months after the end of a course of even bitemporal sine-wave ECT, scores are largely back to baseline, except for recall of recent personal events close to the time of ECT. Of note, the test for television shows could not assess very recent impersonal data, as television shows were not learned in the days and weeks preceding ECT. In other words, the tests of impersonal memories were probably insensitive to very recently learned data and thus could not assess this area of retrograde memory function.

A group led by Dr. Richard Weiner at Duke University published a series of studies in the 1980s that outlined the retrograde memory function advantage of brief-pulse, square-wave electrical stimulation versus sine-wave stimulation as well as unilateral versus bilateral electrode placement. Two of these studies (Daniel et al. 1982, 1983) were described earlier in this chapter and dealt with recall of information provided just before ECT treatments. In a more extensive data set examining memory for personal and impersonal information, Weiner et al. (1982, 1986) randomly allocated ECT patients to receive unilateral or bitemporal electrode placement and sine-wave or brief-pulse waveform. A non-ECT control group was also included. The investigators developed questions about personal and public events and tested at baseline, 2–3 days after the last treatment, and 6 months later. At 2–3 days after last treatment session, there were significant main effects of waveform (sine-wave causing more forgetting than brief-pulse) and electrode placement (bitemporal causing more forgetting than right unilateral). At 6 months, there was substantial recovery of memories, with the bitemporally treated patients still scoring lower than the unilaterally treated patients. Interestingly, the non-ECT control subjects forgot 25% of the baseline information at the second session (which was acute post-ECT for the treated patients), in comparison to 45% forgetting for the brief-pulse bitemporal patients and 20% for the brief-pulse unilateral patients. Thus, these data underscore the fact that not all forgetting in ECT-treated patients can be attributed to the treatments, and most of the baseline information is in fact not forgotten, at least for brief-pulse-treated patients (the bitemporal sine-wave patients had forgetting scores in the acute post-ECT period of 60%). At 6 months, the bitemporal, brief-pulse patients had forgetting scores of 30% in comparison to 18% for the unilateral brief-pulse patients and 17% for the controls. Thus, there is evidence from this well-controlled trial that bitemporal ECT can cause long-lasting (i.e., duration of at least 6 months) recall deficits for personal and impersonal information. However, this effect is relatively small in comparison to normal controls, and still, most baseline information is remembered. Thus, there is no evidence of a "memory wipeout" from ECT.

Another highly significant and influential series of studies has been led by Professor Harold Sackeim and associates at Columbia University. The therapeutic aspects of these studies and the implications for electrode placement and stimulus dosing in clinical practice from that standpoint have been discussed in Chapters 6 and 7. Discussed here are the tests for retrograde memory function performed as part of these studies. These investigators introduced two autobiographical memory tests, the details of which have been published. The first was called the Autobiographical Memory Interview (McElhiney et al. 1995), which consisted of 281 items and typically took several hours to perform. Because of the unwieldy nature of this tedious instrument, the Columbia group developed the Autobiographical Memory Interview—Short Form (McElhiney et al. 2001), which consisted of 30 questions. These are abbreviated as the Columbia AMI and Columbia AMI-SF, respectively, henceforth. These instruments have no norms established and are not copyrighted or commercially available, though they can be downloaded from the internet.

There have been six trials by the Columbia University Consortium using either of these autobiographical memory instruments: the comparison of low-electrical-dose unilateral versus bitemporal electrode placement ECT (Sackeim et al. 1987a); the comparison of low- and moderately high-dose, with either unilateral or bitemporal placement (Sackeim et al. 1993); the comparison of three doses of unilateral with one high-dose bitemporal placement (Sackeim et al. 2000); the large-scale naturalistic trial involving ECT patients treated in several New York area hospitals (Prudic et al. 2004; Sackeim et al. 2007); the ultrabrief stimulus dose trial (Sackeim et al. 2008); and the OPT-ECT acute-phase trial, comparing unilateral and bitemporal placements along with placebo, venlafaxine, or nortriptyline cotreatment (Sackeim et al. 2009). As indicated, each of these primarily therapeutic efficacy studies used extensive cognitive batteries, the results of which for retrograde amnesia have been summarized primarily in 10 publications and will be reviewed below.

Data from the first Columbia trial (low-electrical-dose unilateral versus low-dose bitemporal) were already discussed earlier in this chapter with regard to greater forgetting of information provided just prior to bitemporal ECT than with unilateral ECT (Sackeim et al. 1986). The second trial compared low and moderate dose with both unilateral and bitemporal ECT (thus, four treatment groups) (Sackeim et al. 1993). In this trial, the Columbia group introduced the AMI long form (e.g., vacations taken, major gift purchases, restaurants or movies attended). The interview was conducted at baseline before ECT and then repeated at later time points, such as during a course of treatments and thereafter. At these later interviews, the patients were only questioned about items they had been able to give a positive response to at baseline. For example, if at baseline a patient is not able to recite the name of any restaurant visited, then that patient would not be asked about restaurants at later assessment points. The percentage of baseline items that are responded to in the same way is taken as the "memory score" for later assessments; alternatively, the percentage of questions yielding a different answer from baseline is taken as the "forgetting score" in some of their studies. In the study by Sackeim et al. (1993), the AMI was repeated the day after a treatment in about the middle of the course of ECT and then again 1 week and 2 months after the series was completed. At the 1-week interval, the memory score—that is, the percentage of baseline items recalled correctly after ECT—was 66% for low-dose bitemporal, 76% for high-dose bitemporal, 81% for low-dose unilateral, and 82% for high-dose unilateral ECT. There was a significant main effect for electrode placement, with the bitemporally treated patients obviously faring worse. However, it is also clear that the majority of items are still recalled just 1 week after ECT, and the absolute difference between the two electrode placements seems rather small (i.e., 76% for high-dose bitemporal as compared with 81% for low-dose unilateral). As for the 2-month testing point, the authors mention "no change" versus the baseline scores but do not provide specific data.

In a further elaboration of data obtained from this study, McElhiney et al. (1995) included data from 16 nondepressed control volunteers who were administered the AMI at time points coincident with baseline pre-ECT, 1 week post-ECT, and 2 months post-ECT for the ECT patients. Interestingly, at the baseline testing session, depressed patients gave 11.5% fewer answers to personal memory questions on the AMI than did nondepressed volunteers, demonstrating the effect of severe depression on memory to begin with. At the post-ECT testing sessions, there was no correlation of percentage of items recalled with depression ratings, and this indicates a dissociation of retrograde memory from antidepressant efficacy of ECT. Information that at baseline was corroborated by family members was more resistant to forgetting than information that could not be corroborated. If patients did not respond well to their first treatment assignment (something that happened more often with unilaterally than with bilaterally treated patients) and had crossover treatments with high-dose bitemporal ECT, then their performance at 2 months on recall was worse than that of patients who had responded well to the first course of treatments. This is a very important finding, for if a given electrode placement–stimulus dose combination tends to cause less memory impairment than other combinations but is less therapeutically effective, then a certain percentage of patients given that combination in fact will go on to do worse than all other treatment groups if they need a more aggressive repeat course of treatments. In other words, one must temper one's optimism about a presumably "memory sparing" technique of ECT if an unacceptable percentage of patients do not respond to it and need a second course of higher-electrical-dose bitemporal treatments.

In yet another analysis of data from this trial, Sobin et al. (1995) found that baseline global cognitive function negatively correlated with later forgetting scores on the AMI (in other words, poorer baseline cognition predicted greater forget-ting with ECT) and also that the longer it took patients to recover orientation im-mediately after a treatment, the greater the forgetting on the AMI. The latter thus provides a relatively easy-to-measure clinical variable that may act as a proxy for later memory impairment and that could potentially be incorporated into clinical decision making. Sobin et al. (1995) also presented the 1-week post-ECT scores for percentage of baseline items for which patients later gave different answers (either "I don't know" or an answer different from baseline) and found no effect of stimulus dosing but greater inconsistency with bitemporal ECT. Thus, a sum-mary of the data from this trial indicates that by 2 months post-ECT, scores on the AMI are back to baseline and do not substantially differ between unilateral and bitemporal electrode placement. Also, most memories are in fact recalled, even at 1 week post-ECT, and the differences at that time point between uni-lateral and bitemporal placement are statistically, but not necessarily clinically, significant.

The final report with retrograde amnesia testing from the Sackeim et al. (1993) trial comparing low- and moderate-dose and unilateral and bitemporal electrode placement was provided by Lisanby et al. (2000). In this complex paper, the authors described a memory instrument separate from the AMI—namely, the Personal and Impersonal Memory Test (PIMT). In the PIMT, infor-mation is solicited from patients and classified as personal (i.e., gifts, illnesses, purchases, trips, and restaurants visited) versus impersonal (i.e., births or deaths related to famous people, political events, publicized court cases, natural disasters, other news stories). Detailed interviewing is conducted to ask patients about a variety of recent and remote personal and impersonal events from these catego-ries, and patients are asked to give as many details as they can recall for one per-sonal and one impersonal event per category, both recent and remote. It is similar to Janis's (1950) methodology only with provisions for quantification and scoring of results. After ECT, the same set of questions is asked, and the an-swers are compared with the baseline answers to check for consistency. The post-ECT testing sessions were conducted 1 week and 2 months after the last treat-ment. The main finding of the study was that recent events are more likely to be forgotten than remote events, and impersonal events are more likely to be forgot-ten than personal ones. At the 2-month post-ECT testing session, the only linger-ing impairment in memory compared with baseline testing was for (especially recent) impersonal events for bitemporally treated patients. Further, the lesser the emotional salience attached to a memory—that is, the less "compelling" the memory for an event is—the more likely it is to be forgotten. This lends support to the contention that in large measure, it is information that eventually will be forgotten anyway that is forgotten with ECT.

The next trial from the Columbia Consortium regarding ECT compared three electrical doses of unilateral electrode placement (1.5, 2.5, and 6 times threshold) with one moderately high dose of bitemporal placement (2.5 times threshold) (Sackeim et al. 2000). In that trial, retrograde amnesia testing was performed at baseline before ECT, the day after the sixth or seventh treatment, a day or two after the last treatment in the series, and 2 months later. Regarding more remote information, the AMI was used as well as a test of public events for the three preceding decades. Though scores were not provided, the authors reported poorer recall of data with bitemporal than with even high-dose unilateral electrode placement.

The next large data set collection from the Columbia group consisted of naturalistically following ECT patients at several New York area hospitals (Sackeim et al. 2007). In this very large data set, the AMI-SF was utilized to collect autobiographical data. This instrument involves standardized questions about various time points in a person's life, going back to childhood. As noted earlier, it is much quicker to administer than their previously used AMI long form, which is very time-consuming and enervating for both subjects and technicians administering it. Testing for this trial occurred at baseline and at 1 week and 6 months after ECT. At 6 months, scores were slightly down for those patients treated with bitemporal brief-pulse-width ECT, while the scores were better for those given brief-pulse unilateral ECT. As with several other of the above-mentioned trials, scores were down from baseline at the 1-week interval but substantially improved by 6 months, indicating recovery of at least some memory during that time.

The next controlled ECT trial from the Columbia group was their investigation of the therapeutic and cognitive aspects of ultrabrief-pulse-width ECT (Sackeim et al. 2008). In that trial, depressed patients were randomly allocated to receive unilateral or bitemporal electrode placement with either a "standard" pulse width of 1.5 milliseconds or an "ultrabrief" pulse width of 0.3 milliseconds. Meanwhile, to control for total electrical dose, the investigators modified the stimulus parameters of train duration and pulse frequency accordingly. Retrograde amnesia testing was conducted at baseline, during the week after the last treatment, and 2 and 6 months later. The testing consisted of the Columbia AMI-SF as well as tests of recall of famous people and events from different decades. Interestingly, both unilaterally and bitemporally treated ultrabrief-pulse patients had virtually no evidence of retrograde amnesia at 2 and 6 months after treatment and, for the unilateral ultrabrief-pulse group, during the week after the last treatment. For the standard-pulse-width groups, the scores at 2 and 6 months were slightly lower than at baseline but equal compared with each other. In fact, the effect of pulse width was so strong that autobiographical testing after completion of ECT showed that the ultrabrief-pulse bitemporally treated patients fared better than did the standard-pulse-width unilaterally treated patients. This is the only controlled trial in the annals of ECT research showing better autobiographical memory performance by a bitemporally treated versus a unilaterally treated group. The caveat, as with earlier data from this group, is that patients not responding to the initial randomized treatment and subsequently crossed over to standard-pulse-width treatment fared the worst of all for autobiographical memory.

The final ECT trial data to date from the Columbia group concern randomization to either unilateral 6 times threshold or bitemporal 2.5 times threshold treatment, all using standard pulse width, and to concurrent pharmacotherapy with placebo, venlafaxine, or nortriptyline (thus, six treatment groups in all). The purpose of the trial, discussed in Chapters 7 and 8, was to see if adding antidepressant medication to ECT enhanced acute remission rates or lessened post-ECT relapse rates. The Columbia AMI-SF was used to assess autobiographical memory and was administered at baseline and a few days after the last treatment. Performance was slightly worse just after ECT with bitemporal placement compared with unilateral placement. Additionally, interestingly, the groups treated with nortriptyline performed significantly better than did the other four groups. This finding is counterintuitive, as nortriptyline has substantial anticholinergic activity, which usually is implicated in worsening, rather than improving, memory function.

In summary, the Columbia University Consortium has published extensively analyzed data on various aspects of retrograde amnesia associated with ECT. General findings are that acutely (in the week or so after the end of a course of ECT), performance on tests of retrograde amnesia shows decrements that are relatively slight—in other words, patients tend to recall more than they have forgotten and there is no evidence of a "wiping out" of recent memory. Also, these effects tend to be exaggerated for bitemporal electrode placement as well as with long electrical pulse width. By several months post-treatment, the acute effects are largely, though not necessarily completely, abated, with a greater chance for continued amnesia in bitemporally treated groups. The information most likely to be forgotten concerns recent, impersonal events.

Some other groups have published findings of retrograde amnesia studies in ECT. McCall et al. (2002) compared depressed patients treated with 8 times threshold unilateral ECT versus 1.5 times threshold bitemporal placement, with both groups being treated with standard pulse width. Utilizing the Columbia AMI as described earlier in this chapter (McElhiney et al. 1995), the investigators tested patients at baseline, 1–3 days after the last treatment, and then again 2 and 4 weeks later. There was no difference in memory performance at any time point between the two groups, both of which showed a modest decrement immediately after ECT compared with baseline (i.e., retention scores of about 60%), with performance partially improving by 2 and 4 weeks (scores of about 74% of baseline).

Peretti et al. (1996) studied patients given bitemporal sine-wave ECT and compared them with a medication-only group. Test questions consisted of items pertaining to the reported symptoms of depression at baseline as well as events of the day of hospitalization. The ECT patients had lower scores at 1-week post-ECT compared with the medication-only patients. This is not a surprising result given how recent the to-be-recalled information was relative to the start of ECT treatment.

Williams et al. (1990) studied five groups of depressed patients: patients before and after a course of unilateral sine-wave ECT; normal control volunteers; non-ECT-treated patients whose depression had remitted; currently depressed non-ECT patients; and currently nondepressed patients who had completed ECT 6 months earlier. The testing consisted of 32 autobiographical memory items. The current ECT patients were tested pre- and 2 weeks post-ECT. All other groups were tested once. Scoring consisted of the number of items in which the patient could give an answer. For the current ECT patients, baseline score was a mean of 26, going down to 23 at 2 weeks after ECT. For the other four groups, the mean score was about 28–29. Thus, in this data set, results point to full return of memories within 6 months after ECT.

Calev et al. (1989) studied 16 bitemporally, brief-pulse-treated ECT patients and 10 imipramine-treated depressed patients. Retrograde memory testing was for famous events and personal events at baseline and a day after treatment number 7 (and the same time interval after starting imipramine in the medication patients). There was no change in scores for the imipramine-treated patients, but there was a sharp drop in recall for famous events and personal events in the ECT patients, especially for recent events. In a later trial, Calev et al. (1991) studied patients given the same technique for ECT at baseline and then again at 3 days, 1 month, and 6 months after ECT, using the same famous and personal events questionnaire. Complete data are only given for famous events recall, which had returned to baseline by the 6-month assessment.

Ng et al. (2000) studied depressed patients given right unilateral brief-pulse ECT at 2.5 times threshold stimulation. They used a personal memory test similar to the one used by Weiner et al. (1986), though the latter has never been published in its entirety. Patients were tested at baseline, a day after six treatments, after the last treatment, and again 1 month later. Mean percent recall of baseline items was 67.5%, 72%, and 86.8% for the post-sixth, post-last, and 1-month periods, respectively. Of note, therapeutic response rate was only 31% in this trial, a result that is not surprising considering the relatively weak form of ECT used (modestly suprathreshold unilateral electrode placement).

Kellner et al. (2010) reported results of their electrode placement study, unilateral versus bitemporal versus bifrontal, and included some data on the AMI-SF, the same test that was used by the Columbia Consortium in some of their studies described earlier. Data were reported for baseline versus 1–3 days after the last treatment. Scores were approximately 40% reduced from baseline at the acute post-treatment testing session for all three electrode placements, with the bifrontally treated patients having the lowest scores. Interestingly, the unilaterally and bitemporally treated patients had identical scores, in contrast to some other studies cited earlier.

McCall et al. (2000) studied a group of depressed patients treated at the first session with a threshold determination utilizing standard pulse width with right unilateral electrode placement. After this treatment, the patients were randomly assigned to receive either a fixed electrical dose of 403 millicoulombs or 2.25 times initial threshold (all patients continued with unilateral placement). The fixed-high-dose patients had a level of suprathreshold value calculated by dividing 403 by the initial threshold, thus yielding a variety of suprathreshold values (going all the way up to 12.6). Utilizing a personal memory questionnaire fashioned after the one described by McElhiney et al. (1995), McCall et al. tested patients at baseline and 1–2 days after the last treatment. There was a robust negative relationship between degree of suprathreshold dosing and percent recall of personal memory items (ranging from a mean of 66.1% recall for 2.25 times threshold to 50.4% recall for those receiving 8.4–12.6 times threshold). This study elegantly demonstrates how higher electrical doses result in more memory impairment in ECT.

Kessler et al. (2014) randomly assigned depressed patients to receive either ECT plus medications or medications alone. The Columbia AMI-SF was administered at baseline and shortly after the end of ECT, and at an equivalent time period in the medication-only group, and the percent retention was 72.9% in the ECT group and 80.8% in the medication group, a difference that is not clinically significant. Interestingly, this study shows lowering of scores in a non-ECT group relative to baseline. Also interesting is the finding that global cognition improved significantly in the ECT group.

Martin et al. (2015) searched for clinical predictors of post-ECT reductions in Columbia AMI-SF scores and found that higher postictal disorientation predicted greater loss of memories. Electrode placement made no difference, but longer pulse width also predicted greater memory loss post-ECT. Overall, pre- to post-ECT consistency on the AMI-SF was about 74% 2–3 days after the last treatment, indicating that memory is mostly preserved after ECT.

Weeks et al. (2013) found, in a group treated with bifrontal ECT, 1-month post-treatment retention scores on the Columbia AMI-SF of 69.9%. Dybedal et al. (2015) reported the results of a trial comparing unilateral and bifrontal placement. Patients were divided into those at baseline with or without cognitive impairment. About half of those with cognitive impairment, which was not due to dementia, "converted" to having no cognitive impairment at 1 month after ECT, again demonstrating how beneficial ECT can be for global cognition. In a further analysis of their data, Dybedal et al. (2014) found no change between baseline and 1 week after ECT on the Columbia AMI-SF, though about 11% of patients did show reductions in scores on a test of recall of public events.

Jelovac et al. (2016) and Semkovska and McLoughlin (2013) have outlined some of the difficulties and sources of error in the traditional approach to studying retrograde amnesia with ECT as exemplified by most of the studies cited earlier in this section, and particularly those utilizing the AMI or AMI-SF, such as not accounting for normal forgetting or the effects of depression itself. The authors critiqued the Weiner et al. (1986) Personal Memory Questionnaire (PMQ), in which only questions of an autobiographical nature that were answered pre-ECT are asked post-ECT, so that scores can at best stay the same or go down. The Columbia extensions of the PMQ (the AMI and AMI-SF) suffer the same problems. Percent reductions in normal control populations also occur and are sometimes of the same magnitude as in ECT populations. Public events questionnaires have the advantage that scores can go up over time as well as down but suffer the disadvantage that the questions rapidly become outdated and the tests must be continually updated. The Kopelman AMI (Kopelman et al. 1990), in contrast to the Columbia AMI and AMI-SF, asks the same questions in every administration of the test, if done serially, and thus scores can improve. Interestingly, two studies have shown improvements in Kopelman AMI scores after ECT (Sienaert et al. 2010; Stoppe et al. 2006).

Because scores on the Columbia AMI or AMI-SF can only go down or stay the same in repeat administrations, it is almost preordained that ECT will "look bad" in terms of patients' memory functions after treatment. Additionally, there is ample evidence that in normal controls given autobiographical tests, repeat testing at intervals roughly corresponding to ECT courses and a few weeks later clearly shows decrements, sometimes as much as in ECT samples (Jelovac et al. 2016). Thus, not all "forgetting" can be attributed to ECT treatment. Also, the effects of depression itself on autobiographical memory are complex. For example, it has been shown that depressed people tend to recall personal information in an overgeneralized manner (King et al. 2010). That is, when asked questions about recent events, depressed people tend to give few episodic details and answer with highly learned semantic information about themselves. For example, when asked about recent restaurant experiences, a healthy person can describe actual episodes of going to restaurants, whereas a depressed person tends to say generic things like "I like restaurants." The latter is semantic, not episodic, information. Thus, depressed people recall semantic autobiographical information better than they recall episodic autobiographical information. In one study (Raes et al. 2008), pre-ECT baseline over general memory in depressed patients predicted higher relapse rates post-treatment.

Fraser et al. (2008) have reviewed autobiographical memory in ECT. Tor et al. (2015) conducted a meta-analysis of right unilateral ultrabrief-pulse versus standard-pulse retrograde amnesia studies and found four that showed better such memory for the ultrabrief group and one study (Spaans et al. 2013b) that showed equal performance. Sackeim et al. (2007), in one of the largest cognitive data sets in ECT history, naturalistically followed 347 people treated with non-randomized ECT technique at seven hospitals in New York City. The Columbia AMI-SF was administered at baseline, a few days after the last treatment, and then 6 months later. Those patients given unilateral ECT had higher scores immediately after ECT and 6 months later, though the bilaterally treated groups performed reasonably well. Incidentally noted by the authors was the improved overall cognitive profile (except retrograde memory) in most patients at 6 months. Sobin et al. (1995), like Martin et al. (2013), found that degree of postictal disorientation was correlated positively with degree of retrograde amnesia with ECT. Of note, in this study, the original Columbia AMI (long form, with almost 300 questions) was used. That instrument is so time-consuming to administer, taking several hours in some patients, that it is virtually unusable in routine clinical care.

Jelovac et al. (2016), in their data set, showed that episodic autobiographical memory scores on the Kopelman AMI (Kopelman et al. 1990) were lower at baseline for depressed ECT patients than for normal controls, but that semantic autobiographical memory scores were equal, providing evidence for overgeneralized memory for depressed people. There were no changes in the Kopelman AMI scores from pre-ECT baseline to 1 week post-treatment and at 3-month follow-up.

O'Connor et al. (2010a), in a nonrandomized comparison of bitemporal and unilateral electrode placement in elderly depressed patients, found slightly greater acute reductions in recall of recent events, as assessed with the Kopelman AMI, in the bitemporal group. No follow-up data were presented.

Several studies have shown that ECT patients whose depression has remitted actually show improvements in their ability to recall episodic information compared with the pre-ECT depressed baseline (Semkovska and McLoughlin 2013; Sienaert et al. 2010; Stoppe et al. 2006). Semkovska et al. (2012) found that non-ECT depressed patients whose depression has remitted show improvements in episode-specific autobiographical memory.

Semkovska et al. (2011) reviewed cognition in right unilateral brief-pulse ECT studies and performed a meta-analysis. Three days after the end of ECT, no differences between unilateral and bilateral ECT could be found on any measure. The authors also found that the longer the time interval from the last ECT treatment until cognitive testing, the better the performance of patients, indicating predictable clearing of acute effects as time passes. The authors did an excellent job of reviewing 16 different cognitive domains, including among others general intelligence, global cognition, processing speed, and anterograde memory function. A particularly reassuring finding was the lack of evidence of prolonged anterograde memory decrements with any form of ECT. The same group (Semkovska and McLoughlin 2010) published an extensive meta-analysis of all objective testing done with ECT, excluding retrograde amnesia testing because of the nonstandardized methods used to test that mode of memory. A total of 84 studies were meta-analyzed. Multiple cognitive domains were assessed, and the authors concluded that by 15 days after the last treatment, there is improvement from baseline in some domains, including processing speed, working memory, anterograde memory, and executive function. A final contribution of this group (Semkovska et al. 2016) is the EFFECT-Dep trial comparing twice-weekly bitemporal brief-pulse versus twice-weekly right unilateral brief-pulse ECT. The clinical results have been presented in Chapter 7. Percent retention (memory) scores on the Columbia AMI-SF from immediately post-treatment to 3 and 6 months post-treatment were slightly higher in the unilateral group. Still, the absolute scores were in line with what has been found in normal control populations in other studies when tested over time.

Spaans et al. (2013b) compared eight times threshold, twice-weekly unilateral, ultrabrief versus standard-pulse-width ECT and found no changes in Kopelman AMI scores or results of a public events questionnaire from baseline to immediately post-treatment. Verwijk et al. (2015) followed these patients at 3 and 6 months and found that Kopelman AMI episodic autobiographical incidents scores went up as well as total scores, and relatively similarly in both groups. Loo et al. (2014) compared eight times threshold ultrabrief-pulse-width with five times threshold, standard-pulse-width ECT, both delivered right unilaterally, and found better post-treatment scores on the Columbia AMI-SF with the ultrabrief group immediately after the final ECT but no difference in any cognitive test between the two groups at 1- and 6-month follow-up. Mayur et al. (2013) compared ultrabrief with standard-pulse unilateral ECT and found no changes in either group post-ECT on the Kopelman AMI at 3 months or acutely.

Verwijk et al. (2012) reviewed the cognitive effects of ultrabrief-pulse-width versus standard-pulse-width unilateral ECT and concluded that standard pulse may be associated with somewhat lower recall scores on tests of retrograde amnesia at 6 months post-treatment. There were no other cognitive differences between these two modalities. Meeter et al. (2011) compared ECT patients' recall of public news events with that of normal control subjects over time and found that the depressed ECT patients scored lower on recall of recent public events than did the controls pre-ECT, an important contribution to the notion that depression itself impairs recall of recent events. Just after treatment, there was a decrement in recall, but by 3 months post-ECT, patients' recall of events from 3 months before ECT was equal to that of normal controls for the same interval.

Sienaert et al. (2010) studied a group of patients randomly assigned to receive ultrabrief-pulse bifrontal versus unilateral electrode placement. The therapeutic results of this trial were discussed in Chapter 7. The retrograde memory test was the Kopelman et al. (1990) AMI used in the Kho et al. (2006) study. It was administered at baseline and at 1 week and 6 months post-ECT. Interestingly, there was no drop in scores with either electrode placement at 1 week or 6 months post-ECT.

As can be appreciated from this fairly exhaustive review, numerous investigators have tried to elaborate the nature of retrograde amnesia with ECT, with special attention to the question of whether there is permanent loss of memories as the result of treatment. The studies have a remarkable homogeneity of findings: testing for recall of information gleaned at baseline reveals reductions in the acute post-ECT period with substantial return of recall by several months later. Whether there is complete return or residual forgetting of prior events or knowledge has been the subject of some debate. It has been argued (Abrams 2002, Chapter 10) that it is "unproved" that ECT can cause permanent retrograde amnesia. Of course, the only way to prove "permanence" is to follow somebody for life, which of course has never been done. If one exchanges "at least several months" for "permanent," then the evidence is substantial that reduced recall for previous life events or knowledge about the world (i.e., personal and impersonal memories, respectively) has been demonstrated in some studies of at least some types of ECT. Factors more likely to be related to prolonged recall impairments relative to baseline include bitemporal or bifrontal electrode placement, sine-wave stimulation, and use of very long pulse widths. Of these, sine-wave stimulation should be considered outmoded.

Interestingly, Ribot's law— that is, the theory that recently learned information is more likely to be forgotten than remotely learned information—has rather robustly been confirmed in this ECT/retrograde amnesia literature. Furthermore, it is impersonal information that is more likely to be forgotten than personal, autobiographical information (Lisanby et al. 2000). Another key finding is that there is no evidence of a complete wiping out of recent memories. In fact, patients routinely score greater than 50% on tests of recall of items answered at the baseline testing session, even with bitemporal ECT.

A few more points are worth considering regarding the retrograde amnesia issue. There is a paucity of ultra-long-term follow-up data of prospectively followed, randomly assigned groups. If there is a non-ECT comparison group, along with one or more ECT groups, in which recall for life events and public knowledge for recent and remote time periods is assessed at baseline and then, say, a year and 2 years later, one wonders if the performance of the non-ECT comparison group subjects for the months just prior to the study would be the same as that of the ECT group, given how much people normally forget of their lives over time. As an example, if at baseline assessment normal volunteers are asked to name recent restaurants visited, they probably can come up with answers. If they are asked to name restaurant visits from 2 years ago, they are less likely to recall those. Thus, much of what seems forgotten acutely with ECT is probably lost normally over time and should not be a problem for most patients. Of course, one forgotten important event may be bothersome to a person, and this is something that should be broached in the informed consent process.

Another point is the well-documented phenomenon that recall, though acutely diminished in the first few days or so after an ECT course, improves over the next few months. Memories seemingly gone acutely with ECT can come back. With enough time, do all of them come back, except those that will be normally forgotten anyway? These are unanswered questions in the ECT research literature. Also unanswered is the question as to whether any seemingly forgotten event is "lost from the brain" or somehow "still there" but just difficult to retrieve. Of course, it is impossible to prove that a memory is biologically wiped out from the brain, but the strong return of memories in the few months after treatment raises the question as to whether there are any types of memory rehabilitative attempts that might allow a patient to recall seemingly forgotten events. This is yet another unexplored possibility in the ECT field.

A final point regarding retrograde amnesia and ECT is that all of the studies cited involved patients receiving a single course of treatments without MECT. It is the patient requiring more than one index course of treatments relatively close together and/or aggressive MECT who seems to have the most forgetting of past life events and memories. This is a relatively understudied area, and the ECT practitioner should be aware of this issue and communicate to patients the probable cumulative effects of highly aggressive treatment schedules.

The assessment of retrograde amnesia has been difficult in research settings as described in this section. It is extremely difficult to assess retrograde amnesia in a standardized, quantifiable manner for routine clinical care. The types of autobiographical memory batteries used in the various studies of retrograde amnesia typically take an hour or more to complete, and sometimes several hours. It is hard to imagine, with the constraints on care provider time in modern psychiatry, who has that much time to invest in baseline and middle-of-treatment assessments. Furthermore, the usefulness of doing so has not been established. The autobiographical interviews utilized in research typically have no age, illness, or gender norms with which to compare an individual patient's performance, and there are no studies showing that modification of ECT technique based on any particular score can improve outcomes. It is helpful simply to ask patients and significant others during the course of treatments if there has been any evident forgetting of recent personal events during conversation. Of course, patients may not recall that they have forgotten something, so input from significant others is particularly helpful. Asking if there has been some recent family event such as a trip that has been forgotten or if there have been any new people the patient has met that he or she cannot recall is easy and practical. Asking patients if they recall meeting the doctor they were referred to prior to ECT, or if they recall being in the office before, similarly is easy. For patients who took a trip away from home to the medical center, asking if they recall the trip is easy as well. If the patient is an inpatient in the hospital and is not having regular family visits, either in person or over the phone, then it may be difficult to assess recent memories. One can ask about public events in the news, but one must be cautious, as there are plenty of people who do not follow such events. It is easy to appreciate that personal memories are unique to each person and that unless the practitioner is privy to what the patient's experiences of late have been, it is tough to assess forgetting of them.

How might this informal assessment of retrograde amnesia help with ECT technique planning? If the degree of forgetting seems distressing to the patient or family/significant others, then this should be discussed. If it does not strike the clinician as over and above what is typically seen, then perhaps just reassurance can be provided, without changing technique and potentially compromising efficacy. Again, the literature is rather unhelpful in providing specific information about what degree or type of forgetting has implications for routine care, so formal rules are inappropriate at this stage of the science.

Impairment of Subjective Memory Function

Subjective memory function has been assessed in the ECT literature. Assessment of subjective memory function usually consists of asking patients their own opinions about how memory is functioning during or after a course of ECT. The most commonly utilized test is the Squire Subjective Memory Quotient (SSMQ) developed by Squire et al. (1979). The routine assessment of subjective memory function is probably the most important of all, even though research has established that it may not correlate well with objectively measured memory changes with ECT (Berman et al. 2008; Brakemeier et al. 2011; Coleman et al. 1996; Prudic et al. 2000). Unless a patient is frankly delirious and is unaware of even basic aspects of where he or she is and what is going on, subjective memory functioning is a good guide for technique, especially if the subjective opinion of significant others is also sought. If the patient and family are feeling confident about memory function, then usually sticking with whatever technique has been started is probably appropriate.

One of the fundamental aspects of good medical care is to ask patients their own opinions and impressions about how they are functioning. This is particularly important with regard to memory function and ECT. Perhaps the most important memory assessment of all for ECT patients is to ask patients and families about subjective memory function. In this manner, any specific concerns can be addressed, and this process definitely aids the doctor-patient relationship.

It is one thing to determine whether a person has a memory of an episodic event in his or her life; it is quite another to know whether the person regularly (or even ever) actually accesses that memory. For example, there may be a particular vacation taken decades ago that if brought up in conversation will be remembered by the patient. However, if never brought up, it may never come to mind and thus be functionally forgotten; if that memory becomes inaccessible because of the ECT, the patient may never know this and thus may not be bothered. On the other hand, if the patient has experienced forgetting events brought up in conversation, he or she may be sensitized to this and be vigilant in his or her stream of consciousness for examples of forgetting other things—what is herein termed "amnesia sensitivity." Furthermore, a person's subjective opinion about his or her own memory function is likely to be influenced by the state of the depression. Several studies in fact have found a correlation between relief from depression with ECT and improvements in subjective self-ratings of memory function, as discussed below.

One of the first studies of subjective memory function with ECT was orchestrated by Cronholm and Ottosson (1963b). Within a few days of completing short courses of bitemporal placement ECT (three or four treatments), patients were asked the following questions: Have you experienced a change in memory, in remembering names of people, events of some months ago, or performance on the tests administered before and after ECT? For each of these, patients rated their memory as unchanged, better, or worse on a scale, with positive scores indicating perceived improvement, negative scores indicating perceived worsening, and a score of zero indicating perceived lack of change. The scores on the four questions were added into a summary score. Overall, 16 patients ended up with positive scores, indicating perceived improvement in memory with ECT, while 13 had negative scores and 6 reported no change. Thus, about one-third of the sample felt their memory was worse a few days following the end of ECT.

Squire et al. (1979) introduced what has become known as the Squire Subjective Memory Quotient. This 18-item scale consists of questions about various aspects of anterograde and retrograde amnesia as well as attention/concentration. For each question, the patient rates perceived functioning in the present versus before illness onset, a difficult task for a patient who has had ECT and has to compare the present to a long time ago. At any rate, on each item, a score of zero indicates no perceived change in function, while negative scores (-1 to -4) indicate varying degrees of perceived worsening, and positive scores ($+1$ to $+4$) indicate similar degrees of perceived improvement, similar to the rating system used by Cronholm and Ottosson (1963b). Sample items include "My ability to recall things that happened a long time ago is..." (then the patient indicates the spot on the scale corresponding to the answer, all the way from "much improved" to "much worse"). This question obviously taps into perceived retrograde amnesia. Another item taps more into attention: "My ability to follow what people are saying is..." The first half of the scale items as originally presented to patients by Squire et al. (1979) (i.e., items 1–9) corresponded mostly to anterograde and retrograde amnesia, while items 10–18 roughly corresponded to attentional functioning. ECT patients given bitemporal electrode placement treatments (and sine-wave electrical stimuli, which are now outmoded because of their cognitive toxicity) had, in the week after completion of the treatment series, decrements in scores on the first half of the 18 items. This indicates that the patients were perceiving amnesia. By several months later, the scores on the first-half items improved but did not return back to baseline, whereas scores on the second-half items improved to better than baseline, a change that corresponds to improvement in the depression with its concomitant enhancement of focus and concentration. In a follow-up study, Squire and Slater (1983) reported on a 3-year follow-up of the bitemporally treated patients and found essentially no change from the profile obtained at 7 months. Patients in particular complained of an inability to recall events from about 6 months prior to ECT until about 2 months after completion of the series. Interestingly, from other objective memory function studies from this group (see section on retrograde amnesia earlier in this chapter), by several months post-treatment, there was little evidence of any ongoing memory disturbance. The authors explained the continued subjective complaints of memory dysfunction by noting that patients experience amnesia in the immediate wake of ECT and sustain a vigilance about their perceived memory impairment, reflecting amnesia sensitivity.

Kho et al. (2006) studied a group of post-ECT patients at variable intervals after completion of ECT (range of 0–5 years, mean of 2 years) with a subjective assessment of retrograde amnesia (i.e., patients' own perceptions of their memory for past events), a famous events questionnaire, and the Kopelman et al. (1990) AMI, which is a copyrighted assessment of memory for past life events that is different from the Columbia Consortium AMI. ECT technique was not controlled for in this naturalistic follow-up study. Results indicated that the only signal of any persisting memory problem was recall for recent famous events. Unfortunately, the range of time since last ECT treatment was so variable (that is, a 5-year range) that it is difficult to make firm conclusions from this study. It is interesting to note that patients' subjective perceptions of recall were fairly positive. Also, in this study, in contrast to all other studies on subjective memory function in ECT, the authors obtained patients' ratings of how annoyed they were with their perceived ECT-induced memory problems and found that the ECT patients were more annoyed than a medication-alone group.

The Columbia University Consortium has published extensively on subjective memory function with ECT. In their first report, Coleman et al. (1996) used the SSMQ before and after ECT and found that scores improved and correlated with improvements in depressive symptoms but not with objective memory test results. Prudic et al. (2000), in a review paper, found that improvements in self-reports of memory largely did, in fact, correlate with reported depressive symptoms. Berman et al. (2008), in a follow-up study of a large number of ECT patients, used the Cognitive Failures Questionnaire (CFQ) and another subjective memory test, referred to as the Global Self Evaluation (GSE). The latter consisted simply of asking the patient what effect if any he or she believed ECT had on memory, rated on a scale from 1 (substantial negative influence of ECT on memory) to 7 (substantial improvement with ECT), with a score of 4 indicating no perceived change. This scale, the reader will notice, is virtually identical to the scale used by Cronholm and Ottosson (1963b). The CFQ was developed by Broadbent et al. (1982) and consists of 25 cognitive self-report items in which respondents rate their function on a scale from "very often" to "never" on items such as "Do you leave important letters unanswered for days?" or "Do you read something and find you haven't been thinking about it and must read it again?" Most of the items on this scale tap into focus and concentration rather than anterograde or retrograde amnesia.

Berman et al. (2008) found that there was a very slight positive correlation with score on the GSE and change scores on the AMI, which was used to test retrograde amnesia. However, review of the scatterplot of these data reveals that most patients who actually had an increase in AMI scores reported GSE scores of 4 or less, while there were several patients having a decrease in AMI scores who reported improvements in memory with ECT. Thus, for clinical utility purposes, the GSE does not, in this author's opinion, correlate well with tests of retrograde amnesia. The final report from this group (Brakemeier et al. 2011) involved assessments of subjective memory function in the study that randomly assigned depressed patients to high- or low-pulse-width and unilateral or bitemporal electrode placement (Sackeim et al. 2008). Outcome measures of subjective memory function included the GSE, CFQ, and SSMQ. The CFQ and SSMQ correlated with depression severity and not with AMI scores, while the GSE tended to correlate with AMI scores but not depression severity. However, perusal of the effects of the four different treatment conditions on the GSE reveals puzzling results. For both bitemporal groups (standard pulse width and ultrabrief pulse width), there was a very small negative effect on the GSE, though in both groups a significant percentage of patients reported improvements in GSE scores. For the unilateral groups, the ultrabrief group reported significant improvements on the GSE, but the standard-pulse-width group reported substantial negative effects of ECT on memory that were of lesser intensity than the very small decrements reported by the patients receiving bitemporal, regular-pulse-width ECT. Why would a unilateral group report worse memory than the corresponding bitemporal group? This finding does not make sense and casts a modicum of suspicion on the overall findings of the study.

To summarize the subjective memory impairment literature, it seems clear that on measures of attention and concentration, ECT patients, on average, rate themselves improved with treatment, and this correlates with improvement in depression. If the subjective memory assessment consists of the simple question "Has ECT made your memory better, worse, or not changed?" then some patients feel it is improved, while others feel it is worse or not changed. Roughly, the results with this question very slightly correlate with actual measured retrograde amnesia, but not to a clinically significant degree. From the standpoint of clinical care, it is a good idea to ask ECT patients during the course of treatments as well as thereafter how they feel their memory is functioning, and then to explore any concerns further with follow-up questioning. Typically, during the course of treatments or shortly thereafter, patients and families will report forgetting of recent events as well as inability to hold onto newly learned information. Over time, after the course of treatments is completed, patients will no longer have anterograde amnesia that was induced by ECT. Complaints of retrograde amnesia vary widely, with some patients not feeling like there is anything significant in their lives forgotten, and others feeling there is a "blank period" covering the weeks or months before treatments up until a few weeks after treatments.

There has been too little research attention given to subjective experiences of memory dysfunction in ECT research. As indicated earlier in this section, the most commonly used subjective memory assessment tool, the SSMQ, is difficult to administer and probably does not pick up the core features of how people feel their memory is working after ECT. A further issue, almost completely ignored in the ECT cognition literature, is the question of how distressed, or how bothered, patients are by perceived ECT-induced memory dysfunction. There are patients who have experienced substantial retrograde amnesia but who are not bothered at all by it. Alternatively, there are patients who only have forgotten relatively trivial amounts of declarative memories but who can be quite bothered by that. How do we predict such patients in advance? Unfortunately, there is no science to guide us in that regard. In what follows, the author offers a theoretical construct, which he has termed "amnesia sensitivity," that might help other ECT practitioners in their clinical approach to patients' complaining of memory problems after ECT.

It becomes apparent to any ECT practitioner that patients talk about their memory after a course of treatments or during MECT. It is important as stated to allow patients to explain their own perceptions of how their memory is functioning and to explore coping mechanisms. As patients discover things they have forgotten through conversations with others and in day-to-day life, they can become disconcerted at these failed memories and become sensitized to forgetting. They may tend to blame any incidental forgetting in daily life on ECT, even though it is normal for everybody to forget a large bulk of life events. Even a long time after the end of treatments, long after there is any discernible anterograde amnesia and the period of forgotten time periods is relatively remote, patients may still complain of not remembering certain time periods. The author calls this phenomenon "amnesia sensitivity." The fundamental elements of this construct consist of the following: First, during index ECT, the patient experiences variable degrees of postictal disorientation, anterograde amnesia, and retrograde amnesia. For some patients, interestingly, postictal disorientation, though very short-lived, is quite distressing. The same can be true for the temporary anterograde amnesia. Second, the patient may have an adverse emotional response to the awareness of these side effects and forgetting, such as anger, panic, or emotional distress. Third, even though the acute cognitive effects wear off, the patient may become vigilant for other episodes of forgetting, and the emotional valence attached to this vigilance may itself cause the patient to overexaggerate his or her own memory performance. Finally, the patient may blame any perceived forgetfulness on ECT. These steps have not been confirmed in scientific research; rather, this is an impression the author has formed in many years of ECT practice.

Amnesia sensitivity does not develop in all, or even a majority of, ECT patients. It most likely develops in younger patients with more active lives occupationally and socially, who tend to notice forgetfulness to a greater degree. Patients with severe personality disorders tend to be more likely to fall under this rubric. For patients who evince these dynamics, it is helpful to offer formal neuropsychological testing to provide reassurance that anterograde memory function is normal. Also, it is helpful to provide reassurance that the longer away from a course of treatments one progresses, the less prominent in day-to-day life any retrograde amnesia will be. This is partly because the patient is successfully making new memories of day-to-day life and some of the older forgotten memories (though not all) are, in fact, coming back. Furthermore, patients can be reassured that it is normal for people to forget large chunks of time in their lives, especially months or years after events occur. Indeed, how many people can honestly say they recall a several-month time period 3 years earlier, especially if nothing of great significance occurred? It is hereby emphasized to the reader that this concept of amnesia sensitivity is in no way meant to imply that patients do not experience memory loss with ECT—of course they do. However, the human psyche is complex, and people are known to have attributional styles that exaggerate cause-and-effect relationships in everyday life, and this occasionally happens with ECT patients.

Vamos (2008) approached the subject of evaluation of patients' self-assessments of the cognitive effects of ECT by conducting extensive, open-ended interviews with eight adult ECT patients well after the ECT was finished. The various statements people made are quite heterogeneous, reflecting how unpredictably patients react to ECT. However, the author identified four broad concerns: disappointment over not enough information having been provided before ECT; the importance of practitioners validating the statements that patients make about how they see their memory function; the impact of memory issues on daily functioning, as in going back to work after ECT; and effects on self-esteem. These are issues the clinician should actively discuss with patients who have had ECT and express concern with memory effects.

Memory Function During Maintenance ECT

All the research reviewed up until this point in this chapter is relevant to the cognitive aspects of a single course of index ECT treatments without accompanying continuation or maintenance ECT. As there are many patients who need such treatment to sustain the benefits of a course of treatments to prevent relapse, the cognitive effects of MECT are very important. Unfortunately, the database of studies is very limited. A number of case reports and small case series have been published showing that individual patients seem to function at an acceptable level cognitively during MECT (Vothknecht et al. 2003). Rami-González et al. (2003) published the first attempt at a systematic study of cognition in MECT patients. Eleven with remitted depression who had received previous index ECT followed by MECT with a mean intertreatment interval of about 52 days (which is a very long interval for MECT) were administered a cognitive battery consisting of tests of attention, complex attention, frontal lobe, and immediate and delayed recall. Unfortunately, the authors did not indicate the mean time since the last ECT treatment (in other words, were patients tested within a short time after the last MECT session or shortly before a session?). Eleven patients with remitted depression who had not received either index ECT or MECT were used as a comparison group and were administered the same cognitive battery. Performance on delayed recall, which of course is a measure of anterograde amnesia, was similar in the two groups. Interestingly, the MECT group performed less well on immediate recall and complex attentional tasks ("frontal lobe" functions), two types of cognitive function that have been shown in other studies not to be affected by ECT adversely. The comparison group consisted of patients who probably had less severe depressive disorders over time, with attendant lesser effects on depression-related cognitive dysfunction such as attention and concentration difficulties. Long-standing depression, even when relatively asymptomatic at the moment, can still have adverse effects on cognition. Also in that study, the very small sample sizes limited the sensitivity of the findings.

A better study of the cognitive effects specific to MECT emanated from the CORE (Consortium for Research on Electroconvulsive Therapy) group (Smith et al. 2010). In a comparison of 6 months of MECT with 6 months of continuation pharmacotherapy after remission with index ECT for major depressive disorder (Kellner et al. 2006), neuropsychological testing was performed after remission with index ECT but before randomization and then again at 3 and 6 months after randomization. The latter two test batteries were administered in the morning before a treatment—that is, a full 28 days after the last treatment, allowing for maximal cognitive recovery from each treatment. This is an important issue because if cognitive testing had been performed say, a day after a treatment rather than right before the treatment, then undoubtedly the MECT patients' performances would have been poorer. The investigators utilized a cognitive battery consisting of tests of subjective memory function, anterograde amnesia for both verbal and nonverbal (i.e., visual) information, and autobiographical memory (assessed with the Columbia AMI). Comparison of performances on the complete test battery between the MECT and pharmacotherapy patients indicated that at the 3-month testing time, there was a substantial improvement in anterograde memory function in both groups equally in comparison to just after completion of the index course of treatments, and in addition, there was improvement in subjective memory function. These findings held true at 6 months as well. For autobiographical memory, there was a slight decline from baseline for the MECT group at 3 months compared with the pharmacotherapy group, a difference that disappeared by 6 months, with scores for both groups being about the same as at baseline right after index ECT. What these data indicate is that when MECT patients are tested a full 4 weeks after their last treatment, their cognitive performance is the same as that for pharmacotherapy patients who also had index ECT. As stated before, however, there were no data on how MECT patients function cognitively within the first few days or so after each of their maintenance treatments.

The management of MECT patients is clinically very challenging. First, as extensively discussed in Chapter 8, these patients tend to have very long-standing, chronic, recurrent, medication-refractory illnesses. Keeping them well is difficult. On top of that, MECT, especially when administered more frequently than monthly, tends to be associated with noticeable ongoing anterograde and retrograde memory problems in many patients. Trying to maintain job, school, or household responsibilities can be a difficult problem for some of these patients, who often experience a relapse if MECT is stopped. It is important to discuss memory issues with MECT patients in an ongoing, regular manner to assess the balance between therapeutic benefits and cognitive difficulties.

Other Cognitive Functions and ECT

Ingram et al. (2008) conducted a review of nonmemory cognitive functions with ECT and generally found a paucity of data, though Semkovska and colleagues (Semkovska and McLoughlin 2010; Semkovska et al. 2011) conducted much more thorough reviews and found no evidence that ECT impairs general intelligence, executive functions, information processing speed, visuospatial functions, or language. *Executive functioning* is a somewhat broad term encompassing frontal lobe tasks like divided attention and freedom from distraction as well as problem solving. These functions have been generally attributed to the frontal lobes of the brain. In a study comparing right unilateral, bitemporal, and bifrontal electrode placement, there was no evidence that any of the electrode placements was associated with any decrease in executive function test performance with ECT (Kellner et al. 2010). *Praxis*, which includes the ability to carry out learned behaviors (e.g., putting on clothes), has been tested with visuoconstructive tests and has not been found to diminish with ECT (Semkovska and McLoughlin 2010; Semkovska et al. 2011).

Work/School Performance and Driving

A common issue is whether to give ECT to a student or employed person. Recent semantic memories are the most vulnerable during ECT, as demonstrated nicely by Lisanby et al. (2000); this is precisely the kind of information that students in school have—that is, a lot of recent semantic memories. Thus, one might hesitate giving ECT to a current student unless absolutely necessary, and only then if the student is explicitly informed of the probability of forgetting information. Such patients would probably have to take a leave of absence for ECT; in fact, usually such patients are already performing poorly and have taken a leave because of psychopathology.

Regarding work performance, the more work duties constitute procedural (implicit) memory, or memory for how to perform highly repeated tasks, the less likely they are to be forgotten. Thus, a truck driver should not forget how to drive a truck, though specific recent routes or sets of instructions may be forgotten. On the other hand, work-related memories that are semantically encoded are more likely to be forgotten. As with the student, when the discussion of treatment options gets to the ECT level, the patient is usually already taking a leave of absence, is close to it, or is at the very least not performing at work at optimal levels. The consent process for a patient who is employed should include a discussion of work duties and what is likely to be forgotten so the patient can make an informed choice to proceed with ECT and also have an appropriate period of convalescence after index ECT is finished before resuming full work duties.

Although ECT does not impair the knowledge of how to drive, it may impair reaction time and hand/eye coordination for a while after each treatment. Also, patients may forget routes and thus get lost while driving, especially in unfamiliar places. Thus, patients should not drive for at least 24 hours after a treatment. Beyond that, recommendations should be individualized depending on ECT technique and the patient's ongoing memory functioning.

Pharmacological Attempts to Reduce ECT-Induced Cognitive Effects

With the large number of pharmacological agents available for testing, it is not surprising that there are numerous studies attempting to show a reduction in ECT amnesia by the addition of a drug to the ECT regimen (Krueger et al. 1992). Some of these attempts are based on rational theories of the mechanism of ECT-associated amnesia, while some appear to be based purely on empirical trials. In this section this literature as it is relevant for the clinician is reviewed.

Several mechanisms have been proposed to affect ECT amnesia (nicely reviewed in Pigot et al. 2008). These include glutamatergic action on the *N*-methyl-D-aspartate (NMDA) receptor, pro-inflammatory mechanisms focusing on the COX-2 enzyme, influx of calcium intracellularly (leading to a theory that calcium channel blockade may lessen cognitive impairment), cholinergic blockade, glucocorticoid toxicity, thyroid hormone modulation, opioidergic action, and nitric oxide neurotoxicity. These have led to attempts or theories to reduce ECT amnesia with, respectively, NMDA receptor blockade (e.g., ketamine), COX-2 inhibition (e.g., celecoxib), calcium channel blockade, procholinergic agents (e.g., physostigmine, galantamine, donepezil), glucocorticoid blockade (mifepristone), thyroid augmentation, opioid blockade, or nitric oxide liberation (e.g., nitroprusside).

There have been a relatively large number of efforts at pharmacological reduction of ECT cognitive effects in human studies. Cohen and Swartz (1990–1991) studied eight depressed patients treated with ECT. For each patient, there were two ECT treatments studied, in which the patient was pretreated with 30–60 mg nimodipine (a calcium channel blocker) or placebo. Cognitive testing consisted of time to orientation, retrograde memory for words presented just prior to treatments, and anterograde memory for words presented after the treatments. There was no difference between nimodipine and placebo. Dubovsky et al. (2001) administered either nicardipine or placebo daily throughout ECT courses and found no effect on cognition of nicardipine.

Ezzat et al. (1985) pretreated half of their research ECT patients with intravenous piracetam before inducing the seizures and measured general memory functioning before the first treatment and a few days after the last one. Patients in the piracetam group performed better on the post-ECT test than did those who did not receive the piracetam. Unfortunately, the results were not broken down into which specific memory function (e.g., orientation, anterograde memory, retrograde memory) improved with piracetam. Bagadia et al. (1980) used piracetam or placebo, beginning after the end of a course of ECT. Testing after several weeks of piracetam or placebo revealed no neuropsychological differences. Tang et al. (2002) administered piracetam daily throughout ECT and for 2 weeks thereafter versus placebo and found no benefit on cognitive function.

Lerer et al. (1983), in a methodology similar to that used by Khan et al. (1994), administered intranasal low-dose vasopressin after one ECT treatment and placebo after another in a series of patients. There were no differences in subsequent neuropsychological testing, which did not include retrograde memory testing. Mattes et al. (1990) administered intranasal vasopressin four times a day throughout the ECT course (up through five treatments) at relatively high doses and found no beneficial effect versus placebo as assessed with a variety of tests, including retrograde amnesia for television shows as well as anterograde tests.

Nasrallah et al. (1986) treated patients with ECT and, after the course was completed, performed neuropsychological testing in a variety of domains, then administered either naloxone or placebo and repeated the tests. In this paradigm, naloxone had no effect. Prudic et al. (1999) studied naloxone in ECT. High-dose therapy with this agent (1.6 mg/kg) appeared to worsen some aspects of retrograde amnesia for items provided just prior to treatments. Otherwise, some aspects of post-treatment cognitive function, such as anterograde memory, appeared to improve with high-dose naloxone administered just prior to the treatments. Levin et al. (1990) in a similar methodology administered intravenous naloxone after one ECT treatment and placebo after another, and then tested orientation, immediate learning, and delayed learning; no difference between drug and placebo was found.

Matthews et al. (2008) studied galantamine, a cholinesterase inhibitor, in ECT. This drug was administered nonblindly to a cohort of nine patients throughout their courses of ECT. Cognitive test results of this cohort after ECT were compared with those in a subsequent non-galantamine-treated cohort. Delayed memory and abstract reasoning appeared to be somewhat better in the galantamine cohort. Levin et al. (1987) used physostigmine or placebo after individual ECT treatments and found that physostigmine was associated with better postictal orientation and immediate memory. Prakash et al. (2006) administered either donepezil or placebo throughout the course of ECT to patients and found better postictal orientation recovery with donepezil.

Stern et al. (1991) used 50 µg daily of triiodothyronine (T_3) throughout ECT versus placebo and found no benefit on cognition. Stern et al. (2000) administered T_3 daily throughout the course of ECT or placebo and found that those patients receiving the active drug performed better on autobiographical memory, especially for childhood events. Zervas et al. (1998) used thyroid-releasing hormone (TRH) in ECT patients versus placebo in a counterbalanced manner for the first and second treatments in a series. Most of the memory battery was unaffected by TRH, but recall 24 hours after the treatment for verbal material was a bit improved with it. Khan et al. (1994) administered a low dose of TRH after one of their patients' ECT treatments and placebo after another in a crossover design. After TRH, patients seemed to wake up more quickly than after placebo. No testing of autobiographical memory was undertaken.

In summary, despite an interestingly large number of heterogeneous agents studied, no consistent cognitive-enhancing benefit for ECT patients has emerged. One of the problems with this line of inquiry is that it is not clear what needs to be done neuropharmacologically for cognitive protection to take place. Does a drug need to be given prior to ECT, during ECT, or after ECT? If prior to ECT, for how long? For some drugs, several weeks of treatment may be needed for a true pharmacodynamic effect to occur. It would be very unwieldy in current practice to delay ECT for that period of time, waiting for a putative protective agent to work. Many of the above-listed studies involved administration of only a single dose of a drug right before a treatment. Is that long enough for the drug's action to take place? Perhaps if some of these drugs had been given daily for some time before ECT commencement, a drug effect would have been detected. The neurobiological basis of prevention of ECT-induced cognitive toxicity may be different from that of speeding recovery of cognition after ECT has already been completed. These fine points of methodology will need to be worked out in future research.

In addition to these trials in which a pharmacological agent was used specifically as an attempt to reduce ECT amnesia, the OPT-ECT trial mentioned in Chapter 7 is also relevant (Sackeim et al. 2009). The reader may recall that in that trial, ECT patients were treated concomitantly with placebo, venlafaxine, or nortriptyline to see if these latter antidepressants augmented ECT response. In-depth neuropsychological testing was performed in that study as well, mainly to see if these agents caused an increase in cognitive side effects of ECT. Surprisingly, the group concomitantly treated with nortriptyline performed better in multiple cognitive domains after ECT than did the groups cotreated with either placebo or venlafaxine (performance in the latter two groups did not differ). Thus, the authors concluded that coadministration of nortriptyline might lessen ECT amnesia. This is all the more surprising given that nortriptyline has rather strong anticholinergic effects, a mechanism that, if anything, considering the above-mentioned literature on procholinergic agents' effects on ECT amnesia, would lead one to predict greater cognitive side effects with ECT with nortriptyline. How can procholinergic and anticholinergic agents both lessen ECT amnesia? This set of discrepant findings awaits explanation.

Finally, there has been intense interest in ketamine and glutamatergic mechanisms in mood disorders of late. Of relevance in this discussion, it has been proposed that if glutamate excess is related to ECT-induced memory effects, then NMDA (a type of glutamate receptor) blockade, such as is accomplished with ketamine, may reduce such effects. However, the addition of ketamine at ECT treatments has not accomplished any sparing of cognitive side effects (Loo et al. 2012a; McGirr et al. 2015; Yen et al. 2015).

In summary, a wide variety of agents have been used to try and lessen ECT amnesia. None of the agents have shown convincing ability to do this in properly controlled and powered trials. It is highly unlikely that any entity (i.e., a drug company) will ever invest the time and resources needed to pursue U.S. Food and Drug Administration approval of a drug for this purpose. At the present time, it is not recommended that practitioners use any of the above-mentioned agents in their practice. The only exception might be nortriptyline concomitantly with ECT as an attempt to bolster efficacy, but one would not add that agent specifically or solely to lessen ECT-induced cognitive impairment. However, as time passes, there may yet be convincing evidence of a cognitive-enhancing effect with a particular agent, and one would encourage practitioners of ECT to maintain some vigilance with this literature as this important and worthy goal is pursued.

Monitoring of Cognitive Function During ECT

In the research studies reviewed in this chapter investigating the neuropsychological effects of ECT, the memory batteries used typically take over an hour to complete and often several hours. Such testing, especially if performed serially during ECT, is simply not practical for routine clinical practice. It is logical, then, to ask, What should be routine memory testing for ECT practice? One of the problems in translating research to clinical practice is that despite the extensive testing done in multiple research studies, none of them attempted to correlate the neuropsychological test findings with functional capacity in day-to-day life. Thus, even if a test of retrograde amnesia during ECT were to be routinely performed, one would not know what to do with the findings. For example, if one were to ask a few baseline questions about recent events in a person's life before ECT and then ask if the patient recalls these events during ECT, what is to be done if the patient cannot recall them? If the questions are asked during the course of treatments, one may speculate that the information gleaned from this type of questioning could be used to alter electrode placement or stimulus dose or stimulus configuration. However, much of what is forgotten during the middle of a course of treatments is ultimately recalled after the course of treatments is complete. This may cause the ECT practitioner to alter treatment technique prematurely and at the cost of efficacy. For the cognitive research in ECT to be more helpful clinically, there need to be studies in which results of standardized tests during the middle of the treatment course lead investigators to, in a randomized design, either continue with the current technique or alter it in some way, presumably to lessen memory impairment, and then follow cognition as well as clinical efficacy. Such studies have not been conducted.

Another issue, alluded to earlier in this chapter, is the question of how much a particular retrograde or anterograde test result, even if lower for one treatment group than another, actually translates into either poorer functional capacity in daily life or higher emotional distress at perceived memory dysfunction. Again, such research has not been done. This leaves the ECT practitioner with not much information about the best way to assess cognition during a course of ECT treatments. One recommendation is that patients and significantly involved family or friends be asked their own opinions about how memory is functioning. Has the patient noticed gaps in memory? Have significant others noticed poor memory for recent events? Broaching the patient's and significant others' observations and concerns is the single most important cognitive assessment that the practitioner can utilize in routine practice. In addition, periodic checks of global cognition with commercially available bedside tests help to assess for gross cognitive dysfunction that would indicate the need for either changing treatment technique or halting the course of treatments for a few days. Examples of such tests include the Mini-Mental State Exam (Folstein et al. 1975), the Montreal Cognitive Assessment (Nasreddine et al. 2005), and the Kokmen Short Test of Mental Status (Kokmen et al. 1987). Each of these has norms and is easy to administer at bedside or in the office. Substantial reductions in scores during the course of treatments would indicate a change in technique or halting of treatments for a day or two. Possible interventions include going from thrice- to twice-weekly treatments, switching from bitemporal or bifrontal to unilateral electrode placement, and using ultrabrief-pulse stimulus dosing technique with unilateral placement (the reader will recall that at this stage of the research, bitemporal ultrabrief pulse technique appears to be relatively inefficacious; see Chapter 7 for discussion). Beyond global cognitive assessments and inquiring about subjective memory function from the patient and significant others, it is not standard of care practice to include any other formal neuropsychological test during a course of ECT treatments, for the reasons outlined above.

After ECT is completed, as reviewed in this chapter, anterograde amnesia will clear within a week or two at most, so testing for this after that time period is not likely to be helpful. Retrograde amnesia may persist, of course, but there is no standardized test for this condition that has been shown to be helpful in clinical care, so it is not considered standard of care to perform this type of measure either (though continued questioning about subjective memory impressions is clearly a good idea). For the occasional patient who bitterly complains of longlasting memory impairment, formal neuropsychological testing may be indicated to help quantify memory function. Finally, it is an important consideration to ask what type of memory assessment should be performed during MECT. The research as discussed in this chapter is relatively scant. For patients who complain particularly of anterograde memory problems during MECT, some formal neuropsychological testing that specifically targets this type of memory function may be a good idea, though there is no research that specifically indicates how to translate the findings into clinical care. If an MECT patient does perform poorly on a standardized test of anterograde memory function, then an alteration in technique, such as treatment frequency or electrode placement, or even stopping MECT, can be discussed with the patient.

Martin et al. (2013) attempted to develop an easy-to-use cognitive test that might predict later cognitive issues with ECT. Using a brief test mostly of concentration tasks at baseline before ECT and a day or so after the third treatment, they analyzed whether the changes during that time period were predictive of cognitive functioning a few days after the last treatment. The screening test did not impressively predict retrograde amnesia scores, but the test results did correlate reasonably well with functions that normalize within a week or so after ECT is done (e.g., anterograde memory function). Thus, the clinical utility of this cognitive assessment is questionable.

Does ECT Cause Brain Damage?

The question of whether ECT causes brain damage is often posed by patients during the consent process. The answer depends on the precise definition of "brain damage." Those who argue that ECT does fundamentally damage the brain in some way would argue that if specific memories have been erased by the procedure (or at least are inaccessible), then that constitutes ipso facto evidence of brain damage, even if the neurobiological changes associated with the memory loss are unknown. Others might argue that "erasure" of a memory without any permanent change in memory function is analogous to erasing a recording from a tape such as a cassette. The tape is still capable of being recorded on without change in function, and so, it is argued, the erasure does not constitute "brain damage." In any case, the debate about the effect of ECT on neurohistology has proceeded for many decades.

In an excellent review of the history of this issue, Devanand et al. (1994) pointed out some of the early presumed evidence of brain-damaging effects of electroconvulsive shock (ECS) in animals. The issue centers on the method of preserving brain tissue after the animal who has been subjected to ECS is killed. In the method of immersion fixation, the brain is removed from the cranium and immersed in fixative material. Unfortunately, the fixative takes a long time to penetrate into the deep areas of the brain, and by that time agonal (i.e., death-related) changes have taken place that are not related to ECS. In the method of perfusion fixation, the freshly scooped-out animal brain is injected via the carotid and vertebral arteries with fixative that penetrates into deep brain structures quickly. In studies of animals given ECS whose brains are subsequently studied with perfusion fixation, there is no evidence of neuronal loss. In addition, as reviewed by Devanand et al. (1994), neuroimaging studies consisting of head computed tomography or magnetic resonance imaging (MRI) show no evidence of ECT-induced structural changes. Particularly enlightening in this regard are the classic MRI studies by Coffey et al. (1991), in which serial head MRI was performed on ECT patients at baseline, just after the end of treatments, and several months later. Neuroradiologists blind to sequencing of scans (i.e., they did not know whether a particular scan was baseline, immediate post-treatment, or several months post-treatment) utilizing precise measurement techniques of various brain regions found no evidence of ECT-induced changes over time. Further animal studies have shown that it takes 1.5–2.0 hours of continuous seizure activity for animals to start showing evidence of neuronal loss, and even longer if muscle relaxation and continuous oxygenation are used as in human ECT (Devanand et al. 1994).

Dwork et al. (2009) administered ECS in a manner identical to that for humans to monkeys and performed very precise histological analyses of frontal and hippocampal brain areas and found no evidence of neuronal loss or any other abnormal pattern. This probably constitutes the best evidence thus far of a lack of structural changes during ECT. Additionally, several investigators have measured serum levels of a variety of putative markers of acute brain injury (e.g., neuron-specific enolase) and have found no increases in such compounds after ECS in animals (Berrouschot et al. 1997; Giltay et al. 2008; Palmio et al. 2010; Zachrisson et al. 2000).

While all this research is very valuable, it will not mollify those in the "anti-ECT" crowd who will always claim ECT is brain damaging. No matter how hard researchers look for evidence of brain damage after ECT in humans or ECS in animals, such people will claim that scientists have not looked hard enough. It is axiomatic in life that it is virtually impossible to prove the absence of a putative phenomenon—those who believe in its existence will simply say previous methods are inadequate to find it. However, from the standpoint of routine clinical care—and, more specifically, regarding patient teaching and the informed consent process—patients and their families can honestly be told that intense scientific efforts to look at brain changes with ECT have failed to find any that are currently measurable. The more practical aspects of the issue of "how ECT affects the brain" can focus on what is known about amnestic side effects.

Key Points

- Memory is the cognitive domain most affected by ECT.

- Intelligence is not affected by ECT.

- Memory side effects can be minimized by good electrical dosing technique and judicious use of unilateral electrode placement in select circumstances.

- Anterograde memory side effects are temporary.

- Retrograde memory side effects may be permanent.

10

ECT Versus Other Neuropsychiatric Treatments

In the preceding chapters the author has discussed aspects of safe, effective delivery of electroconvulsive therapy (ECT). However, there are other neuropsychiatric treatment modalities available to the modern psychiatric clinician, as well as a few experimental ones that might be on the horizon. In this chapter the clinical decision making relevant to choosing ECT as opposed to these other modalities is discussed along with some speculations about newer technologies. As a general principle, when a medical clinician is faced with choosing between two treatment modalities, the factors to consider include efficacy, adverse effects, cost, and inconvenience. Efficacy is obviously a major consideration, because clinicians would prefer to choose the most efficacious treatment for their patients. However, adverse effects may preclude doing so in certain situations. For example, ECT is commonly thought of as the best antidepressant treatment available, yet it is not given to mildly depressed patients who have not yet been treated with other modalities, largely because of adverse effects on memory as well as cost and inconvenience. A treatment as expensive as ECT would not be considered cost-effective for a mildly depressed patient who has not yet had any treatment at all. Finally, convenience is an important but oft-missed consideration. This refers to the amount of time needed to administer the treatment in question (separate from cost or adverse side effects). A treatment may be efficacious, safe, and cost-effective, yet its use may be precluded by high inconvenience (i.e., it may be too time-consuming or its availability may cause too much inconvenience to receive). These four factors in comparing other treatments to ECT will be considered below.

The neuropsychiatric treatment alternatives to ECT that will be discussed herein can be classified as electrical versus magnetic, convulsive versus nonconvulsive, and internally (i.e., surgically) versus externally applied. ECT is a type of convulsive, externally administered, electrical stimulus treatment. Transcranial magnetic stimulation (TMS) is a magnetic, externally applied, nonconvulsive form of treatment. Magnetic seizure therapy (MST) is a magnetic, convulsive, externally applied treatment. Transcranial direct current stimulation (tDCS) is an electrical, externally applied, nonconvulsive treatment. Focal electrically administered therapy (FEAT) is a type of tDCS, while focal electrically administered seizure therapy (FEAST) is a type of ECT. Occasionally, all externally applied electrical treatments (i.e., ECT, tDCS, FEAT, FEAST) are referred to collectively as *repetitive transcranial electrical stimulation*, or rTES (after Borckardt et al. 2009). Vagus nerve stimulation (VNS) and deep brain stimulation (DBS) are electrical, nonconvulsive, surgically applied modalities. The reader should note that comparisons of ECT with pharmacotherapy were discussed in Chapter 2 and will not be repeated here. Also, the modalities discussed in this chapter are used for depression, so mania, catatonia, and schizophrenia do not pertain herein.

Transcranial Magnetic Stimulation

Transcranial magnetic stimulation has received a lot of press in the recent past. Back in the 1990s, when research on TMS for depression was first discussed, some of its fervent early advocates were predicting that TMS would eventually replace ECT. Over two decades later, nothing of the sort has transpired. The efficacy of TMS is simply too weak. However, it is approved by government regulatory agencies in the United States and many other countries for treatment of some depressive patients, and clinicians should at least have some type of plan regarding when to refer for TMS, if they choose to do so, and when to refer for ECT.

As a brief review, TMS involves the generation of a magnetic force by a machine that is powered electrically. The magnetic force is applied to the patient's head with a large coil that is shaped like a figure 8. The use of this configuration allows for a certain amount of focality in directing the magnetic force, which passes unabated through the skull and into the cerebral cortex, causing changes in cortical cells. TMS treatments are administered as a series much like ECT treatments. Because there is a lack of side effects on cognition (there is no anesthesia used), TMS treatments can be given daily until sufficient clinical response is appreciated. A typical course of TMS is 30 treatments given 5 days a week for 6 weeks. This obviously is a substantial time commitment for the patient. During a TMS session, the strength of the magnetic force can be varied and is quantified as a percentage of the amount needed to elicit a muscle contraction in the thumb contralateral to the side of stimulation. If too much magnetic force is used, the risk for eliciting a seizure is heightened. The magnetic pulses are administered, and the frequency of pulses can be manipulated, as well as the duration of pulse trains and intertrain intervals, all leading to the quantification of total number of pulses per session. A typical TMS session may last half an hour after the practitioner determines the precise location of where to apply the figure 8 coil. TMS machines make a loud noise, so patients need to apply earplugs. Headaches are also common.

There have been a very large number of reports published since the mid-1990s on the efficacy of TMS in depression. However, the bulk of clinically useful scientific data emanate from two well-controlled trials in which depressed patients were randomly assigned to receive either real TMS sessions or sham TMS, the latter a placebo treatment in which application of the figure 8 coil and noise made were identical to real TMS except that no magnetic pulses were applied to the brain. Thus, these were good placebo-controlled trials. One of them was funded by the company seeking government approval for TMS (O'Reardon et al. 2007), while the other was funded by the National Institute of Mental Health (George et al. 2010). The results were remarkably similar—in fact, virtually identical. Precise criteria for remission based on the 24-item Hamilton Rating Scale for Depression were used. The chances of remission in the real TMS groups in the two studies were 17.4% and 14.1% (O'Reardon et al. 2007, and George et al. 2010, respectively), while the chances of remission for sham TMS were 8.2% and 5.1% for the same respective studies. The reader can decide whether this speaks well for TMS or not. Those who support TMS—in large part practitioners who are consultants being paid by the company that makes the machine—emphasize the difference between real and sham TMS (e.g., "real TMS has about double the remission rate that sham TMS has," a statement that superficially sounds impressive). More skeptical observers, including this author, tend to emphasize the rather pitiful absolute rate of remission (i.e., about 15%) with real TMS. Furthermore, this outcome was in patients who tended not to be highly medication refractory. In fact, in the George et al. (2010) trial, most subjects who experienced remission had low antidepressant medication resistance.

There are some interesting trials comparing TMS and ECT head to head, reviewed by Rasmussen (2011b). In that paper, the author reviewed the six then-extant comparisons of ECT versus TMS in depression and concluded that the overall response rate in ECT patients was 58.8% versus 38% in TMS patients, a highly clinically significant difference. In a study published subsequently to that review, Hansen et al. (2011) found that right unilateral electrode placement at relatively low electrical doses resulted in substantially more improvement in depression at 3 weeks but not at 7 weeks in comparison to TMS. Some formal meta-analyses of ECT versus TMS conclude that efficacy is greater for ECT (Ren et al. 2014; Slotema et al. 2010). These trials involved primarily nonpsychotic depressed patients who were also not catatonic or melancholic, or if melancholic, not so severely melancholic that they could not take part in the consent process. Patients who are not behaviorally cooperative with TMS cannot receive that treatment, whereas agitated or behaviorally disruptive patients can easily be given ECT with anesthesia. It is hard to imagine agitated manic patients, stuporous catatonic, or psychomotorically agitated or retarded melancholic patients receiving TMS.

If TMS is somewhat less effective than ECT for depression, then how do these two treatments compare regarding side effects, cost, and convenience? ECT clearly causes memory impairment, whereas TMS does not, though the latter can cause headaches or facial pain. As far as cost goes, on a per-treatment basis, TMS is cheaper than ECT, but if an average course of TMS lasts 6 weeks, while a typical course of ECT is 3 weeks (and ECT is thrice weekly, while TMS is five times weekly), then the costs are not much different. At the very least, TMS is drastically more costly than antidepressant medication. Regarding convenience issues, TMS patients can drive their cars and do not have to take extra days off from work, but because of the time involved getting to the TMS suite, waiting for one's turn, getting the treatment, and then going back to work, probably most of one day will be taken for most people. Thus, if an acute course of TMS consists of 6 weeks of 5-days-a-week treatments, that amounts to a lot of time lost at work.

In sum, it appears the efficacy of TMS in predominantly nonpsychotic depressed patients is less than that for ECT. Additionally, efficacy is not established for psychotically depressed patients or those with mania, catatonia, or schizophrenia. Because of TMS's lower side effect profile, some patients may prefer that treatment modality. Because of its high cost, TMS is used mostly as a second-line treatment after multiple drug trial failures, and that population of medication-resistant patients has been shown not to respond to TMS well (George et al. 2010). Thus, TMS is predominantly the refuge of chronically ill patients with nonpsychotic depression. Such patients are often attracted to the newest, latest treatments, of which TMS is the main one in modern psychiatry. It also tends to be chosen by patients who can easily afford the high cost.

It also must be stated that the technology of TMS is progressing, and it is possible that in the future, there will be TMS methods that duplicate the efficacy of ECT. For example, TMS researchers can alter the location of stimulation (right vs. left vs. bilateral, or dorsolateral prefrontal cortex vs. ventrolateral prefrontal cortex). Also, more intensive forms of stimulation, such as one called "theta burst stimulation" (e.g., Bakker et al. 2015) or the Hesel-coil deep TMS method (Nordenskjöld et al. 2016), have been tried, thus far without evidence of increased efficacy for depression versus traditionally applied TMS. However, with further technological development, the future of TMS therapy may offer better treatment than what is now available.

Magnetic Seizure Therapy

In the early days of TMS, it was noted that a small number of patients had a seizure during the treatment sessions. These of course were unintended, and precautionary TMS parameter algorithms were developed to prevent this unwanted side effect. However, some groups of investigators have developed TMS technology with the purpose of intentionally inducing seizures as with ECT. This tentative treatment has been termed *magnetic seizure therapy*. According to theory, MST devices, which amount to TMS devices modified to give much stronger magnetic stimulations, provide more focal brain stimulation with resultant seizures that are less generalized than ECT seizures and might target the brain regions involved in the antidepressant activity of ECT while sparing the brain areas involved with the amnestic aspects of ECT (Lisanby and Deng 2015). The goal with MST research is to develop a procedure that has the same efficacy as ECT has without cognitive side effects.

Thus far there has been an impressive series of studies comparing ECS (electroconvulsive shock in animals) with MST in primates (e.g., macaques). These studies have shown weaker electroencephalographic expression (Lisanby et al. 2003), less cognitive impairment (Moscrip et al. 2006; Spellman et al. 2008), less heart rate response (Rowny et al. 2009), and less ictal power (Cycowicz et al. 2009) with MST than with ECS in animals. But what about humans?

The MST literature began with single case reports acting as a proof-of-concept introduction, one in a primate (Lisanby et al. 2001a) and another in a human (Lisanby et al. 2001b). The latter case report documented that seizures could be induced with magnetic pulses, and the patient in question, a middle-aged depressed woman, seemed to obtain clinical benefit from the treatments. A smattering of other case reports of a similar nature have been published over the years (Hoy and Fitzgerald 2010; Kayser et al. 2009; Kosel et al. 2003). A few larger case series and small controlled studies have also been published. Kayser et al. (2011) randomly assigned 20 nonpsychotic depressed patients to receive twice-weekly MST or three-times-threshold, ultrabrief-pulse right unilateral ECT. Patients were treated twice weekly for 6 weeks. Outcome measures consisted of several depression rating scales. Criteria for remission were met in 3 of the MST patients and 4 of the ECT patients, results that represented not very impressive efficacy and that were not surprising for ECT considering the weak form of treatment given (i.e., three-times-threshold unilateral placement). Reorientation postictally was a few minutes faster for MST, and this also conferred a mild advantage in anterograde memory testing later in the day of a treatment. If MST is ultimately to be an advantageous treatment, remission rates will need to be greater than 30%. As far as cognition goes, there will also need to be a better profile of longer-term retrograde amnesia, and not just better acute anterograde memory, which returns to normal in ECT within days to a few weeks after treatment. In a review of cognitive aspects of MST, preliminary data indicate better reorientation times by an average of a few minutes and perhaps better acute performance on some cognitive tests in the immediate posttreatment time period (Moreines et al. 2011). This does not inspire confidence, however, that there would be a clinically significant cognitive advantage of MST in humans vis-à-vis right unilateral ultrabrief ECT.

Kirov et al. (2008) treated 11 patients who were receiving courses of ECT with one MST treatment during the series and measured postictal orientation, which turned out to be 15 minutes earlier with MST than with ECT (about 7 minutes vs. about 22 minutes, respectively). However, in one of the 11 patients, a seizure could not be elicited with the MST machine.

Lisanby et al. (2003) reported on 10 patients given one threshold treatment each with MST and ECT and one suprathreshold treatment with each (thus, a total of four treatments). Retrograde amnesia was tested for information provided just prior to a treatment and was slightly better with MST. From the same research group, White et al. (2006) provided data on depression ratings with MST in 10 patients versus 10 age- and gender-matched ECT patients (treatment was not randomized) and found lesser reductions with MST than with ECT. MST patients required less muscle-paralyzing drug doses because of the relatively weaker motor seizure manifestations, lending support to the notion that MST seizures are weaker than ECT seizures.

In summary, there has been an impressive preclinical literature documenting some neurophysiological differences between MST and ECS in animals and some very preliminary data in humans. What is somewhat perplexing at this point is that more than a decade and a half as of this writing has transpired since the first case report—where is the randomized, multisite comparison between MST and ECT that should take place for further clinical development in humans? One would think such a study would have been conducted and its findings published by now. One possible explanation concerns the very demanding technical requirements and electricity usage of MST machines (Zyss et al. 2010). Overheating of hardware apparently has been a problem, and this would be prohibitive if MST machines are called on to treat many patients a day as ECT machines can reliably do. One wonders about the eventual cost of MST machines should they be approved for clinical use. Finally, with the data that have been published regarding the apparent lack of retrograde amnesia with ultrabrief pulse ECT (see Chapter 9 for review), one wonders if there really will be an advantage with MST. The field awaits new data, but it will likely be many years before this technology is commercially available if at all or cost-effective.

Transcranial Direct Current Stimulation

A technology was developed several decades ago whereby direct current stimulation could be applied externally to a patient's head without causing a seizure. Use of such a current has been termed *transcranial direct current stimulation*. A good older review is provided by Lolas (1977). Up to that time, the technique consisted of applying one or more electrodes to the head and another on the leg, a technique no longer utilized. Thus, the older literature is of historical significance only. In modern times, the tDCS technique consists of applying two electrodes, one an anode and the other a cathode. The machine generates a unidirectional current, which flows from the anode to the cathode. Typically, the anode is placed on the left dorsolateral prefrontal cortex (DLPFC) on the scalp and the cathode is placed on the right supraorbital area. A current of 1–2 milliamps is passed continuously between these two electrodes for 20 minutes. A seizure is not elicited with such a tiny current (the reader may recall that with ECT machines, a current of 800–900 milliamps is used in modern devices). Recent reviews discussing tDCS technique and studies are those by Dell'Osso et al. (2011), Murphy et al. (2009), Nitsche et al. (2009), and Rau et al. (2007). Broaching the concern that very little of the tDCS current actually makes its way to the brain, Miranda et al. (2006) used a model of a human head to study intracerebral current and estimated that about one-half of a typical tDCS current makes its way to the brain, with relatively widespread distribution.

Boggio et al. (2008) randomly assigned 39 patients to different treatment groups: 20 patients were given anodal left DLPFC stimulation; 9 patients were given anodal left occipital stimulation; and 10 patients were given sham stimulation with electrodes placed as in the first group. In all three groups, the cathodal electrode was placed over the right supraorbital region (there of course was no stimulation in the sham group). There were 5 sessions per week for 2 weeks (thus, 10 sessions), with each session consisting of 20 minutes of continuous stimulation utilizing a 2-milliamp current. Percent reduction in depression rating scale scores, blindly evaluated, was 40% for the anodal left DLPFC group, 21.3% for the anodal left occipital group, and 10.4% for the sham group. There was a 25% remission rate for the anodal left DLPFC group.

Using data from this trial, Boggio et al. (2007) also performed a cognitive task known as the "go–no go" test with these groups. In this type of cognitive test, subjects must perform a certain motor task under one type of stimulus condition and inhibit that motor activity under other stimulus conditions. In the trial, only the patients given anodal left DLPFC stimulation had improved performance on this task after the end of a session. In another sham-controlled, albeit very small, study, Fregni et al. (2006) gave 10 depressed patients 5 days of tDCS with 1-milliamp current, 20-minute sessions every other day for five sessions, and left DLPFC anodal stimulation. There were four responders in the active treatment group and none in the sham-treated group. One cannot help but wonder if in these "sham-controlled" trials the patients were able to discern, based on presence or absence of skin sensations, whether they were in the real or sham groups. If larger trials of tDCS are to be conducted and taken seriously by the clinical psychiatric community, the investigators would need to ensure that the double-blind is intact. In a sham-controlled trial, Loo et al. (2010) randomly assigned 40 depressed patients to anodal left DLPFC tDCS using a 1-milliamp current for 20 minutes every other day for five sessions versus sham and found no difference in depression ratings. Reductions in Montgomery-Åsberg Depression Rating Scale scores from about 30 to about 20 in both groups occurred over 10 days (i.e., five treatments every other day).

There are some open-label trials as well. Ferrucci et al. (2009) gave depressed patients a 5-day trial of tDCS twice daily utilizing 2-milliamp currents for 20 minutes per session. They found a 30% reduction in depression scores with this short-term study. Dell'Osso et al. (2011) gave left DLPFC anodal stimulation utilizing 2-milliamp currents for 20 minutes twice daily for five days to 23 depressed patients. Mean Hamilton Rating Scale for Depression scores fell from a baseline of approximately 20 to 13 in this short-term study. Brunoni et al. (2011), using a methodology for anodal placement and stimulus parameters and frequency similar to those used by Dell'Osso et al. (2011), compared antidepressant responses in patients with unipolar versus bipolar depression and found similar posttreatment scores, which were in the upper teens for both groups. Finally, there is a single case report of a depressed patient responding to tDCS (Palm et al. 2009).

Regarding safety of tDCS, Poreisz et al. (2007) reported their experience with 567 tDCS sessions in their research lab utilizing normal control subjects and patients with migraines, poststroke status, or tinnitus. Common side effects were tingling and itching. No serious adverse events occurred. Nitsche et al. (2009) also discussed electrical safety issues of tDCS and concluded that the technique is quite safe. Two more-recent reviews have found only modest evidence for the efficacy of tDCS, with these results derived from patient populations comprising predominantly nonpsychotic outpatients, with evidence for much lower efficacy in patients with medication-resistant conditions (Palm et al. 2016; Shiozawa et al. 2014). Perhaps with further development of technical enhancements, the efficacy of tDCS will be increased. For now, tDCS is not a viable option in fulminantly acutely ill patients, patients for whom ECT is especially efficacious (i.e., patients with psychotic depression, mania, catatonia, or schizophrenia).

At this early stage of tDCS development, it is not possible to give a detailed comparison with ECT. In fact, tDCS is not even U.S. Food and Drug Administration (FDA) approved. It certainly appears to be easy to deliver, lacks serious adverse effects, and would probably be relatively cheap from a cost standpoint. Whether it delivers impressive efficacy comparable to that of ECT awaits controlled trials. In particular, if the efficacy of tDCS depends on the strength of the current delivered, then one wonders whether the currents needed for efficacy are of such high amperage that the risk of inducing a seizure becomes significant.

Focal Electrically Administered Therapy

A group from Columbia University (Borckardt et al. 2009) published an article on a technique they refer to as "focal electrically administered therapy," or FEAT. This is a type of repetitive transcranial electrical stimulation (rTES, as defined in the introduction to this chapter) in which alternating current may be used instead of direct current as in tDCS. Thus, FEAT can be classified as a type of transcranial alternating current stimulation (tACS) in such cases. It is nonconvulsive. In a study of 19 normal control humans, these investigators placed two electrodes over the forehead and passed pulsed electrical current between them, meanwhile varying systematically the following variables: left anode/right cathode or left cathode/right anode, unidirectional (tDCS) versus bidirectional (tACS) currents, current intensity, and electrode size (e.g., large anode/small cathode vs. small anode/large cathode). The subjects' perceptions of skin sensations and pain were assessed. Results indicated that perceptions of current location and pain depended on the variables listed above. The authors speculate that manipulation of these variables also may result in differential neurobiological effects in the brain and may have implications for antidepressant efficacy. FEAT thus far is at a very early stage of development.

Focal Electrically Administered Seizure Therapy

A group at Columbia University has also published on a technique they refer to as "focal electrically administered seizure therapy," or FEAST (Spellman et al. 2009). This is simply a form of ECT in which an electrical current is applied externally to induce a seizure. However, this group of investigators has added three new variables to study: unidirectional current flow (as opposed to the standard bidirectional flow in currently available ECT machines); control of location of current flow (i.e., positioning of the anode and cathode in varying locations); and asymmetric electrode size. For example, current flows, by definition, from anode to cathode. If the anode is relatively large and the cathode small, then current starts out relatively widely spaced in the brain but ends up being concentrated in cortical regions just below where the small cathode is located. Alternatively, if the anode is small and the cathode large, then current is relatively more widely spaced under the cathode. The authors speculate this type of difference may have therapeutic implications for how ECT is delivered. In a study of rhesus monkeys (Spellman et al. 2009), it was found that the animals had lower seizure thresholds with unidirectional versus bidirectional current flows and with an electrode configuration consisting of small anterior/large posterior placement versus the usual bitemporal equal-size placement. Anterior anode/posterior cathode current direction was associated with different electroencephalographic expression than anterior cathode/posterior anode. This group has also described, in two open-label case series of FEAST in humans, using right anterior frontal small anode–right posterior frontal large cathode configurations to achieve seemingly therapeutic courses of treatment with no detectable cognitive disturbances (Nahas et al. 2013; Sahlem et al. 2016).

Further research in humans is needed to see if these findings have clinical implications for ECT practice. One obstacle to such a line of research is that with regulatory restraints in place regarding FDA approval of new types of devices, getting approval may be a prohibitively expensive proposition for constructing machines with these capabilities.

Vagus Nerve Stimulation

The above-mentioned technologies involve stimulation applied externally to the cranium. Two internal, surgically implanted forms of stimulation for psychiatric disorders have been developed. The first to be discussed here is *vagus nerve stimulation*. On each side of the neck courses a large nerve, extending from the midbrain to the periphery, called the *vagus nerve*, from the Latin *vagus*, meaning "wandering," which refers to the widespread distribution of the vagus nerve to heart, lungs, gut, and other tissues. About one-third of the vagus nerve fibers are efferent parasympathetic fibers emanating from the midbrain and coursing to the peripheral organs for innervation. About two-thirds of the vagus nerve fibers are afferent fibers emanating from the peripheral organs and providing input into the brain. It was discovered some years ago that tonic stimulation of the left vagus nerve could stop seizure activity. Presumably, the connections of the nerve in the midbrain and then progressively on up to the cortex were responsible for this finding. A technology was developed whereby an electrical generator about the size of a cardiac pacemaker could be surgically implanted into a patient's chest cavity and connected to a wire that was tunneled up into the neck and wrapped around the vagus nerve. The generator could be programmed to provide varying amounts of electrical stimulation to the vagus nerve, and clinical trials established efficacy in epilepsy, leading to FDA approval for this condition for the VNS system. Later observations seemed to indicate a possible antidepressant effect of the VNS system, and trials were undertaken for this indication. The electrical stimulus to the vagus nerve in VNS has four parameters: pulse frequency (e.g., 20 Hz); pulse width (e.g., 500 microseconds); current (e.g., 3.5 milliamps); and on/off cycle, which refers to the amount of stimulation time ("on" time) and amount of time without stimulation ("off" time) in between "on" cycles (e.g., typical "on" times might be 30 seconds, with "off" cycles of 5 minutes). If patients ever experience intolerable side effects, such as voice hoarseness, they can turn the device off with an externally applied magnet until such time as a physician can alter the parameters in the office. During "on"-time stimulation, the current of the electrical stimulus can be manipulated to provide stronger or weaker current. This is accomplished with a special wand that can be placed over the chest wall on the spot where the generator was placed and does not require further embarrassment of skin integrity.

Initially, findings from an open-label trial in 30 chronically depressed patients were reported (Rush et al. 2000). Median length of the current depressed episode was 4.7 years, indicating very chronically depressed patients. Detailed ongoing evaluations included depression ratings serially while the level of electrical stimulation was titrated for each patient. The results indicated that 40% of the patients met criteria for response after 10 weeks of stimulation. Common side effects included hoarse voice during times of active stimulation. Sackeim et al. (2001) extended these open-label data with 29 more patients, yielding a total initial open-label sample of 59 patients receiving VNS. With this larger sample, there was a 30.5% response rate at 10 weeks, with response being defined as an at least 50% reduction in depression rating scale scores. For those patients who had been treated with at least seven adequate antidepressant treatments before VNS in the current depressive episode (13 in all), none of them responded to VNS.

On the basis of what was perceived as good success in the initial open-label trial, a controlled trial was planned (Rush et al. 2005a). This consisted of implanting the generator and connecting the wire to the left vagus nerve in 222 patients. Of note, the left vagus is always used because the right vagus nerve is more involved with cardiac function, and stimulation of that nerve might cause arrhythmias. After implantation in the controlled trial, patients were randomly assigned to receive active stimulation over the course of 10 weeks, while the other half, in a double-blind manner, received no stimulation (thus, the latter constituted a sham or placebo group). After the end of the double-blind, sham-controlled phase, all patients proceeded with nonblinded active stimulation. At the end of the double-blind phase, depression ratings indicated no difference between the active and the sham group in six of seven outcome measures. In one outcome measure, the 30-item version of the Index of Depressive Symptoms—Subject Rating (IDS-SR$_{30}$), which is a patient self-report scale, there was a 17% response rate with active VNS versus 7.3% with sham VNS at 10 weeks. This difference was statistically significant. However, the primary outcome measures of the study, the Montgomery-Åsberg Depression Rating Scale and the Hamilton Rating Scale for Depression, showed no significant difference at the end of 10 weeks.

Rush et al. (2005b) reported on the yearlong open-label follow-up phase after the sham-controlled trial. Thus, all patients in the follow-up phase had the VNS device turned on in a nonblinded manner. For the 181 patients thus evaluated, the mean baseline Hamilton Rating Scale for Depression score was 28.0, while mean score at 12 months was 19.6, a significant but rather modest decline, because a score of 19.6 still indicates very significant depressive symptoms. The same group of investigators (George et al. 2005) compared this open-label VNS cohort with another cohort of depressive patients followed in a different study, in which patients were treated naturalistically with pharmacotherapy and psychotherapy. This latter mode is referred to as "treatment as usual" (TAU). Thus, a TAU group was compared with a VNS-plus-TAU group (of note, the VNS-treated patients also received TAU at the hands of their primary psychiatrists). At 12 months, there was a small but statistically significant difference in mean IDS-SR$_{30}$ scores in the VNS-plus-TAU group. The main drawback to this analysis, of course, is that the two groups were not randomly assigned or blindly evaluated for the outcome assessments—two critical aspects of properly scientific clinical trials.

Finally, in a 2-year follow-up of this cohort of VNS-plus-TAU patients, Nahas et al. (2005) reported a 42% response rate at 2 years and a 22% remission rate. Eighty-one percent of the original cohort was still being treated with VNS at the 2-year mark, which means that almost one in five patients originally implanted with the device had elected to have it removed by 2 years. Nierenberg et al. (2008) reported on the benefits of VNS in unipolar versus bipolar depressed patients from this cohort and found no differences in responding. Marangell et al. (2008) found that among nine rapid-cycling bipolar patients treated with VNS, there was a 38% improvement in mood symptoms at the 40-week mark. In a European cohort, Corcoran et al. (2006) reported that in 11 depressed patients implanted with VNS, 6 had responded to treatment at 1 year and 3 had experienced remission of their depression by that time point. Of note, the sample was similarly middle-aged and very chronically depressed as were the other cohorts noted above. George et al. (2008) implanted VNS devices in 7 patients with obsessive-compulsive disorder, 1 patient with panic disorder, and 2 patients with posttraumatic stress disorder, all of whom were very chronically ill and whose illnesses had been refractory to multiple standard treatments. These authors found that 4 years later, 4 of the original 10 were still receiving VNS and seemed to benefit. George et al. proposed that more research be conducted in VNS for patients with anxiety disorders.

The various authors of the above-mentioned studies, almost all of which were sponsored by the device manufacturer, had the impression that there seemed to be significant efficacy that took several months to occur in most patients. The population studied comprised chronically ill patients with highly medication-refractory illnesses. Thus, the backers of these trials argued that even though efficacy did not appear highly impressive, since this was in a group of patients who were "end stage" in their depressions, it still constituted gains impressive enough to convince the FDA to approve VNS for clinical use. That occurred in 2005. More recently, long-term open-label case series in 15 patients (Cristancho et al. 2011) and 41 patients (Christmas et al. 2013) found 1-year response rates commensurate with those in earlier series, ranging from about 30% to 40%.

Suffice it to say that since VNS was approved in 2005, it has not exactly taken the psychiatric community by storm. There has been the perception that VNS has, at best, weak efficacy that, even if it occurs, takes months to a year to unfold. Obviously, then, this would not be an ideal treatment option for a patient with a fulminant episode of an illness who needs acute treatment. ECT would be much more suited to those scenarios, such as acute episodes of melancholia, mania, catatonia, or nonaffective psychosis. The implantation of a device has implications for permanency, since even though the generator itself may be removed, the wire connection to the vagus nerve may have to stay in place because of scar tissue development. Thus, implanting these devices is not a trivial issue. VNS for depression will undoubtedly fade in popularity (it already has) and probably in a decade or so will for all practical purposes vanish. For now, some patients with very chronic depressive psychopathology (i.e., years long) who have taken a large number of medications and who even have had ECT may wish to try a VNS system. Finding a surgeon competent to perform the procedure and obtaining funding for the expensive device and operation are barriers for most patients.

Deep Brain Stimulation

Similar to VNS, deep brain stimulation involves the implantation of an electrical generator in the chest, except that the attached wire is tunneled up under the neck, then the scalp, and then inserted through a hole drilled into the top of the skull and inserted down into deep brain tissues. DBS has been approved for usage in Parkinson's disease, tremor, and, as part of a compassionate-use protocol only, dystonia and obsessive-compulsive disorder. It is in experimental trials for use in depression, though small data sets do exist.

Several implantation locations in the brain have been used to investigate antidepressant actions of DBS, including the ventral capsule/ventral striatum (also called the anterior branch of the capsula interna), Brodmann area 25, the nucleus accumbens, the superior branch of the medial forebrain bundle, and the posterior gyrus rectus (Accolla et al. 2016; Schlaepfer 2015). There have been many open-label case series and one sham-controlled trial published thus far. Some reviews are worth reading (Kuhn and Huff 2010; Mayberg 2009).

Lozano et al. (2008) described 20 patients, including the 6 patients from that group's original publication (Mayberg et al. 2005). Bilateral burr holes were drilled into the frontal bones of patients' skulls, pulse generators were implanted in the anterior chest wall, and wires containing quadripolar electrodes (meaning four electrodes at the tip of the wire) were inserted into each burr hole, with the tips tunneled down into the subcallosal cingulate gyrus (SCG) utilizing stereotactic methods to ensure proper placement. For each set of electrodes, one was placed at the bottom bank of gray matter in the SCG, one was placed at the top bank of gray matter in the SCG, and the remaining two were placed in the intervening white matter. Electrical stimulation, once begun, was continuous, with pulse frequency set at 130 Hz, pulse width set at 90 microseconds, and intensity of stimulation modified via voltage, which varied between 3.5 and 5.0 volts. For each wire tip with four electrodes, two of the electrodes were chosen to have stimulation.

Hamilton Rating Scale for Depression score was followed as the main outcome variable, with assessments performed monthly for a year. Baseline demographics of the sample of 20 patients revealed 9 males and 11 females, mean age about 45, and a mean duration of episode of 7 years, with most patients having had ECT as well as numerous antidepressant medication trials and psychotherapy. The mean depression rating scale score at baseline was about 25. These data are quite revealing. These are middle-aged chronically depressed patients who are nonpsychotic and report subjective depressive symptoms but probably otherwise have normal mental status examinations (i.e., they do not have pseudodementia and they are not profoundly psychomotorically impaired, psychotic, or unable to participate in the consent process due to severe ruminations). The reader will recall that the studies on most of the above-mentioned new neurostimulation techniques involve similar patients. These tend not to be the best ECT candidates, as discussed in Chapter 2, because they tend not to obtain great improvement with index ECT, and even when they do, they need ongoing maintenance ECT, which is often not tolerated well because of ongoing anterograde amnesia.

In the Lozano et al. (2008) sample of 20 such patients with chronic depression, by 1 month of DBS, about 35% had had a response and 10% had achieved remission of their illness , while at 6 months the response rate was 60% and the remission rate was 35%. Interestingly, these response and remission rates are similar to those reported in the original sample of VNS patients discussed earlier, who were similarly chronically depressed patients with highly treatment-refractory illnesses.

Other research groups have conducted DBS trials with stimulation to areas other than the SCG. Sartorius et al. (2010) implanted bilateral DBS leads into the lateral habenula in a chronically recurrent depressed patient who had responded well to index courses of ECT but who had always relapsed during maintenance treatments. The patient appeared to enjoy sustained improvement with DBS, although it took several months of stimulation for the improvement to become evident. Malone et al. (2009) and Malone (2010) implanted DBS leads into the ventral capsule/ventral striatum in 17 patients and reported remission rates of approximately 35% at a mean of 37 months of treatment. Schlaepfer et al. (2008) implanted DBS leads into the nucleus accumbens in 3 patients and noticed modest improvements in depressive symptoms.

Dougherty et al. (2015) published the only sham-controlled DBS trial thus far for depression. The ventral capsule/ventral striatum was chosen as the DBS implantation site. The response rate in those given active stimulation, at 16 weeks, was 20%, while the rate for those in the sham (placebo) group at the same time point was 14.3%, a nonsignificant difference. Thus, in the only sham-controlled trial for DBS for depression thus far, active stimulation failed to separate from sham stimulation.

After all the reports of patients given DBS in the various regions of stimulation are reviewed, it becomes clear that the types of patients potentially benefiting from this modality will be quite different from the classic ECT-responsive patients. The latter are those with acute, fulminant psychopathological syndromes like melancholia, mania, catatonia, and psychosis (whether schizophrenia-like or affective) as well as some acute neurological delirious states. As far as patients who receive implanted devices go, these will likely not be the patients given such treatments. It is hard to imagine a patient with an acute psychotic depression given such a long-term permanent device when a course of ECT or perhaps medication will result in remission. It is only chronically ill patients who, in all likelihood, may be candidates for the implanted devices. It is a good question whether such patients originally started out having the same illness as the acutely ill patients and then progressed for whatever reason to chronicity with ever-evolving psychopathological features or whether they have had an entirely different illness from the beginning. In the Lozano et al. (2008) series, the mean age at onset of the depressive illness was mid-20s, current age was mid-40s, current episode duration was 7 years, and mean number of prior episodes was about 4. Thus, for all intents and purposes, these are middle-age people who have been miserable and unhappy almost continuously for two decades. Similar demographics were noted in the Dougherty et al. (2015) report. Another point worth mentioning is that the Lozano et al. (2008) group excluded patients with comorbid Axis I conditions, which are far more common than not in these chronic patients, as well as Cluster A Axis II patients (i.e., borderline, narcissistic, and histrionic patients) and suicidal patients. Thus, one cannot help but wonder what types of response/remission rates they would have seen had they attempted to treat these other "high maintenance" patients, who are far more common than the purely depressed chronically ill patient. DBS will ultimately only be appropriate and available for a tiny fraction of all psychiatric patients. However, the study of DBS will teach important lessons about how the brain functions and can help lead to cheaper, easier, more widely available treatments.

In summary, a few case reports detail apparent clinical improvement in depression with DBS. This treatment will require highly technical neurosurgical expertise, something likely never to be widespread. Thus, DBS will be available to only a few people in wealthy countries and will not represent a good public health intervention. Also, one must consider the psychological aspects of having an implanted surgical device (and yes, even in the age of neural circuitry, it will be important to understand psychological factors in patient behavior). Having an implanted device essentially reifies and "validates" a person's role as "medical patient." Some types of patients will flock to having VNS or DBS, with deep psychological needs to have the patient role validated and more firmly established in their lives. It might have the effect of making disability claims more substantial. Also, it does not seem likely that patients with acute, fulminant psychopathological episodes would be good candidates for something that is essentially lifelong. How long to keep the electrodes in place is an unanswered question. As of this writing, DBS does not represent a viable alternative to ECT for severe depressive states.

ECT: A View to the Future

As it now stands, ECT is the most effective neuropsychiatric treatment modality, better for more clinical circumstances than medications or any one of the above-listed neuromodulatory alternatives being investigated. The neurosurgically implanted techniques (i.e., VNS and DBS) are thus far unimpressive in terms of efficacy and probably never will be widely available to a large number of mentally ill people. Further, surgical approaches will also probably never be appropriate for treatment of fulminant, acute episodes of mood disorders or psychoses, in contrast to ECT. The nonconvulsive modalities (i.e., TMS and tDCS/tACS), while quite safe and virtually lacking in adverse effects, are simply too weak in efficacy to replace ECT. Convulsive therapy will undoubtedly be a major psychiatric intervention for many years to come.

In terms of future technological development of convulsive modalities, there seems to be somewhat of a "competition" of sorts going on between MST and fine-tuned advancements in electrically induced seizure therapy (e.g., FEAST). MST machines generate huge amounts of energy in order to cause seizures, leading to risks of spontaneous combustion of the machines and failure to induce seizures, especially if several treatments are to be delivered in one day. Also, such machines, if ever commercially available, are likely to be extremely expensive, as they constitute modified TMS machines, the latter being already available and often five times as expensive as ECT machines. Further, it is yet to be demonstrated that the unwieldy technique of MST can yield the efficacy expected of ECT while causing clinically significantly less memory impairment than, say, right unilateral ultrabrief ECT, which already is known to cause very little such impairment. On the other hand, further refinements of ECT technique such as seen in FEAST are much more likely to be financially cheaper. It is the author's prediction that, over the coming decades, MST is unlikely to come to fruition as a commercially available therapeutic modality. In contrast, enhancements of ECT electrical stimulus delivery, such as in FEAST, are much more viable.

Key Points

- No other neurostimulatory modality as yet developed matches the efficacy of ECT.

- Transcranial magnetic stimulation, while well tolerated, is weak in efficacy.

- Magnetic seizure therapy is still in the developmental stage and likely will never outperform ECT.

- Refinements in ECT electrical stimulus delivery will likely reduce ECT cognitive side effects while preserving its well-known efficacy.

References

Aarsland D, Larsen JP, Waage O, et al: Maintenance electroconvulsive therapy for Parkinson's disease. Convuls Ther 13(4):274–277, 1997 9437571

Abbasinazari M, Adib-Eshgh L, Rostami A, et al: Memantine in the prevention or alleviation of electroconvulsive therapy induces cognitive disorders: a placebo-controlled trial. Asian J Psychiatr 15:5–9, 2015 25998093

Abbott CC, Lemke NT, Gopal S, et al: Electroconvulsive therapy response in major depressive disorder: a pilot functional network connectivity resting state FMRI investigation. Front Psychiatry 4:10, 2013 23459749

Abdallah CG, Fasula M, Kelmendi B, et al: Rapid antidepressant effect of ketamine in the electroconvulsive therapy setting. J ECT 28(3):157–161, 2012 22847373

Abdollahi MH, Izadi A, Hajiesmaeili MR, et al: Effect of etomidate versus thiopental on major depressive disorder in electroconvulsive therapy, a randomized double-blind controlled clinical trial. J ECT 28(1):10–13, 2012 21983758

Abou-Saleh MT: How long should drug therapy for depression be maintained? (letter) Am J Psychiatry 144(9):1247–1248, 1987 3631338

Abraham G, Milev R, Delva N, et al: Clinical outcome and memory function with maintenance electroconvulsive therapy: a retrospective study. J ECT 22(1):43–45, 2006 16633206

Abrams R: Daily administration of unilateral ECT. Am J Psychiatry 124(3):384–386, 1967 6039994

Abrams R: ECT for Parkinson's disease (editorial). Am J Psychiatry 146(11):1391–1393, 1989 2817111

Abrams R: Electroconvulsive Therapy, 4th Edition. New York, Oxford University Press, 2002

Abrams R, Fink M: Clinical experiences with multiple electroconvulsive treatments. Compr Psychiatry 13(2):115–121, 1972 5010591

Abrams R, Taylor MA: Anterior bifrontal ECT: a clinical trial. Br J Psychiatry 122(570):587–590, 1973 4717031

Abrams R, Vedak C: Prediction of ECT response in melancholia. Convuls Ther 7(2):81–84, 1991 11941106

Accolla EA, Aust S, Merkl A, et al: Deep brain stimulation of the posterior gyrus rectus region for treatment resistant depression. J Affect Disord 194:33–37, 2016 26802505

Adityanjee: Concurrent use of lithium and ECT (letter). J Clin Psychiatry 50(8):307–308, 1989

Adityanjee, Jayaswal SK, Chan TM, et al: Temporary remission of tardive dystonia following electroconvulsive therapy. Br J Psychiatry 156:433–435, 1990 2346849

Ahmed SK, Stein GS: Negative interaction between lithium and ECT (letter). Br J Psychiatry 151:419–420, 1987 3427307

Akcaboy ZN, Akcaboy EY, Yigitbasl B, et al: Effects of remifentanil and alfentanil on seizure duration, stimulus amplitudes and recovery parameters during ECT. Acta Anaesthesiol Scand 49(8):1068–1071, 2005 16095445

Albin SM, Rasmussen KG: ECT in patients taking prednisone. J ECT 23(1):53, 2007

Albin SM, Stevens SR, Rasmussen KG: Blood pressure before and after electroconvulsive therapy in hypertensive and nonhypertensive patients. J ECT 23(1):9–10, 2007 17435564

Alexander RC, Salomon M, Ionescu-Pioggia M, et al: Convulsive therapy in the treatment of mania: McLean Hospital in 1973–1986. Convuls Ther 4(2):115–125, 1988 11940951

Alizadeh NS, Maroufi A, Jamshidi M, et al: Effect of memantine on cognitive performance in patients undergoing electroconvulsive therapy: a double-blind randomized clinical trial. Clin Neuropharmacol 38(6):236–240, 2015 26536019

American Psychiatric Association: Diagnostic and Statistical Manual of Mental Disorders, 3rd Edition. Washington, DC, American Psychiatric Association, 1980

American Psychiatric Association: Diagnostic and Statistical Manual of Mental Disorders, 4th Edition. Washington, DC, American Psychiatric Association, 1994

American Psychiatric Association: Diagnostic and Statistical Manual of Mental Disorders, 5th Edition. Arlington, VA, American Psychiatric Association, 2013

American Psychiatric Association Committee on Electroconvulsive Therapy: Electroconvulsive Therapy: Recommendations for Treatment, Training, and Privileging, 2nd Edition. Washington, DC, American Psychiatric Publishing, 2001

Amiri S, Ghorishizadeh MA, Hekmatura S: Comparison of bifrontal and bitemporal electroconvulsive therapy in patients with major depressive disorder. Iran J Psychiatry 4:13–16, 2009

Andersen K, Balldin J, Gottfries CG, et al: A double-blind evaluation of electroconvulsive therapy in Parkinson's disease with "on-off" phenomena. Acta Neurol Scand 76(3):191–199, 1987 2446463

Andreescu C, Mulsant BH, Peasley-Miklus C, et al; STOP-PD Study Group: Persisting low use of antipsychotics in the treatment of major depressive disorder with psychotic features. J Clin Psychiatry 68(2):194–200, 2007 17335316

Asnis GM, Leopold MA: A single-blind study of ECT in patients with tardive dyskinesia. Am J Psychiatry 135(10):1235–1237, 1978 696908

Atiku L, Gorst-Unsworth C, Khan BU, et al: Improving relapse prevention after successful electroconvulsive therapy for patients with severe depression: completed audit cycle involving 102 full electroconvulsive therapy courses in West Sussex, United Kingdom. J ECT 31(1):34–36, 2015 25029538

Ayhan Y, Akbulut BB, Karahan S, et al: Etomidate is associated with longer seizure duration, lower stimulus intensity, and lower number of failed trials in electroconvulsive therapy compared with thiopental. J ECT 31(1):26–30, 2015 24901431

Baeza I, Flamarique I, Garrido JM, et al: Clinical experience using electroconvulsive therapy in adolescents with schizophrenia spectrum disorders. J Child Adolesc Psychopharmacol 20(3):205–209, 2010 20578933

Bagadia VN, Gada MT, Mundra VK, et al: A double blind trial of piracetam (UCB 6215) and placebo in cases of post-ECT cognitive deficiency. J Postgrad Med 26(2):116–120, 1980 7012328

Bagadia VN, Abhyankar RR, Doshi J, et al: A double blind controlled study of ECT vs chlorpromazine in schizophrenia. J Assoc Physicians India 31(10):637–640, 1983 6671932

Baghai TC, Marcuse A, Brosch M, et al: The influence of concomitant antidepressant medication on safety, tolerability and clinical effectiveness of electroconvulsive therapy. World J Biol Psychiatry 7(2):82–90, 2006 16684680

Bailine S, Kremen N, Kohen I, et al: Bitemporal electroconvulsive therapy for depression in a Parkinson disease patient with a deep-brain stimulator. J ECT 24(2):171–172, 2008 18580566

Bailine SH, Rifkin A, Kayne E, et al: Comparison of bifrontal and bitemporal ECT for major depression. Am J Psychiatry 157(1):121–123, 2000 10618025

Bailine S, Fink M, Knapp R, et al: Electroconvulsive therapy is equally effective in unipolar and bipolar depression. Acta Psychiatr Scand 121(6):431–436, 2010 19895623

Bakker N, Shahab S, Giacobbe P, et al: rTMS of the dorsomedial prefrontal cortex for major depression: safety, tolerability, effectiveness, and outcome predictors for 10 Hz versus intermittent theta-burst stimulation. Brain Stimul 8(2):208–215, 2015 25465290

Balke LD, Varma A: A case of long-term maintenance ECT in a 78-year-old with depression and possible Parkinson's disease. CNS Spectr 12(5):325–326, 2007 17585431

Balldin J, Granérus A-K, Lindstedt G, et al: Predictors for improvement after electroconvulsive therapy in parkinsonian patients with on-off symptoms. J Neural Transm (Vienna) 52(3):199–211, 1981 7310392

Bang J, Price D, Prentice G, et al: ECT treatment for two cases of dementia-related pathological yelling. J Neuropsychiatry Clin Neurosci 20(3):379–380, 2008 18806251

Barekatain M, Jahangard L, Haghighi M, et al: Bifrontal versus bitemporal electroconvulsive therapy in severe manic patients. J ECT 24(3):199–202, 2008 18772704

Barton JL, Mehta S, Snaith RP: The prophylactic value of extra ECT in depressive illness. Acta Psychiatr Scand 49(4):386–392, 1973 4746007

Battersby M, Ben-Tovim D, Eden J: Electroconvulsive therapy: a study of attitudes and attitude change after seeing an educational video. Aust N Z J Psychiatry 27(4):613–619, 1993 8135686

Beale MD, Bernstein HJ, Kellner CH: Maintenance electroconvulsive therapy for geriatric depression: a one-year follow up. Clin Gerontol 16:86–90, 1996

Beall EB, Malone DA, Dale RM, et al: Effects of electroconvulsive therapy on brain functional activation and connectivity in depression. J ECT 28(4):234–241, 2012 22820953

Bennett AE: Preventing traumatic complications in convulsive shock therapy by curare. JAMA 114:322–324, 1940

Bergsholm P, Gran L, Bleie H: Seizure duration in unilateral electroconvulsive therapy: the effect of hypocapnia induced by hyperventilation and the effect of ventilation with oxygen. Acta Psychiatr Scand 69(2):121–128, 1984 6422704

Berman RM, Prudic J, Brakemeier E-L, et al: Subjective evaluation of the therapeutic and cognitive effects of electroconvulsive therapy. Brain Stimul 1(1):16–26, 2008 20633366

Berrouschot J, Rolle K, Kühn H-J, et al: Serum neuron-specific enolase levels do not increase after electroconvulsive therapy. J Neurol Sci 150(2):173–176, 1997 9268247

Besson JAO, Palin AN: Tardive dyskinesia, depression and ECT (letter). Br J Psychiatry 159:446, 1991 1958968

Bidder TG, Strain JJ, Brunschwig L: Bilateral and unilateral ECT: follow-up study and critique. Am J Psychiatry 127(6):737–745, 1970 5482867

Birkenhäger TK, Renes J-W, Pluijms EM: One-year follow-up after successful ECT: a naturalistic study in depressed inpatients. J Clin Psychiatry 65(1):87–91, 2004 14744175

Birkenhäger TK, van den Broek WW, Mulder PG, et al: One-year outcome of psychotic depression after successful electroconvulsive therapy. J ECT 21(4):221–226, 2005 16301881

Bjølseth TM, Engedal K, Benth JS, et al: Clinical efficacy of formula-based bifrontal versus right unilateral electroconvulsive therapy (ECT) in the treatment of major depression among elderly patients: a pragmatic, randomized, assessor-blinded, controlled trial. J Affect Disord 175:8–17, 2015 25590761

Black DW, Winokur G, Nasrallah A: ECT in unipolar and bipolar disorders: a naturalistic evaluation of 460 patients. Convuls Ther 2(4):231–237, 1986 11940870

Black DW, Winokur G, Nasrallah A: Treatment of mania: a naturalistic study of electroconvulsive therapy versus lithium in 438 patients. J Clin Psychiatry 48(4):132–139, 1987 3104316

Blanch J, Martínez-Pallí G, Navinés R, et al: Comparative hemodynamic effects of urapidil and labetalol after electroconvulsive therapy. J ECT 17(4):275–279, 2001 11731729

Bloch Y, Levcovitch Y, Bloch AM, et al: Electroconvulsive therapy in adolescents: similarities to and differences from adults. J Am Acad Child Adolesc Psychiatry 40(11):1332–1336, 2001 11699808

Boggio PS, Bermpohl F, Vergara AO, et al: Go-no-go task performance improvement after anodal transcranial DC stimulation of the left dorsolateral prefrontal cortex in major depression. J Affect Disord 101(1–3):91–98, 2007 17166593

Boggio PS, Rigonatti SP, Ribeiro RB, et al: A randomized, double-blind clinical trial on the efficacy of cortical direct current stimulation for the treatment of major depression. Int J Neuropsychopharmacol 11(2):249–254, 2008 17559710

Bonds C, Frye MA, Coudreaut MF, et al: Cost reduction with maintenance ECT in refractory bipolar disorder. J ECT 14(1):36–41, 1998 9661092

Borckardt JJ, Linder KJ, Ricci R, et al: Focal electrically administered therapy: device parameter effects on stimulus perception in humans. J ECT 25(2):91–98, 2009 19092677

Bouckaert F, Sienaert P, Obbels J, et al: ECT: its brain enabling effects: a review of electroconvulsive therapy-induced structural brain plasticity. J ECT 30(2):143–151, 2014 24810772

Bourgon LN, Kellner CH: Relapse of depression after ECT: a review. J ECT 16(1):19–31, 2000 10735328

Bourne H: Convulsion dependence (letter). Lancet 267(6850):1193–1196, 1954 13213158

Brakemeier EL, Berman R, Prudic J, et al: Self-evaluation of the cognitive effects of electroconvulsive therapy. J ECT 27(1):59–66, 2011 20926956

Brakemeier EL, Merkl A, Wilbertz G, et al: Cognitive-behavioral therapy as continuation treatment to sustain response after electroconvulsive therapy in depression: a randomized controlled trial (Erratum appears in Biol Psychiatry 2014 Sep 1; 76[5]:430). Biol Psychiatry 76(3):194–202, 2014 24462229

Brandon S, Cowley P, McDonald C, et al: Electroconvulsive therapy: results in depressive illness from the Leicestershire trial. Br Med J (Clin Res Ed) 288(6410):22–25, 1984 6418300

Brandon S, Cowley P, McDonald C, et al: Leicester ECT trial: results in schizophrenia. Br J Psychiatry 146:177–183, 1985 3884080

Bright-Long LE, Fink M: Reversible dementia and affective disorder: the Rip Van Winkle syndrome. Convuls Ther 9(3):209–216, 1993 11941215

Broadbent DE, Cooper PF, FitzGerald P, et al: The Cognitive Failures Questionnaire (CFQ) and its correlates. Br J Clin Psychol 21 (Pt 1):1–16, 1982 7126941

Brown ED, Lee H, Scott D, et al: Efficacy of continuation/maintenance electroconvulsive therapy for the prevention of recurrence of a major depressive episode in adults with unipolar depression: a systematic review. J ECT 30(3):195–202, 2014 24979654

Brunoni AR, Ferrucci R, Bortolomasi M, et al: Transcranial direct current stimulation (tDCS) in unipolar vs. bipolar depressive disorder. Prog Neuropsychopharmacol Biol Psychiatry 35(1):96–101, 2011 20854868

Bryson EO, Ahle GM, Liebman LS, et al: Dosing and effectiveness of ketamine anesthesia for electroconvulsive therapy (ECT): a case series. Australas Psychiatry 22(5):467–469, 2014 25135435

Buchan H, Johnstone E, McPherson K, et al: Who benefits from electroconvulsive therapy? Combined results of the Leicester and Northwick Park trials. Br J Psychiatry 160:355–359, 1992 1562861

Bunney WE Jr, Davis JM: Norepinephrine in depressive reactions: a review. Arch Gen Psychiatry 13(6):483–494, 1965 5320621

Burgut FT, Kellner CH: Electroconvulsive therapy (ECT) for dementia with Lewy bodies. Med Hypotheses 75(2):139–140, 2010 20538415

Burgut FT, Popeo D, Kellner CH: ECT for agitation in dementia: is it appropriate? (editorial) Med Hypotheses 75(1):5–6, 2010 20434848

Calarge CA, Crowe RR, Gergis SD, et al: The comparative effects of sevoflurane and methohexital for electroconvulsive therapy. J ECT 19(4):221–225, 2003 14657775

Calev A, Ben-Tzvi E, Shapira B, et al: Distinct memory impairments following electroconvulsive therapy and imipramine. Psychol Med 19(1):111–119, 1989 2727201

Calev A, Nigal D, Shapira B, et al: Early and long-term effects of electroconvulsive therapy and depression on memory and other cognitive functions. J Nerv Ment Dis 179(9):526–533, 1991 1919554

Canbek O, Ipekcioglu D, Menges OO, et al: Comparison of propofol, etomidate, and thiopental in anesthesia for electroconvulsive therapy: a randomized, double-blind clinical trial. J ECT 31(2):91–97, 2015 25268043

Carlyle W, Killick L, Ancill R: ECT: an effective treatment in the screaming demented patient (letter). J Am Geriatr Soc 39(6):637–639, 1991 2037760

Carney MWP, Sheffield BF: Depression and Newcastle scales: their relationship to Hamilton's scale. Br J Psychiatry 121(560):35–40, 1972 5047168

Carney MWP, Roth M, Garside RF: The diagnosis of depressive syndromes and the prediction of ECT response. Br J Psychiatry 111:659–674, 1965 14337413

Castelli I, Steiner LA, Kaufmann MA, et al: Comparative effects of esmolol and labetalol to attenuate hyperdynamic states after electroconvulsive therapy. Anesth Analg 80(3):557–561, 1995 7864425

Chacko RC, Root L: ECT and tardive dyskinesia: two cases and a review. J Clin Psychiatry 44(7):265–266, 1983 6134719

Chanpattana W: Continuation electroconvulsive therapy in schizophrenia: a pilot study. J Med Assoc Thai 80(5):311–318, 1997 9175375

Chanpattana W: Maintenance ECT in schizophrenia: a pilot study. J Med Assoc Thai 81(1):17–24, 1998 9470317

Chanpattana W: Combined ECT and clozapine in treatment-resistant mania. J ECT 16(2):204–207, 2000 10868331

Chanpattana W, Chakrabhand ML: Combined ECT and neuroleptic therapy in treatment-refractory schizophrenia: prediction of outcome. Psychiatry Res 105(1–2):107–115, 2001 11740980

Chanpattana W, Sackeim HA: Electroconvulsive therapy in treatment-resistant schizophrenia: prediction of response and the nature of symptomatic improvement. J ECT 26(4):289–298, 2010 20375701

Chanpattana W, Chakrabhand ML, Kirdcharoen N, et al: The use of the stabilization period in electroconvulsive therapy research in schizophrenia, II: implementation. J Med Assoc Thai 82(6):558–568, 1999a 10443077

Chanpattana W, Chakrabhand ML, Kitaroonchai W, et al: Effects of twice- versus thrice-weekly electroconvulsive therapy in schizophrenia. J Med Assoc Thai 82(5):477–483, 1999b 10443097

Chanpattana W, Chakrabhand ML, Kongsakon R, et al: Short-term effect of combined ECT and neuroleptic therapy in treatment-resistant schizophrenia. J ECT 15(2):129–139, 1999c 10378152

Chanpattana W, Chakrabhand ML, Sackeim HA, et al: Continuation ECT in treatment-resistant schizophrenia: a controlled study. J ECT 15(3):178–192, 1999d 10492856

Chanpattana W, Chakrabhand ML, Buppanharun W, et al: Effects of stimulus intensity on the efficacy of bilateral ECT in schizophrenia: a preliminary study. Biol Psychiatry 48(3):222–228, 2000 10924665

Charlson F, Siskind D, Doi SAR, et al: ECT efficacy and treatment course: a systematic review and meta-analysis of twice vs thrice weekly schedules. J Affect Disord 138(1–2):1–8, 2012 21501875

Chater SN, Simpson KH: Effect of passive hyperventilation on seizure duration in patients undergoing electroconvulsive therapy. Br J Anaesth 60(1):70–73, 1988 3122811

Chen ST: Remifentanil: a review of its use in electroconvulsive therapy. J ECT 27(4):323–327, 2011 21673589

Childers RT Jr: Comparison of four regimens in newly admitted female schizophrenic patients. Am J Psychiatry 120:1010–1011, 1964 14138834

Childers RT Jr, Therrien R: A comparison of the effectiveness of trifluoperazine and chlorpromazine in schizophrenia. Am J Psychiatry 118:552–554, 1961 13878978

Chou KL, Hurtig HI, Jaggi JL, et al: Electroconvulsive therapy for depression in a Parkinson's disease patient with bilateral subthalamic nucleus deep brain stimulators. Parkinsonism Relat Disord 11(6):403–406, 2005 15994113

Christ M, Michael N, Hihn H, et al: Auditory processing of sine tones before, during and after ECT in depressed patients by fMRI. J Neural Transm (Vienna) 115(8):1199–1211, 2008 18317681

Christmas D, Steele JD, Tolomeo S, et al: Vagus nerve stimulation for chronic major depressive disorder: 12-month outcomes in highly treatment-refractory patients. J Affect Disord 150(3):1221–1225, 2013 23816447

Ciapparelli A, Dell'Osso L, Tundo A, et al: Electroconvulsive therapy in medication-nonresponsive patients with mixed mania and bipolar depression. J Clin Psychiatry 62(7):552–555, 2001 11488367

Clarke TB, Coffey CE, Hoffman GW Jr, et al: Continuation therapy for depression using outpatient electroconvulsive therapy. Convuls Ther 5(4):330–337, 1989 11941031

Coffey CE, Figiel GS, Weiner RD, et al: Caffeine augmentation of ECT. Am J Psychiatry 147(5):579–585, 1990 2183632

Coffey CE, Weiner RD, Djang WT, et al: Brain anatomic effects of electroconvulsive therapy: a prospective magnetic resonance imaging study. Arch Gen Psychiatry 48:1013–1021, 1991 1747016

Cohen MR, Swartz CM: Absence of nimodipine premedication effect on memory after electroconvulsive therapy. Neuropsychobiology 24(4):165–168, 1990–1991 2135706

Coleman EA, Sackeim HA, Prudic J, et al: Subjective memory complaints prior to and following electroconvulsive therapy. Biol Psychiatry 39(5):346–356, 1996 8704066

Colenda CC, McCall WV: A statistical model predicting the seizure threshold for right unilateral ECT in 106 patients. Convuls Ther 12(1):3–12, 1996 8777650

Consoli A, Benmiloud M, Wachtel L, et al: Electroconvulsive therapy in adolescents with the catatonia syndrome: efficacy and ethics. J ECT 26(4):259–265, 2010 21099377

Conway CR, Nelson LA: The combined use of bupropion, lithium, and venlafaxine during ECT: a case of prolonged seizure activity. J ECT 17(3):216–218, 2001 11528316

Coppen A, Abou-Saleh MT, Milln P, et al: Lithium continuation therapy following electroconvulsive therapy. Br J Psychiatry 139:284–287, 1981 6799032

Corcoran CD, Thomas P, Phillips J, et al: Vagus nerve stimulation in chronic treatment-resistant depression: preliminary findings of an open-label study. Br J Psychiatry 189:282–283, 2006 16946367

Cristancho P, Cristancho MA, Baltuch GH, et al: Effectiveness and safety of vagus nerve stimulation for severe treatment-resistant major depression in clinical practice after FDA approval: outcomes at 1 year. J Clin Psychiatry 72(10):1376–1382, 2011 21295002

Cronholm B, Ottosson J-O: "Countershock" in electroconvulsive therapy. Influence on retrograde amnesia. Arch Gen Psychiatry 4:254–258, 1961 13696558

Cronholm B, Ottosson J-O: Ultrabrief stimulus technique in electroconvulsive therapy, I: influence on retrograde amnesia of treatments with the Elther ES electroshock apparatus, Siemens Konvulsator III and of lidocaine-modified treatment. J Nerv Ment Dis 137:117–123, 1963a 14047818

Cronholm B, Ottosson J-O: Ultrabrief stimulus technique in electroconvulsive therapy, II: comparative studies of therapeutic effects and memory disturbances in treatment of endogenous depression with the Elther ES electroshock apparatus and Siemens Konvulsator III. J Nerv Ment Dis 137:268–276, 1963b 14051942

Cycowicz YM, Luber B, Spellman T, et al: Neurophysiological characterization of high-dose magnetic seizure therapy: comparisons with electroconvulsive shock and cognitive outcomes. J ECT 25(3):157–164, 2009 19300292

Daly JJ, Prudic J, Devanand DP, et al: ECT in bipolar and unipolar depression: differences in speed of response. Bipolar Disord 3(2):95–104, 2001 11333069

Damm J, Eser D, Schüle C, et al: Influence of age on effectiveness and tolerability of electroconvulsive therapy. J ECT 26(4):282–288, 2010 20357671

Daniel WF, Crovitz HF, Weiner RD, Rogers HJ: The effects of ECT modifications on autobiographical and verbal memory. Biol Psychiatry 17(8):919–924, 1982 7115840

Daniel WF, Weiner RD, Crovitz HF: Autobiographical amnesia with ECT: an analysis of the roles of stimulus wave form, electrode placement, stimulus energy, and seizure length. Biol Psychiatry 18(1):121–126, 1983 6830921

Dare FY, Rasmussen KG: Court-approved electroconvulsive therapy in patients unable to provide their own consent: a case series. J ECT 31(3):147–149, 2015 25222527

DeBattista C, Mueller K: Is electroconvulsive therapy effective for the depressed patient with comorbid borderline personality disorder? J ECT 17(2):91–98, 2001 11417933

Decina P, Guthrie EB, Sackeim HA, et al: Continuation ECT in the management of relapses of major affective episodes. Acta Psychiatr Scand 75(6):559–562, 1987 3618276

d'Elia G, Widepalm K: Comparison of frontoparietal and temporoparietal unilateral electroconvulsive therapy. Acta Psychiatr Scand 50(2):225–232, 1974 4604251

Dell'Osso B, Priori A, Altamura AC: Efficacy and safety of transcranial direct current stimulation in major depression. Biol Psychiatry 69(8):e23–e24, 2011 21310394

DePaulo JR Jr, Folstein MF, Correa EI: The course of delirium due to lithium intoxication. J Clin Psychiatry 43(11):447–449, 1982 7174620

DeQuardo JR, Tandon R: Concurrent lithium therapy prevents ECT-induced switch to mania (letter). J Clin Psychiatry 49(4):167–168, 1988 3356676

DeQuardo JR, Tandon R: Drs. DeQuardo and Tandon reply (letter). J Clin Psychiatry 50(8):307–308, 1989

Devanand DP, Dwork AJ, Hutchinson ER, et al: Does ECT alter brain structure? Am J Psychiatry 151(7):957–970, 1994 8010381

Devanand DP, Polanco P, Cruz R, et al: The efficacy of ECT in mixed affective states. J ECT 16(1):32–37, 2000 10735329

de Vreede IM, Burger H, van Vliet IM: Prediction of response to ECT with routinely collected data in major depression. J Affect Disord 86(2–3):323–327, 2005 15935255

Dinan TG, Barry S: A comparison of electroconvulsive therapy with a combined lithium and tricyclic combination among depressed tricyclic nonresponders. Acta Psychiatr Scand 80(1):97–100, 1989 2504034

Di Pauli J, Conca A: Impact of seizure duration in maintenance electroconvulsive therapy. Psychiatry Clin Neurosci 63(6):769–771, 2009 20021631

Dodd ML, Dolenc TJ, Karpyak VM, et al: QTc dispersion in patients referred for electroconvulsive therapy. J ECT 24(2):131–133, 2008 18580556

Dodwell D, Goldberg D: A study of factors associated with response to electroconvulsive therapy in patients with schizophrenic symptoms. Br J Psychiatry 154:635–639, 1989 2597856

Dolenc TJ, Rasmussen KG: The safety of electroconvulsive therapy and lithium in combination: a case series and review of the literature. J ECT 21(3):165–170, 2005 16127306

Dolenc TJ, Barnes RD, Hayes DL, et al: Electroconvulsive therapy in patients with cardiac pacemakers and implantable cardioverter defibrillators. Pacing Clin Electrophysiol 27(9):1257–1263, 2004a 15461716

Dolenc TJ, Habl SS, Barnes RD, et al: Electroconvulsive therapy in patients taking monoamine oxidase inhibitors. J ECT 20(4):258–261, 2004b 15591861

Dombrovski AY, Mulsant BH, Haskett RF, et al: Predictors of remission after electroconvulsive therapy in unipolar major depression. J Clin Psychiatry 66(8):1043–1049, 2005 16086621

Donahue AB: Electroconvulsive therapy and memory loss: a personal journey. J ECT 16(2):133–143, 2000 10868323

Dougherty DD, Rezai AR, Carpenter LL, et al: A randomized sham-controlled trial of deep brain stimulation of the ventral capsule/ventral striatum for chronic treatment-resistant depression. Biol Psychiatry 78(4):240–248, 2015 25726497

Douyon R, Serby M, Klutchko B, et al: ECT and Parkinson's disease revisited: a "naturalistic" study. Am J Psychiatry 146(11):1451–1455, 1989 2817117

Dubin WR, Jaffe R, Roemer R, et al: The efficacy and safety of maintenance ECT in geriatric patients. J Am Geriatr Soc 40(7):706–709, 1992 1607587

Dubovsky SL, Buzan R, Thomas M, et al: Nicardipine improves the antidepressant action of ECT but does not improve cognition. J ECT 17(1):3–10, 2001 11281512

Dudley WH Jr, Williams JG: Electroconvulsive therapy in delirium tremens. Compr Psychiatry 13(4):357–360, 1972 5035611

Dukakis K, Tye L: Shock. New York, Avery, 2007

Dukart J, Regen F, Kherif F, et al: Electroconvulsive therapy-induced brain plasticity determines therapeutic outcome in mood disorders. Proc Natl Acad Sci USA 111(3):1156–1161, 2014 24379394

Dunne RA, McLoughlin DM: Systematic review and meta-analysis of bifrontal electroconvulsive therapy versus bilateral and unilateral electroconvulsive therapy in depression. World J Biol Psychiatry 13(4):248–258, 2012 22098115

Dybedal GS, Tanum L, Sundet K, et al: Cognitive side-effects of electroconvulsive therapy in elderly depressed patients. Clin Neuropsychol 28(7):1071–1090, 2014 25220219

Dybedal GS, Tanum L, Sundet K, et al: The role of baseline cognitive function in the neurocognitive effects of electroconvulsive therapy in depressed elderly patients. Clin Neuropsychol 29(4):487–508, 2015 26029851

Dwork AJ, Christensen JR, Larsen KB, et al: Unaltered neuronal and glial counts in animal models of magnetic seizure therapy and electroconvulsive therapy. Neuroscience 164(4):1557–1564, 2009 19782728

El-Mallakh RS: Lithium and ECT interaction (letter). Convuls Ther 3(4):309, 1987 11940935

el-Mallakh RS: Complications of concurrent lithium and electroconvulsive therapy: a review of clinical material and theoretical considerations. Biol Psychiatry 23(6):595–601, 1988 3281716

Endler NS: Holiday of Darkness: A Psychologist's Journey Out of His Depression. New York, Wiley, 1982

Enns M, Peeling J, Sutherland GR: Hippocampal neurons are damaged by caffeine-augmented electroshock seizures. Biol Psychiatry 40(7):642–647, 1996 8886298

Erdil F, Begeç Z, Kayhan GE, et al: Effects of sevoflurane or ketamine on the QTc interval during electroconvulsive therapy. J Anesth 29(2):180–185, 2015 25085036

Eschweiler GW, Vonthein R, Bode R, et al: Clinical efficacy and cognitive side effects of bifrontal versus right unilateral electroconvulsive therapy (ECT): a short-term randomised controlled trial in pharmaco-resistant major depression. J Affect Disord 101(1–3):149–157, 2007 17196664

Euba R: Electroconvulsive therapy and ethnicity. J ECT 28(1):24–26, 2012 21983756

Ezzat DH, Ibraheem MM, Makhawy B: The effect of piracetam on ECT—induced memory disturbances. Br J Psychiatry 147:720–721, 1985 3913489

Faber R, Trimble MR: Electroconvulsive therapy in Parkinson's disease and other movement disorders. Mov Disord 6(4):293–303, 1991 1758447

Fall P-A, Granérus A-K: Maintenance ECT in Parkinson's disease. J Neural Transm (Vienna) 106(7–8):737–741, 1999 10907732

Farzan F, Boutros NN, Blumberger DM, et al: What does the electroencephalogram tell us about the mechanisms of action of ECT in major depressive disorders? J ECT 30(2):98–106, 2014 24810774

Fenton L, Fasula M, Ostroff R, et al: Can cognitive behavioral therapy reduce relapse rates of depression after ECT? A preliminary study. J ECT 22(3):196–198, 2006

Ferrucci R, Bortolomasi M, Vergari M, et al: Transcranial direct current stimulation in severe, drug-resistant major depression. J Affect Disord 118(1–3):215–219, 2009 19286265

Feske U, Mulsant BH, Pilkonis PA, et al: Clinical outcome of ECT in patients with major depression and comorbid borderline personality disorder. Am J Psychiatry 161(11):2073–2080, 2004 15514409

Fink M: ECT for Parkinson's disease? (editorial). Convuls Ther 4(3):189–191, 1988 11940963

Fink M: Electroconvulsive Therapy: A Guide for Professionals and Their Patients. New York, Oxford University Press, 2009

Fink M, Sackeim HA: Convulsive therapy in schizophrenia? Schizophr Bull 22(1):27–39, 1996 8685661

Fink M, Rush AJ, Knapp R, et al; Consortium for Research in ECT (CORE) Study Group: DSM melancholic features are unreliable predictors of ECT response: a CORE publication. J ECT 23(3):139–146, 2007 17804986

First MB, Spitzer RL, Gibbon M, et al: Structured Clinical Interview for DSM IV Axis I Disorders. Washington, DC, American Psychiatric Press, 1996

Flescher G: Retrograde amnesia following electric shock: a contribution to the general problem of amnesia. Schweiz Arch Neurol Psychiatr 48:1–28, 1941

Flint AJ, Rifat SL: Two-year outcome of psychotic depression in late life. Am J Psychiatry 155(2):178–183, 1998 9464195

Flint V, Hill-Johnes S: How effective is ECT for those with borderline personality disorder? Nurs N Z 14(9):12–14, 2008 18959290

Folkerts HW, Michael N, Tölle R, et al: Electroconvulsive therapy vs. paroxetine in treatment-resistant depression—a randomized study. Acta Psychiatr Scand 96(5):334–342, 1997 9395150

Folstein MF, Folstein SE, McHugh PR: "Mini-mental state": a practical method for grading the cognitive state of patients for the clinician. J Psychiatr Res 12(3):189–198, 1975 1202204

Fox HA: Extended continuation and maintenance ECT for long-lasting episodes of major depression. J ECT 17(1):60–64, 2001 11281519

Frank E, Prien RF, Jarrett RB, et al: Conceptualization and rationale for consensus definitions of terms in major depressive disorder: remission, recovery, relapse, and recurrence. Arch Gen Psychiatry 48(9):851–855, 1991 1929776

Fraser LM, O'Carroll RE, Ebmeier KP: The effect of electroconvulsive therapy on autobiographical memory: a systematic review. J ECT 24(1):10–17, 2008 18379329

Freeman CPL, Basson JV, Crighton A: Double-blind controlled trial of electroconvulsive therapy (E.C.T.) and simulated E.C.T. in depressive illness. Lancet 1(8067):738–740, 1978 76748

Fregni F, Boggio PS, Nitsche MA, et al: Treatment of major depression with transcranial direct current stimulation (letter). Bipolar Disord 8(2):203–204, 2006 16542193

Friedel RO: The combined use of neuroleptics and ECT in drug resistant schizophrenic patients. Psychopharmacol Bull 22(3):928–930, 1986 3797594

Fromm GH: Observations on the effect of electroshock treatment on patients with parkinsonism. Bull Tulane Univ Med Fac 18(2):71–73, 1959 13629283

Gagné GG Jr, Furman MJ, Carpenter LL, et al: Efficacy of continuation ECT and antidepressant drugs compared to long-term antidepressants alone in depressed patients. Am J Psychiatry 157(12):1960–1965, 2000 11097961

Gangadhar BN, Kapur RL, Kalyanasundaram S: Comparison of electroconvulsive therapy with imipramine in endogenous depression: a double blind study. Br J Psychiatry 141:367–371, 1982 6756530

Gangadhar BN, Janakiramaiah N, Subbakrishna DK, et al: Twice versus thrice weekly ECT in melancholia: a double-blind prospective comparison. J Affect Disord 27(4):273–278, 1993 8509527

Garcia RF, Dias AG, de Freitas AR, et al: Short-lived response of cervical dystonia to electroconvulsive therapy. J ECT 25(2):135–136, 2009 19145211

Geoghegan JJ, Stevenson GH: Prophylactic electroshock. Am J Psychiatry 105(7):494–496, 1949 18121767

George MS, Rush AJ, Marangell LB, et al: A one-year comparison of vagus nerve stimulation with treatment as usual for treatment-resistant depression. Biol Psychiatry 58(5):364–373, 2005 16139582

George MS, Ward HE Jr, Ninan PT, et al: A pilot study of vagus nerve stimulation (VNS) for treatment-resistant anxiety disorders. Brain Stimul 1(2):112–121, 2008 20633378

George MS, Lisanby SH, Avery D, et al: Daily left prefrontal transcranial magnetic stimulation for major depressive disorder: a sham-controlled randomized trial. Arch Gen Psychiatry 67(5):507–516, 2010 20439832

Gerring JP, Shields HM: The identification and management of patients with a high risk for cardiac arrhythmias during modified ECT. J Clin Psychiatry 43(4):140–143, 1982 7068545

Giltay EJ, Kho KH, Blansjaar BA: Serum markers of brain-cell damage and C-reactive protein are unaffected by electroconvulsive therapy. World J Biol Psychiatry 9(3):231–235, 2008 17853285

Go CL, Rosales RL, Caraos RJ, et al: The current prevalence and factors associated with tardive dyskinesia among Filipino schizophrenic patients. Parkinsonism Relat Disord 15(9):655–659, 2009 19346155

Goldberg RJ, Badger JM: Major depressive disorder in patients with the implantable cardioverter defibrillator: two cases treated with ECT. Psychosomatics 34(3):273–277, 1993 8493312

Golla F, Walter WG, Fleming GW: Electrically induced convulsions. Proc R Soc Med 33(5):261–267, 1940 19992197

Good MS, Dolenc TJ, Rasmussen KG: Electroconvulsive therapy in a patient with glaucoma. J ECT 20(1):48–49, 2004 15087998

Gordon HL: Fifty shock therapy theories. Mil Surg (Wash) 103(5):397–401, 1948

Gosek E, Weller RA: Improvement of tardive dyskinesia associated with electroconvulsive therapy. J Nerv Ment Dis 176(2):120–122, 1988 2892889

Grant JE, Mohan SN: Treatment of agitation and aggression in four demented patients using ECT. J ECT 17(3):205–209, 2001 11528314

Graveland PE, Wierdsma AI, van den Broek WW, et al: A retrospective comparison of the effects of propofol and etomidate on stimulus variables and efficacy of electroconvulsive therapy in depressed inpatients. Prog Neuropsychopharmacol Biol Psychiatry 45:230–235, 2013 23774194

Greenhalgh J, Knight C, Hind D, et al: Clinical and cost-effectiveness of electroconvulsive therapy for depressive illness, schizophrenia, catatonia and mania: systematic reviews and economic modelling studies. Health Technol Assess 9(9):1–156, iii–iv, 2005 15774232

Gregory S, Shawcross CR, Gill D: The Nottingham ECT Study: a double-blind comparison of bilateral, unilateral and simulated ECT in depressive illness. Br J Psychiatry 146:520–524, 1985 3893601

Griesemer DA, Kellner CH, Beale MD, et al: Electroconvulsive therapy for treatment of intractable seizures: initial findings in two children. Neurology 49(5):1389–1392, 1997 9371927

Grisso T, Appelbaum PS, Hill-Fotouhi C: The MacCAT-T: a clinical tool to assess patients' capacities to make treatment decisions. Psychiatr Serv 48(11):1415–1419, 1997 9355168

Gruber NP, Dilsaver SC, Shoaib AM, et al: ECT in mixed affective states: a case series. J ECT 16(2):183–188, 2000 10868328

Grunhaus L, Pande AC, Haskett RF: Full and abbreviated courses of maintenance electroconvulsive therapy. Convuls Ther 6(2):130–138, 1990 11941054

Grunhaus L, Hirschman S, Dolberg OT, et al: Coadministration of melatonin and fluoxetine does not improve the 3-month outcome following ECT. J ECT 17(2):124–128, 2001 11417923

Grunhaus L, Schreiber S, Dolberg OT, et al: Response to ECT in major depression: are there differences between unipolar and bipolar depression? Bipolar Disord 4 (suppl 1):91–93, 2002 12479688

Gujavarty K, Greenberg LB, Fink M: Electroconvulsive therapy and neuroleptic medication in therapy-resistant positive-symptom psychosis. Convuls Ther 3(3):185–195, 1987 11940915

Gupta S, Austin R, Devanand DP: Lithium and maintenance electroconvulsive therapy. J ECT 14(4):241–244, 1998 9871844

Gupta S, Tobiansky R, Bassett P, et al: Efficacy of maintenance electroconvulsive therapy in recurrent depression: a naturalistic study. J ECT 24(3):191–194, 2008 18772702

Hagen D: (Untitled letter.) Convulsive Therapy Bulletin 1(2):11, 1976

Haghighi M, Bajoghli H, Bigdelou G, et al: Assessment of cognitive impairments and seizure characteristics in electroconvulsive therapy with and without sodium valproate in manic patients. Neuropsychobiology 67(1):14–24, 2013 23221898

Hallam KT, Smith DI, Berk M: Differences between subjective and objective assessments of the utility of Electroconvulsive therapy in patients with bipolar and unipolar depression. J Affect Disord 112(1–3):212–218, 2009 18501434

Hamilton M: A rating scale for depression. J Neurol Neurosurg Psychiatry 23:56–62, 1960 14399272

Hanin B, Lerner Y, Srour N: An unusual effect of ECT on drug-induced parkinsonism and tardive dystonia. Convuls Ther 11(4):271–274, 1995 8919580

Hansen PEB, Ravnkilde B, Videbech P, et al: Low-frequency repetitive transcranial magnetic stimulation inferior to electroconvulsive therapy in treating depression. J ECT 27(1):26–32, 2011 20351570

Haq AU, Sitzmann AF, Goldman ML, et al: Response of depression to electroconvulsive therapy: a meta-analysis of clinical predictors. J Clin Psychiatry 76(10):1374–1384, 2015 26528644

Harris JA, Robin AA: A controlled trial of phenelzine in depressive reactions. J Ment Sci 106:1432–1437, 1960 13711745

Hartigan GP: The use of lithium salts in affective disorders. Br J Psychiatry 109:810–814, 1963 14080575

Haskett RF: Electroconvulsive therapy's mechanism of action: neuroendocrine hypotheses. J ECT 30(2):107–110, 2014 24800689

Hausner L, Damian M, Sartorius A, et al: Efficacy and cognitive side effects of electroconvulsive therapy (ECT) in depressed elderly inpatients with coexisting mild cognitive impairment or dementia. J Clin Psychiatry 72(1):91–97, 2011 21208587

Hay DP, Hay L, Blackwell B, et al: ECT and tardive dyskinesia. J Geriatr Psychiatry Neurol 3(2):106–109, 1990 1976309

Heijnen WT, Birkenhäger TK, Wierdsma AI, et al: Antidepressant pharmacotherapy failure and response to subsequent electroconvulsive therapy: a meta-analysis. J Clin Psychopharmacol 30(5):616–619, 2010 20814336

Heikman P, Kalska H, Katila H, et al: Right unilateral and bifrontal electroconvulsive therapy in the treatment of depression: a preliminary study. J ECT 18(1):26–30, 2002 11925518

Heshe J, Röder E, Theilgaard A: Unilateral and bilateral ECT: a psychiatric and psychological study of therapeutic effect and side effects. Acta Psychiatr Scand Suppl (275):1–180, 1978 281863

Hickie I, Parsonage B, Parker G: Prediction of response to electroconvulsive therapy: preliminary validation of a sign-based typology of depression. Br J Psychiatry 157:65–71, 1990 1975760

Hiremani RM, Thirthalli J, Tharayil BS, et al: Double-blind randomized controlled study comparing short-term efficacy of bifrontal and bitemporal electroconvulsive therapy in acute mania. Bipolar Disord 10(6):701–707, 2008 18837864

Hobson RF: Prognostic factors in electric convulsive therapy. J Neurol Neurosurg Psychiatry 16(4):275–281, 1953 13109543

Hodgson RE, Dawson P, Hold AR, et al: Anaesthesia for electroconvulsive therapy: a comparison of sevoflurane with propofol. Anaesth Intensive Care 32(2):241–245, 2004 15957723

Hoenig J, Chaulk R: Delirium associated with lithium therapy and electroconvulsive therapy. Can Med Assoc J 116(8):837–838, 1977 851921

Höflich G, Kasper S, Burghof K-W, et al: Maintenance ECT for treatment of therapy-resistant paranoid schizophrenia and Parkinson's disease. Biol Psychiatry 37(12):892–894, 1995 7548464

Holcomb HH, Sternberg DE, Heninger GR: Effects of electroconvulsive therapy on mood, parkinsonism, and tardive dyskinesia in a depressed patient: ECT and dopamine systems. Biol Psychiatry 18(8):865–873, 1983 6615944

Howie MB, Black HA, Zvara D, et al: Esmolol reduces autonomic hypersensitivity and length of seizures induced by electroconvulsive therapy. Anesth Analg 71(4):384–388, 1990 1975995

Hoy KE, Fitzgerald PB: Introducing magnetic seizure therapy: a novel therapy for treatment resistant depression. Aust N Z J Psychiatry 44(7):591–598, 2010 20560846

Hoyer C, Kranaster L, Janke C, et al: Impact of the anesthetic agents ketamine, etomidate, thiopental, and propofol on seizure parameters and seizure quality in electroconvulsive therapy: a retrospective study. Eur Arch Psychiatry Clin Neurosci 264(3):255–261, 2014 23835527

Husain MM, Meyer DE, Muttakin MH, Weiner MF: Maintenance ECT for treatment of recurrent mania. Am J Psychiatry 150(6):985, 1993 8494084

Husain MM, Rush AJ, Fink M, et al: Speed of response and remission in major depressive disorder with acute electroconvulsive therapy (ECT): a Consortium for Research in ECT (CORE) report. J Clin Psychiatry 65(4):485–491, 2004 15119910

Husain MM, McClintock SM, Rush AJ, et al: The efficacy of acute electroconvulsive therapy in atypical depression. J Clin Psychiatry 69(3):406–411, 2008 18278988

Hustig H, Onilov R: ECT rekindles pharmacological response in schizophrenia. Eur Psychiatry 24(8):521–525, 2009 19556109

Huston PE, Locher LM: Involutional psychosis; course when untreated and when treated with electric shock. Arch Neurol Psychiatry 59(3):385–394, 1948a 18874270

Huston PE, Locher LM: Manic-depressive psychosis; course when treated and untreated with electric shock. Arch Neurol Psychiatry 60(1):37–48, 1948b 18111203

Huuhka K, Viikki M, Tammentie T, et al: One-year follow-up after discontinuing maintenance electroconvulsive therapy. J ECT 28(4):225–228, 2012 22531209

Imlah NW, Ryan E, Harrington JA: The influence of antidepressant drugs on the response to electroconvulsive therapy and on subsequent relapse rates. Neuropsychopharmacology 4:438–442, 1965

Inglis J: Electrode placement and the effect of E.C.T. on mood and memory in depression. Can Psychiatr Assoc J 14(5):463–471, 1969 4903548

Ingram A, Saling MM, Schweitzer I: Cognitive side effects of brief pulse electroconvulsive therapy: a review. J ECT 24(1):3–9, 2008 18379328

Jaffe R, Dubin W, Shoyer B, et al: Outpatient electroconvulsive therapy: efficacy and safety. Convuls Ther 6(3):231–238, 1990 11941073

Jaffe RL, Rives W, Dubin WR, et al: Problems in maintenance ECT in bipolar disorder: replacement by lithium and anticonvulsants. Convuls Ther 7(4):288–294, 1991 11941135

Jagadeesh HN, Gangadhar BN, Janakiramaiah N, et al: Time dependent therapeutic effects of single electroconvulsive therapy (ECT) in endogenous depression. J Affect Disord 24(4):291–295, 1992 1578085

Jahangard L, Haghighi M, Bigdelou G, et al: Comparing efficacy of ECT with and without concurrent sodium valproate therapy in manic patients. J ECT 28(2):118–123, 2012 22531205

Jalota L, Kalira V, George E, et al; Perioperative Clinical Research Core: Prevention of pain on injection of propofol: systematic review and meta-analysis. BMJ 342:d1110, 2011 21406529

Janakiramaiah N, Channabasavanna SM, Murthy NS: ECT/chlorpromazine combination versus chlorpromazine alone in acutely schizophrenic patients. Acta Psychiatr Scand 66(6):464–470, 1982 7180565

Janakiramaiah N, Motreja S, Gangadhar BN, et al: Once vs. three times weekly ECT in melancholia: a randomized controlled trial. Acta Psychiatr Scand 98(4):316–320, 1998 9821454

Janicak PG, Davis JM, Gibbons RD, et al: Efficacy of ECT: a meta-analysis. Am J Psychiatry 142(3):297–302, 1985 3882006

Janis IL: Psychologic effects of electric convulsive treatments, I: post-treatment amnesias. J Nerv Ment Dis 111(5):359–382, 1950 15412352

Janke C, Bumb JM, Aksay SS, et al: Ketamine as anesthetic agent in electroconvulsion therapy [in German]. Anaesthesist 64(5):357–364, 2015 25943498

Janouschek H, Nickl-Jockschat T, Haeck M, et al: Comparison of methohexital and etomidate as anesthetic agents for electroconvulsive therapy in affective and psychotic disorders. J Psychiatr Res 47(5):686–693, 2013 23399487

Järventausta K, Chrapek W, Kampman O, et al: Effects of S-ketamine as an anesthetic adjuvant to propofol on treatment response to electroconvulsive therapy in treatment-resistant depression: a randomized pilot study. J ECT 29(3):158–161, 2013 23475029

Jarvis MR, Zorumski CF, Goewert AJ, et al: Maintenance electroconvulsive therapy and seizure duration. Convuls Ther 9(1):8–13, 1993 11941186

Jelovac A, Kolshus E, McLoughlin DM: Relapse following successful electroconvulsive therapy for major depression: a meta-analysis. Neuropsychopharmacology 38(12):2467–2474, 2013 23774532

Jelovac A, O'Connor S, McCarron S, McLoughlin DM: Autobiographical memory specificity in major depression treated with electroconvulsive therapy. J ECT 32(1):38–43, 2016 26252557

Jenkins LC, Graves HB: Potential hazards of psychoactive drugs in association with anaesthesia. Can Anaesth Soc J 12:121–128, 1965 14311657

Jephcott G, Kerry RJ: Lithium: an anaesthetic risk. Br J Anaesth 46(5):389–390, 1974 4471016

Jha AK, Stein GS, Fenwick P: Negative interaction between lithium and electroconvulsive therapy—a case-control study. Br J Psychiatry 168(2):241–243, 1996 8837918

Johnstone EC, Deakin JFW, Lawler P, et al: The Northwick Park electroconvulsive therapy trial. Lancet 2(8208–8209):1317–1320, 1980 6109147

Joshi SH, Espinoza RT, Pirnia T, et al: Structural plasticity of the hippocampus and amygdala induced by electroconvulsive therapy in major depression. Biol Psychiatry 79(4):282–292, 2016 25842202

Kales HC, Dequardo JR, Tandon R: Combined electroconvulsive therapy and clozapine in treatment-resistant schizophrenia. Prog Neuropsychopharmacol Biol Psychiatry 23(3):547–556, 1999 10378236

Kalinowsky L: Electric convulsive therapy, with emphasis on importance of adequate treatment. Arch Neurol Psychiatry 50:652–660, 1943

Kamel H, Cornes SB, Hegde M, et al: Electroconvulsive therapy for refractory status epilepticus: a case series. Neurocrit Care 12(2):204–210, 2010 19809802

Karliner W, Wehrheim HK: Maintenance convulsive treatments. Am J Psychiatry 121:1113–1115, 1965 14283312

Kayser S, Bewernick B, Axmacher N, et al: Magnetic seizure therapy of treatment-resistant depression in a patient with bipolar disorder. J ECT 25(2):137–140, 2009 19057399

Kayser S, Bewernick BH, Grubert C, et al: Antidepressant effects, of magnetic seizure therapy and electroconvulsive therapy, in treatment-resistant depression. J Psychiatr Res 45(5):569–576, 2011 20951997

Kellner CH, Monroe RR Jr, Pritchett J, et al: Weekly ECT in geriatric depression. Convuls Ther 8(4):245–252, 1992 11941174

Kellner CH, Fink M, Knapp R, et al: Relief of expressed suicidal intent by ECT: a consortium for research in ECT study. Am J Psychiatry 162(5):977–982, 2005 15863801

Kellner CH, Knapp RG, Petrides G, et al: Continuation electroconvulsive therapy vs pharmacotherapy for relapse prevention in major depression: a multisite study from the Consortium for Research in Electroconvulsive Therapy (CORE). Arch Gen Psychiatry 63(12):1337–1344, 2006 17146008

Kellner CH, Knapp R, Husain MM, et al: Bifrontal, bitemporal and right unilateral electrode placement in ECT: randomised trial. Br J Psychiatry 196(3):226–234, 2010 20194546

Kellner CH, Husain MM, Knapp RG, et al; CORE/PRIDE Work Group: Right unilateral ultrabrief pulse ECT in geriatric depression: phase 1 of the PRIDE study. Am J Psychiatry 173(11):1101–1109, 2016a 27418379

Kellner CH, Husain MM, Knapp RG, et al; CORE/PRIDE Work Group: A novel strategy for continuation ECT in geriatric depression: phase 2 of the PRIDE study. Am J Psychiatry 173(11):1110–1118, 2016b 27418381

Kendell RE: The classification of depressions: a review of contemporary confusion. Br J Psychiatry 129:15–28, 1976 938800

Kessler U, Schoeyen HK, Andreassen OA, et al: The effect of electroconvulsive therapy on neurocognitive function in treatment-resistant bipolar disorder depression. J Clin Psychiatry 75(11):e1306–e1313, 2014 25470096

Khan A, Mirolo MH, Claypoole K, et al: Effects of low-dose TRH on cognitive deficits in the ECT postictal state. Am J Psychiatry 151(11):1694–1696, 1994 7943463

Kho KH, van Vreeswijk MF, Simpson S, et al: A meta-analysis of electroconvulsive therapy efficacy in depression. J ECT 19(3):139–147, 2003 12972983

Kho KH, Blansjaar BA, de Vries S, et al: Electroconvulsive therapy for the treatment of clozapine nonresponders suffering from schizophrenia—an open label study. Eur Arch Psychiatry Clin Neurosci 254(6):372–379, 2004 15538604

Kho KH, Zwinderman AH, Blansjaar BA: Predictors for the efficacy of electroconvulsive therapy: chart review of a naturalistic study. J Clin Psychiatry 66(7):894–899, 2005 16013905

Kho KH, VanVreeswijk MF, Murre JMJ: A retrospective controlled study into memory complaints reported by depressed patients after treatment with electroconvulsive therapy and pharmacotherapy or pharmacotherapy only. J ECT 22(3):199–205, 2006 16957537

Kiloh LG: Pseudo-dementia. Acta Psychiatr Scand 37(4):336–351, 1961 14455934

Kiloh LG, Child JP, Latner G: A controlled trial of iproniazid in the treatment of endogenous depression. J Ment Sci 106:1139–1144, 1960a 13755968

Kiloh LG, Child JP, Latner G: Endogenous depression treated with iproniazid—a follow-up study. J Ment Sci 106:1425–1428, 1960b 13755969

Kimball JN, Rosenquist PB, Dunn A, McCall V: Prediction of antidepressant response in both 2.25xthreshold RUL and fixed high dose RUL ECT. J Affect Disord 112(1-3):85–91, 2009 18539340

Kindler S, Shapira B, Hadjez J, et al: Factors influencing response to bilateral electroconvulsive therapy in major depression. Convuls Ther 7(4):245–254, 1991 11941129

King MJ, MacDougall AG, Ferris SM, et al: A review of factors that moderate autobiographical memory performance in patients with major depressive disorder. J Clin Exp Neuropsychol 32(10):1122–1144, 2010 20544462

Kirov G, Ebmeier KP, Scott AIF, et al: Quick recovery of orientation after magnetic seizure therapy for major depressive disorder. Br J Psychiatry 193(2):152–155, 2008 18670002

Kokmen E, Naessens JM, Offord KP: A short test of mental status: description and preliminary results. Mayo Clin Proc 62(4):281–288, 1987 3561043

König P, Glatter-Götz U: Combined electroconvulsive and neuroleptic therapy in schizophrenia refractory to neuroleptics. Schizophr Res 3(5–6):351–354, 1990 1980828

Kopelman M, Wilson B, Baddeley A: The Autobiographical Memory Interview. London, Thames Valley Test Company, Harcourt Assessment, 1990

Kosel M, Frick C, Lisanby SH, et al: Magnetic seizure therapy improves mood in refractory major depression. Neuropsychopharmacology 28(11):2045–2048, 2003 12942146

Kovac AL, Goto H, Arakawa K, et al: Esmolol bolus and infusion attenuates increases in blood pressure and heart rate during electroconvulsive therapy. Can J Anaesth 37(1):58–62, 1990 1967227

Kovac AL, Goto H, Pardo MP, et al: Comparison of two esmolol bolus doses on the haemodynamic response and seizure duration during electroconvulsive therapy. Can J Anaesth 38(2):204–209, 1991 1673645

Kramer BA: A naturalistic review of maintenance ECT at a university setting. J ECT 15(4):262–269, 1999 10492862

Kranaster L, Kammerer-Ciernioch J, Hoyer C, et al: Clinically favourable effects of ketamine as an anaesthetic for electroconvulsive therapy: a retrospective study. Eur Arch Psychiatry Clin Neurosci 261(8):575–582, 2011 21400226

Kranaster L, Hoyer C, Janke C, et al: Preliminary evaluation of clinical outcome and safety of ketamine as an anesthetic for electroconvulsive therapy in schizophrenia. World J Biol Psychiatry 15(3):242–250, 2014 22397616

Krishna NR, Taylor MA, Abrams R: Response to lithium carbonate. Biol Psychiatry 13(5):601–606, 1978 31948

Krueger RB, Sackeim HA, Gamzu ER: Pharmacological treatment of the cognitive side effects of ECT: a review. Psychopharmacol Bull 28(4):409–424, 1992 1296219

Krystal AD: Ictal electroencephalographic response, in Clinical Manual of Electroconvulsive Therapy. Edited by Mankad MV, Beyer JL, Weiner RD, et al. Washington, DC, American Psychiatric Publishing, 2010, pp 105–128

Krystal AD, Watts BV, Weiner RD, et al: The use of flumazenil in the anxious and benzodiazepine-dependent ECT patient. J ECT 14(1):5–14, 1998 9661088

Kuhn J, Huff W: Will deep-brain stimulation be as successful in major depression as it has been in Parkinson's disease? Expert Rev Neurother 10(9):1363–1365, 2010 20819005

Kukopulos A, Reginaldi D, Tondo L, et al: Spontaneous length of depression and response to ECT. Psychol Med 7(4):625–629, 1977 594243

Kukopulos A, Tundo A, Foggia D, et al: Electroconvulsive therapy, in Depression and Mania: Modern Lithium Therapy. Edited by Johnson FN. Oxford, UK, IRL Press, 1988, pp 177–179

Kutcher S, Robertson HA: Electroconvulsive therapy in treatment-resistant bipolar youth. J Child Adolesc Psychopharmacol 5(3):167–175, 1995

Kwentus JA, Schulz SC, Hart RP: Tardive dystonia, catatonia, and electroconvulsive therapy. J Nerv Ment Dis 172(3):171–173, 1984 6142087

Lambourn J, Gill D: A controlled comparison of simulated and real ECT. Br J Psychiatry 133:514–519, 1978 367479

Lancaster NP, Steinert RR, Frost I: Unilateral electro-convulsive therapy. J Ment Sci 104(434):221–227, 1958 13514463

Langsley DG, Enterline JD, Hickerson GX Jr: A comparison of chlorpromazine and EST in treatment of acute schizophrenic and manic reactions. AMA Arch Neurol Psychiatry 81(3):384–391, 1959 13626291

Lapid MI, Rummans TA, Poole KL, et al: Decisional capacity of severely depressed patients requiring electroconvulsive therapy. J ECT 19(2):67–72, 2003 12792453

Lauritzen L, Odgaard K, Clemmesen L, et al: Relapse prevention by means of paroxetine in ECT-treated patients with major depression: a comparison with imipramine and placebo in medium-term continuation therapy. Acta Psychiatr Scand 94(4):241–251, 1996 8911559

Lauterbach EC, Moore NC: Parkinsonism-dystonia syndrome and ECT (letter). Am J Psychiatry 147(9):1249–1250, 1990 2386259

Lawson JS, Inglis J, Delva NJ, et al: Electrode placement in ECT: cognitive effects. Psychol Med 20(2):335–344, 1990 2356258

Lebovitz AE: (Untitled letter.) Convulsive Therapy Bulletin 1(2):11, 1976

Lebowitz P: Etomidate is still a valid anesthetic for electroconvulsive therapy (letter). J ECT 30(4):261–262, 2014 25010029

Lerer B, Zabow T, Egnal N, et al: Effect of vasopressin on memory following electroconvulsive therapy. Biol Psychiatry 18(7):821–824, 1983 6615939

Lerer B, Shapira B, Calev A, et al: Antidepressant and cognitive effects of twice- versus three-times-weekly ECT. Am J Psychiatry 152(4):564–570, 1995 7694905

Lesse S: Electroshock therapy and tranquilizing drugs. J Am Med Assoc 170(15):1791–1795, 1959 13672773

Letemendia FJ, Delva NJ, Rodenburg M, et al: Therapeutic advantage of bifrontal electrode placement in ECT. Psychol Med 23(2):349–360, 1993 8332652

Levin Y, Elizur A, Korczyn AD: Physostigmine improves ECT-induced memory disturbances. Neurology 37(5):871–875, 1987 3574695

Levin Y, Salganik I, Etzion T, et al: Naloxone fails to improve memory and cognitive disturbances after electroconvulsive therapy. Brain Dysfunct 3:193–196, 1990

Lévy-Rueff M, Jurgens A, Lôo H, et al: Maintenance electroconvulsive therapy and treatment of refractory schizophrenia [in French]. Encephale 34(5):526–533, 2008 19068343

Lévy-Rueff M, Gourevitch R, Lôo H, et al: Maintenance electroconvulsive therapy: an alternative treatment for refractory schizophrenia and schizoaffective disorders. Psychiatry Res 175(3):280–283, 2010 20034675

Lewis AB: ECT in drug-refractory schizophrenic patients. Hillside J Clin Psychiatry 4:141–154, 1982

Liberson WT: Brief stimulus therapy; physiological and clinical observations. Am J Psychiatry 105(1):28–39, 1948 18874254

Lim L-M: A practice audit of maintenance electroconvulsive therapy in the elderly (letter). Int Psychogeriatr 18(4):751–754, 2006 17026780

Lippmann SB, El-Mallakh R: Can electroconvulsive therapy be given during lithium treatment? Lithium 5:205–209, 1994

Lippmann SB, Tao CA: Electroconvulsive therapy and lithium: safe and effective treatment. Convuls Ther 9(1):54–57, 1993 11941193

Lisanby SH, Deng Z-D: Magnetic seizure therapy for the treatment of depression, in Brain Stimulation: Methodologies and Interventions. Edited by Reti IM. Hoboken, NJ, Wiley Blackwell, 2015, pp 123–148

Lisanby SH, Maddox JH, Prudic J, et al: The effects of electroconvulsive therapy on memory of autobiographical and public events. Arch Gen Psychiatry 57(6):581–590, 2000 10839336

Lisanby SH, Luber B, Finck AD, et al: Deliberate seizure induction with repetitive transcranial magnetic stimulation in nonhuman primates. Arch Gen Psychiatry 58(2):199–200, 2001a 11177122

Lisanby SH, Schlaepfer TE, Fisch H-U, et al: Magnetic seizure therapy of major depression. Arch Gen Psychiatry 58(3):303–305, 2001b 11231838

Lisanby SH, Moscrip T, Morales O, et al: Neurophysiological characterization of magnetic seizure therapy (MST) in non-human primates, in Transcranial Magnetic Stimulation and Transcranial Direct Current Stimulation (supplements to Clinical Neurophysiology, Vol 56). Edited by Paulus W, Tergau F, Nitsche MA, et al. New York, Elsevier Science, 2003, pp 81–99

Lohr WD, Figiel GS, Hudziak JJ, et al: Maintenance electroconvulsive therapy in schizophrenia (letter). J Clin Psychiatry 55(5):217–218, 1994 8071275

Lolas F: Brain polarization: behavioral and therapeutic effects. Biol Psychiatry 12(1):37–47, 1977 300033

Loo C, Sheehan P, Pigot M, et al: A report on mood and cognitive outcomes with right unilateral ultrabrief pulsewidth (0.3 ms) ECT and retrospective comparison with standard pulsewidth right unilateral ECT. J Affect Disord 103(1–3):277–281, 2007 17706790

Loo CK, Sainsbury K, Sheehan P, et al: A comparison of RUL ultrabrief pulse (0.3 ms) ECT and standard RUL ECT. Int J Neuropsychopharmacol 11(7):883–890, 2008 18752719

Loo CK, Sachdev P, Martin D, et al: A double-blind, sham-controlled trial of transcranial direct current stimulation for the treatment of depression. Int J Neuropsychopharmacol 13(1):61–69, 2010 19671217

Loo CK, Mahon M, Katalinic N, et al: Predictors of response to ultrabrief right unilateral electroconvulsive therapy. J Affect Disord 130(1–2):192–197, 2011

Loo CK, Katalinic N, Garfield JBB, et al: Neuropsychological and mood effects of ketamine in electroconvulsive therapy: a randomised controlled trial. J Affect Disord 142(1–3):233–240, 2012a 22858219

Loo CK, Katalinic N, Martin D, et al: A review of ultrabrief pulse width electroconvulsive therapy. Ther Adv Chronic Dis 3(2):69–85, 2012b 23251770

Loo CK, Garfield JBB, Katalinic N, et al: Speed of response in ultrabrief and brief pulse width right unilateral ECT. Int J Neuropsychopharmacol 16(4):755–761, 2013 22963997

Loo CK, Katalinic N, Smith DJ, et al: A randomized controlled trial of brief and ultrabrief pulse right unilateral electroconvulsive therapy. Int J Neuropsychopharmacol 18(1):1–8, 2014 25522389

Loughnan T, McKenzie G, Leong S: Sevoflurane versus propofol for induction of anaesthesia for electroconvulsive therapy: a randomized crossover trial. Anaesth Intensive Care 32(2):236–240, 2004 15957722

Lozano AM, Mayberg HS, Giacobbe P, et al: Subcallosal cingulate gyrus deep brain stimulation for treatment-resistant depression. Biol Psychiatry 64(6):461–467, 2008 18639234

Lu PH, Boone KB, Cozolino L, et al: Effectiveness of the Rey-Osterrieth Complex Figure Test and the Meyers and Meyers recognition trial in the detection of suspect effort. Clin Neuropsychol 17(3):426–440, 2003 14704893

Lunde ME, Lee EK, Rasmussen KG: Electroconvulsive therapy in patients with epilepsy. Epilepsy Behav 9(2):355–359, 2006 16876485

Magid M, Lapid MI, Sampson SM, et al: Use of electroconvulsive therapy in a patient 10 days after myocardial infarction. J ECT 21(3):182–185, 2005 16127311

Mak PH, Campbell RC, Irwin MG; American Society of Anesthesiologists: The ASA Physical Status Classification: inter-observer consistency. Anaesth Intensive Care 30(5):633–640, 2002 12413266

Malone DA Jr: Use of deep brain stimulation in treatment-resistant depression. Cleve Clin J Med 77 (suppl 3):S77–S80, 2010 20622083

Malone DA Jr, Dougherty DD, Rezai AR, et al: Deep brain stimulation of the ventral capsule/ventral striatum for treatment-resistant depression. Biol Psychiatry 65(4):267–275, 2009 18842257

Mandel MR, Madsen J, Miller AL, et al: Intoxication associated with lithium and ECT. Am J Psychiatry 137(9):1107–1109, 1980 7425167

Manning M: Undercurrents: A Life Beneath the Surface. New York, HarperOne, 1995

Manteghi A, Hojjat SK, Javanbakht A: Remission of tardive dystonia with electroconvulsive therapy (letter). J Clin Psychopharmacol 29(3):314–315, 2009 19440098

Marangell LB, Suppes T, Zboyan HA, et al: A 1-year pilot study of vagus nerve stimulation in treatment-resistant rapid-cycling bipolar disorder. J Clin Psychiatry 69(2):183–189, 2008 18211128

Marcuse LV, Fields M, Yoo J: Rowan's Primer of EEG, 2nd Edition. New York, Elsevier, 2016

Martin BA, Bean GJ: Competence to consent to electroconvulsive therapy. Convuls Ther 8(2):92–102, 1992 11659635

Martin BA, Kramer PM: Clinical significance of the interaction between lithium and a neuromuscular blocker. Am J Psychiatry 139(10):1326–1328, 1982 6812439

Martin DM, Katalinic N, Ingram A, et al: A new early cognitive screening measure to detect cognitive side-effects of electroconvulsive therapy? J Psychiatr Res 47(12):1967–1974, 2013 24074514

Martin DM, Galvez V, Loo CK: Predicting retrograde autobiographical memory changes following electroconvulsive therapy: relationships between individual, treatment, and early clinical factors. Int J Neuropsychopharmacol 18(12):pii: pyv067, 2016 26091817

Martinez MW, Rasmussen KG, Mueller PS, et al: Troponin elevations after electro-convulsive therapy: the need for caution. Am J Med 124(3):229–234, 2011 21396506

Martínez-Amorós E, Cardoner N, Gálvez V, et al: Effectiveness and pattern of use of continuation and maintenance electroconvulsive therapy. Rev Psiquiatr Salud Ment 5(4):241–253, 2012a 23021297

Martínez-Amorós E, Cardoner N, Soria V, et al: Long-term treatment strategies in major depression: a 2-year prospective naturalistic follow-up after successful electroconvulsive therapy. J ECT 28(2):92–97, 2012b 22531201

Martiny K, Larsen ER, Licht RW, et al; Danish University Antidepressant Group (DUAG): Relapse prevention in major depressive disorder after successful electroconvulsive treatment: a 6-month double-blind comparison of three fixed dosages of escitalopram and a fixed dose of nortriptyline—lessons from a failed randomised trial of the Danish University Antidepressant Group (DUAG-7). Pharmacopsychiatry 48(7):274–278, 2015 26529118

Matheson SL, Green MJ, Loo C, et al: Quality assessment and comparison of evidence for electroconvulsive therapy and repetitive transcranial magnetic stimulation for schizophrenia: a systematic meta-review. Schizophr Res 118(1–3):201–210, 2010 20117918

Mattes JA, Pettinati HM, Stephens S, et al: A placebo-controlled evaluation of vasopressin for ECT-induced memory impairment. Biol Psychiatry 27(3):289–303, 1990 2405915

Matthews JD, Blais M, Park L, et al: The impact of galantamine on cognition and mood during electroconvulsive therapy: a pilot study. J Psychiatr Res 42(7):526–531, 2008 17681545

May PR, Tuma AH, Yale C, et al: Schizophrenia—a follow-up study of results of treatment. Arch Gen Psychiatry 33(4):481–486, 1976 938185

May PR, Tuma AH, Dixon WJ, et al: Schizophrenia: a follow-up study of the results of five forms of treatment. Arch Gen Psychiatry 38(7):776–784, 1981 6113821

Mayberg HS: Targeted electrode-based modulation of neural circuits for depression. J Clin Invest 119(4):717–725, 2009 19339763

Mayberg HS, Lozano AM, Voon V, et al: Deep brain stimulation for treatment-resistant depression. Neuron 45(5):651–660, 2005 15748841

Mayur P: Ictal electroencephalographic characteristics during electroconvulsive therapy: a review of determination and clinical relevance. J ECT 22(3):213–217, 2006 16957539

Mayur P, Bray A, Fernandes J, et al: Impact of hyperventilation on stimulus efficiency during the early phase of an electroconvulsive therapy course: a randomized double-blind study. J ECT 26(2):91–94, 2010

Mayur PM, Gangadhar BN, Janakiramaiah N: Factors influencing ratio of motor and EEG seizure duration in ECT (letter). Can J Psychiatry 44(2):191, 1999 10097847

Mayur PM, Gangadhar BN, Subbakrishna DK, et al: Discontinuation of antidepressant drugs during electroconvulsive therapy: a controlled study. J Affect Disord 58(1):37–41, 2000 10760556

Mayur P, Byth K, Harris A: Autobiographical and subjective memory with right unilateral high-dose 0.3-millisecond ultrabrief-pulse and 1-millisecond brief-pulse electroconvulsive therapy: a double-blind, randomized controlled trial. J ECT 29(4):277–282, 2013 24263273

McAllister DA, Perri MG, Jordan RC, et al: Effects of ECT given two vs. three times weekly. Psychiatry Res 21(1):63–69, 1987 3602221

McCabe MS: ECT in the treatment of mania: a controlled study. Am J Psychiatry 133(6):688–691, 1976 1275099

McCabe MS, Norris B: ECT versus chlorpromazine in mania. Biol Psychiatry 12(2):245–254, 1977 870095

McCall WV, Shelp FE, Weiner RD, et al: Effects of labetalol on hemodynamics and seizure duration during ECT. Convuls Ther 7(1):5–14, 1991 11941090

McCall WV, Zvara D, Brooker R, et al: Effect of esmolol pretreatment on EEG seizure morphology in RUL ECT. Convuls Ther 13(3):175–180, 1997 9342133

McCall WV, Sparks W, Jane J, et al: Variation of ictal electroencephalographic regularity with low-, moderate-, and high-dose stimuli during right unilateral electroconvulsive therapy. Biol Psychiatry 43(8):608–611, 1998 9564446

McCall WV, Reboussin DM, Weiner RD, et al: Titrated moderately suprathreshold vs fixed high-dose right unilateral electroconvulsive therapy: acute antidepressant and cognitive effects. Arch Gen Psychiatry 57(5):438–444, 2000 10807483

McCall WV, Dunn A, Rosenquist PB, et al: Markedly suprathreshold right unilateral ECT versus minimally suprathreshold bilateral ECT: antidepressant and memory effects. J ECT 18(3):126–129, 2002 12394530

McCall WV, Prudic J, Olfson M, et al: Health-related quality of life following ECT in a large community sample. J Affect Disord 90(2–3):269–274, 2006 16412519

McCully RB, Karon BL, Rummans TA, et al: Frequency of left ventricular dysfunction after electroconvulsive therapy. Am J Cardiol 91(9):1147–1150, 2003 12714169

McDonald WM, Phillips VL, Figiel GS, et al: Cost-effective maintenance treatment of resistant geriatric depression. Psychiatr Ann 28(1):47–52, 1998

McDonald WM, Weiner RD, Fochtmann LJ, et al: The FDA and ECT. J ECT 32(2):75–77, 2016 27191123

McElhiney MC, Moody BJ, Steif BL, et al: Autobiographical memory and mood: effects of electroconvulsive therapy. Neuropsychology 9(4):501–517, 1995

McElhiney MC, Moody BJ, Sackeim HA: The Autobiographical Memory Interview—Short Form. New York, Department of Biological Psychiatry, New York State Psychiatric Institute, 2001

McGirr A, Berlim MT, Bond DJ, et al: A systematic review and meta-analysis of randomized controlled trials of adjunctive ketamine in electroconvulsive therapy: efficacy and tolerability. J Psychiatr Res 62:23–30, 2015 25684151

McNeill DL: Phenothiazine resistance (letter). BMJ 2(6079):127–128, 1977 17450

Medda P, Perugi G, Zanello S, et al: Response to ECT in bipolar I, bipolar II and unipolar depression. J Affect Disord 118(1–3):55–59, 2009 19223079

Medda P, Perugi G, Zanello S, et al: Comparative response to electroconvulsive therapy in medication-resistant bipolar I patients with depression and mixed state. J ECT 26(2):82–86, 2010 19710623

Medda P, Mauri M, Fratta S, et al: Long-term naturalistic follow-up of patients with bipolar depression and mixed state treated with electroconvulsive therapy. J ECT 29(3):179–188, 2013 23899721

Medda P, Toni C, Mariani MG, et al: Electroconvulsive therapy in 197 patients with a severe, drug-resistant bipolar mixed state: treatment outcome and predictors of response. J Clin Psychiatry 76(9):1168–1173, 2015 25938268

Meeter M, Murre JMJ, Janssen SMJ, et al: Retrograde amnesia after electroconvulsive therapy: a temporary effect? J Affect Disord 132(1–2):216–222, 2011 21450347

Meldrum BS: Neuropathological consequences of chemically and electrically induced seizures. Ann N Y Acad Sci 462:186–193, 1986 3085568

Mendels J: Electroconvulsive therapy and depression, I: the prognostic significance of clinical factors. Br J Psychiatry 111:675–681, 1965a 14337414

Mendels J: Electroconvulsive therapy and depression, III: a method for prognosis. Br J Psychiatry 111:687–690, 1965b 14337416

Mendels J: The prediction of response to electroconvulsive therapy. Am J Psychiatry 124(2):153–159, 1967 4951568

Meyers BS, Klimstra SA, Gabriele M, et al: Continuation treatment of delusional depression in older adults. Am J Geriatr Psychiatry 9(4):415–422, 2001 11739068

Meyers BS, Flint AJ, Rothschild AJ, et al: A double-blind randomized controlled trial of olanzapine plus sertraline vs olanzapine plus placebo for psychotic depression: the Study of Pharmacotherapy of Psychotic Depression (STOP-PD). Arch Gen Psychiatry 66(8):838–847, 2009 19652123

Michael N, Erfurth A, Ohrmann P, et al: Metabolic changes within the left dorsolateral prefrontal cortex occurring with electroconvulsive therapy in patients with treatment resistant unipolar depression. Psychol Med 33(7):1277–1284, 2003a 14580081

Michael N, Erfurth A, Ohrmann P, et al: Neurotrophic effects of electroconvulsive therapy: a proton magnetic resonance study of the left amygdalar region in patients with treatment-resistant depression. Neuropsychopharmacology 28(4):720–725, 2003b 12655317

Milstein V, Small JG, Klapper MH, et al: Uni- versus bilateral ECT in the treatment of mania. Convuls Ther 3(1):1–9, 1987 11940883

Minelli A, Abate M, Zampieri E, et al: Seizure adequacy markers and the prediction of electroconvulsive therapy response. J ECT 32(2):88–92, 2016 26397151

Minnai GP, Salis PG, Oppo R, et al: Effectiveness of maintenance electroconvulsive therapy in rapid-cycling bipolar disorder. J ECT 27(2):123–126, 2011 20559148

Miranda PC, Lomarev M, Hallett M: Modeling the current distribution during transcranial direct current stimulation. Clin Neurophysiol 117(7):1623–1629, 2006 16762592

Mohan TSP, Tharyan P, Alexander J, et al: Effects of stimulus intensity on the efficacy and safety of twice-weekly, bilateral electroconvulsive therapy (ECT) combined with antipsychotics in acute mania: a randomised controlled trial. Bipolar Disord 11(2):126–134, 2009 19267695

Monroe RR Jr: Maintenance electroconvulsive therapy. Psychiatr Clin North Am 14(4):947–960, 1991 1771156

Montgomery SA, Åsberg M: A new depression scale designed to be sensitive to change. Br J Psychiatry 134(4):382–389, 1979 444788

Moore NP: The maintenance treatment of chronic psychotics by electrically induced convulsions. J Ment Sci 89:257–269, 1943

Moreines JL, McClintock SM, Holtzheimer PE: Neuropsychologic effects of neuro-modulation techniques for treatment-resistant depression: a review. Brain Stimul 4(1):17–27, 2011 21255751

Moscarillo FM, Annunziata CM: ECT in a patient with a deep brain-stimulating electrode in place. J ECT 16(3):287–290, 2000 11005051

Moscrip TD, Terrace HS, Sackeim HA, et al: Randomized controlled trial of the cog-nitive side-effects of magnetic seizure therapy (MST) and electroconvulsive shock (ECS). Int J Neuropsychopharmacol 9(1):1–11, 2006 16045810

Mueller PS, Schak KM, Barnes RD, et al: Safety of electroconvulsive therapy in pa-tients with asthma. Neth J Med 64(11):417–421, 2006 17179572

Mueller PS, Barnes RD, Varghese R, et al: The safety of electroconvulsive therapy in patients with severe aortic stenosis. Mayo Clin Proc 82(11):1360–1363, 2007 17976355

Mueller PS, Albin SM, Barnes RD, et al: Safety of electroconvulsive therapy in pa-tients with unrepaired abdominal aortic aneurysm: report of 8 patients. J ECT 25(3):165–169, 2009 19730028

Mukherjee S: Combined ECT and lithium therapy. Convuls Ther 9(4):274–284, 1993 11941223

Mukherjee S, Debsikdar V: Absence of neuroleptic-induced parkinsonism in psy-chotic patients receiving adjunctive electroconvulsive therapy. Convuls Ther 10(1):53–58, 1994 7914462

Mukherjee S, Sackeim HA, Lee C: Unilateral ECT in the treatment of manic epi-sodes. Convuls Ther 4(1):74–80, 1988 11940944

Mukherjee S, Sackeim HA, Schnur DB: Electroconvulsive therapy of acute manic ep-isodes: a review of 50 years' experience. Am J Psychiatry 151(2):169–176, 1994 8296883

Muller D: 1. Nardil (phenelzine) as a potentiator of electroconvulsive therapy (ECT). 2. A survey of outpatient E.C.T. J Ment Sci 107:994–996, 1961 14477115

Munk-Olsen T, Laursen TM, Videbech P, et al: All-cause mortality among recipients of electroconvulsive therapy: register-based cohort study. Br J Psychiatry 190:435–439, 2007 17470959

Murphy DN, Boggio P, Fregni F: Transcranial direct current stimulation as a thera-peutic tool for the treatment of major depression: insights from past and recent clinical studies. Curr Opin Psychiatry 22(3):306–311, 2009 19339889

Nahas Z, Marangell LB, Husain MM, et al: Two-year outcome of vagus nerve stimu-lation (VNS) for treatment of major depressive episodes. J Clin Psychiatry 66(9):1097–1104, 2005 16187765

Nahas Z, Short B, Burns C, et al: A feasibility study of a new method for electrically producing seizures in man: focal electrically administered seizure therapy (FEAST). Brain Stimul 6(3):403–408, 2013 23518262

Nascimento AL, Appolinario JC, Segenreich D, et al: Maintenance electroconvulsive therapy for recurrent refractory mania. Bipolar Disord 8(3):301–303, 2006 16696835

Nasrallah HA, Varney N, Coffman JA, et al: Opiate antagonism fails to reverse post-ECT cognitive deficits. J Clin Psychiatry 47(11):555–556, 1986 3771502

Nasreddine ZS, Phillips NA, Bédirian V, et al: The Montreal Cognitive Assessment, MoCA: a brief screening tool for mild cognitive impairment. J Am Geriatr Soc 53(4):695–699, 2005 15817019

National Institutes of Health: Consensus conference. Electroconvulsive therapy. JAMA 254(15):2103–2108, 1985 4046138

Navarro V, Gastó C, Torres X, et al: Continuation/maintenance treatment with nortriptyline versus combined nortriptyline and ECT in late-life psychotic depression: a two-year randomized study. Am J Geriatr Psychiatry 16(6):498–505, 2008 18515694

Nelson JC, Mazure C: Ruminative thinking: a distinctive sign of melancholia. J Affect Disord 9(1):41–46, 1985 3160746

Nelson JP, Benjamin L: Efficacy and safety of combined ECT and tricyclic antidepressant drugs in the treatment of depressed geriatric patients. Convuls Ther 5(4):321–329, 1989 11941030

Netzel PJ, Mueller PS, Rummans TA, et al: Safety, efficacy, and effects on glycemic control of electroconvulsive therapy in insulin-requiring type 2 diabetic patients. J ECT 18(1):16–21, 2002 11925516

Ng C, Schweitzer I, Alexopoulos P, et al: Efficacy and cognitive effects of right unilateral electroconvulsive therapy. J ECT 16(4):370–379, 2000 11314875

Nguyen TT, Chhibber AK, Lustik SJ, et al: Effect of methohexitone and propofol with or without alfentanil on seizure duration and recovery in electroconvulsive therapy. Br J Anaesth 79(6):801–803, 1997 9496217

Niemantsverdriet L, Birkenhäger TK, van den Broek WW: The efficacy of ultrabrief-pulse (0.25 millisecond) versus brief-pulse (0.50 millisecond) bilateral electroconvulsive therapy in major depression. J ECT 27(1):55–58, 2011 21343712

Nierenberg AA, Alpert JE, Gardner-Schuster EE, et al: Vagus nerve stimulation: 2-year outcomes for bipolar versus unipolar treatment-resistant depression. Biol Psychiatry 64(6):455–460, 2008 18571625

Nishikawa K, Higuchi M, Kawagishi T, et al: Effect of divided supplementation of remifentanil on seizure duration and hemodynamic responses during electroconvulsive therapy under propofol anesthesia. J Anesth 25(1):29–33, 2011 21116659

Nitsche MA, Boggio PS, Fregni F, et al: Treatment of depression with transcranial direct current stimulation (tDCS): a review. Exp Neurol 219(1):14–19, 2009 19348793

Nobuhara K, Matsuda S, Okugawa G, et al: Successful electroconvulsive treatment of depression associated with a marked reduction in the symptoms of tardive dyskinesia. J ECT 20(4):262–263, 2004 15591862

Nordanskog P, Dahlstrand U, Larsson MR, et al: Increase in hippocampal volume after electroconvulsive therapy in patients with depression: a volumetric magnetic resonance imaging study. J ECT 26(1):62–67, 2010 20190603

Nordenskjöld A, von Knorring L, Engström I: Predictors of time to relapse/ recurrence after electroconvulsive therapy in patients with major depressive disorder: a population-based cohort study. Depress Res Treat 2011:470985, 2011a 22110913

Nordenskjöld A, von Knorring L, Engström I: Rehospitalization rate after continued electroconvulsive therapy—a retrospective chart review of patients with severe depression. Nord J Psychiatry 65(1):26–31, 2011b 20482461

Nordenskjöld A, von Knorring L, Ljung T, et al: Continuation electroconvulsive therapy with pharmacotherapy versus pharmacotherapy alone for prevention of relapse of depression: a randomized controlled trial. J ECT 29(2):86–92, 2013 23303421

Nordenskjöld A, Mårtensson B, Pettersson A, et al: Effects of Hesel-coil deep transcranial magnetic stimulation for depression—a systematic review. Nord J Psychiatry 70(7):492–497, 2016 27093104

Nothdurfter C, Eser D, Schüle C, et al: The influence of concomitant neuroleptic medication on safety, tolerability and clinical effectiveness of electroconvulsive therapy. World J Biol Psychiatry 7(3):162–170, 2006 16861142

Nuttall GA, Bowersox MR, Douglass SB, et al: Morbidity and mortality in the use of electroconvulsive therapy. J ECT 20(4):237–241, 2004 15591857

O'Brien PD, Berrios GE: Concurrent psychotropic medication has no negative influence on the outcome of electroconvulsive therapy. Encephale 19(4):347–349, 1993 7903929

O'Connor CJ, Rothenberg DM, Soble JS, et al: The effect of esmolol pretreatment on the incidence of regional wall motion abnormalities during electroconvulsive therapy. Anesth Analg 82(1):143–147, 1996 8712391

O'Connor DW, Gardner B, Eppingstall B, et al: Cognition in elderly patients receiving unilateral and bilateral electroconvulsive therapy: a prospective, naturalistic comparison. J Affect Disord 124(3):235–240, 2010a 20053457

O'Connor DW, Gardner B, Presnell I, et al: The effectiveness of continuation-maintenance ECT in reducing depressed older patients' hospital re-admissions. J Affect Disord 120(1–3):62–66, 2010b 19411112

O'Connor MK, Knapp R, Husain M, et al: The influence of age on the response of major depression to electroconvulsive therapy: a C.O.R.E. report. Am J Geriatr Psychiatry 9(4):382–390, 2001 11739064

O'Connor M, Lebowitz BK, Ly J, et al: A dissociation between anterograde and retrograde amnesia after treatment with electroconvulsive therapy: a naturalistic investigation. J ECT 24(2):146–151, 2008 18580560

Odeberg H, Rodriguez-Silva B, Salander P, et al: Individualized continuation electroconvulsive therapy and medication as a bridge to relapse prevention after an index course of electroconvulsive therapy in severe mood disorders: a naturalistic 3-year cohort study. J ECT 24(3):183–190, 2008 18695624

O'Flaherty D, Husain MM, Moore M, et al: Circulatory responses during electroconvulsive therapy: the comparative effects of placebo, esmolol and nitroglycerin. Anaesthesia 47(7):563–567, 1992 1352662

Okamoto H, Shimizu E, Ozawa K, et al: Lithium augmentation in milnacipran-refractory depression for the prevention of relapse following electroconvulsive therapy. Aust N Z J Psychiatry 39(1–2):108, 2005 15660714

Okamoto N, Nakai T, Sakamoto K, et al: Rapid antidepressant effect of ketamine anesthesia during electroconvulsive therapy of treatment-resistant depression: comparing ketamine and propofol anesthesia. J ECT 26(3):223–227, 2010 19935085

O'Leary DA, Lee AS: Seven year prognosis in depression: mortality and readmission risk in the Nottingham ECT cohort. Br J Psychiatry 169(4):423–429, 1996 8894191

Oltman JE, Friedman S: Analysis of temporal factors in manic-depressive psychosis, with particular reference to the effect of shock therapy. Am J Psychiatry 107(1):57–68, 1950 15419335

Ona CM, Onoye JM, Goebert D, et al: Sociodemographic characterization of ECT utilization in Hawaii. J ECT 30(1):43–46, 2014 24080537

O'Reardon JP, Solvason HB, Janicak PG, et al: Efficacy and safety of transcranial magnetic stimulation in the acute treatment of major depression: a multisite randomized controlled trial. Biol Psychiatry 62(11):1208–1216, 2007 17573044

Ottosson J-O: Experimental studies of memory impairment after electroconvulsive therapy. The role of the electrical stimulation and of the seizure studied by variation of stimulus intensity and modification by lidocaine of seizure discharge. Acta Psychiatr Scand Suppl 35(145):103–131, 1960 14429445

Ottosson J-O, Fink M: Ethics in Electroconvulsive Therapy. New York, Brunner-Routledge, 2004

Owens JA: Psychopharmacology, in The American Psychiatric Publishing Textbook of Psychosomatic Medicine: Psychiatric Care of the Medically Ill, 2nd Edition. Edited by Levenson JL. Washington, DC, American Psychiatric Publishing, 2011, pp 976–1019

Pagnin D, de Queiroz V, Pini S, et al: Efficacy of ECT in depression: a meta-analytic review. J ECT 20(1):13–20, 2004 15087991

Palm U, Keeser D, Schiller C, et al: Transcranial direct current stimulation in a patient with therapy-resistant major depression. World J Biol Psychiatry 10(4 Pt 2):632–635, 2009 19995213

Palm U, Hasan A, Strube W, et al: tDCS for the treatment of depression: a comprehensive review. Eur Arch Psychiatry Clin Neurosci 266(8):681–694, 2016 26842422

Palmer DM, Sprang HE, Hans CL: Electroshock therapy in schizophrenia; a statistical survey of 455 cases. J Nerv Ment Dis 114(2):162–171, 1951 14861659

Palmio J, Huuhka M, Laine S, et al: Electroconvulsive therapy and biomarkers of neuronal injury and plasticity: serum levels of neuron-specific enolase and S-100b protein. Psychiatry Res 177(1–2):97–100, 2010 20378182

Pande AC, Shea J, Shettar S, et al: Effect of hyperventilation on seizure length during electroconvulsive therapy. Biol Psychiatry 27(7):799–801, 1990 2109642

Pearlman C: Lithium-ECT interaction (letter). Convuls Ther 4(2):182, 1988 11940961

Penland HR, Ostroff RB: Combined use of lamotrigine and electroconvulsive therapy in bipolar depression: a case series. J ECT 22(2):142–147, 2006 16801832

Penney JF, Dinwiddie SH, Zorumski CF, et al: Concurrent and close temporal administration of lithium and ECT. Convuls Ther 6(2):139–145, 1990 11941055

Peretti CS, Danion JM, Grangé D, Mobarek N: Bilateral ECT and autobiographical memory of subjective experiences related to melancholia: a pilot study. J Affect Disord 41(1):9–15, 1996 8938200

Perrin JS, Merz S, Bennett DM, et al: Electroconvulsive therapy reduces frontal cortical connectivity in severe depressive disorder. Proc Natl Acad Sci USA 109(14):5464–5468, 2012 22431642

Perry CL, Lindell EP, Rasmussen KG: ECT in patients with arachnoid cysts (Erratum appears in J ECT. 2007; 23(2):136). J ECT 23(1):36–37, 2007 17435574

Perry P, Tsuang MT: Treatment of unipolar depression following electroconvulsive therapy: relapse rate comparisons between lithium and tricyclics therapies following ECT. J Affect Disord 1(2):123–129, 1979 162494

Peterchev AV, Krystal AD, Rosa MA, et al: Individualized low-amplitude seizure therapy: minimizing current for electroconvulsive therapy and magnetic seizure therapy. Neuropsychopharmacology 40(9):2076–2084, 2015 25920013

Petrides G: Continuation ECT: a review. Psychiatr Ann 28:517–523, 1998

Petrides G, Fink M: Atrial fibrillation, anticoagulation, and electroconvulsive therapy. Convuls Ther 12(2):91–98, 1996 8744168

Petrides G, Dhossche D, Fink M, et al: Continuation ECT: relapse prevention in affective disorders. Convuls Ther 10(3):189–194, 1994 7834255

Petrides G, Fink M, Husain MM, et al: ECT remission rates in psychotic versus nonpsychotic depressed patients: a report from CORE. J ECT 17(4):244–253, 2001 11731725

Petrides G, Tobias KG, Kellner CH, et al: Continuation and maintenance electroconvulsive therapy for mood disorders: review of the literature. Neuropsychobiology 64(3):129–140, 2011 21811083

Pettinati HM, Mathisen KS, Rosenberg J, et al: Meta-analytical approach to reconciling discrepancies in efficacy between bilateral and unilateral electroconvulsive therapy. Convuls Ther 2(1):7–17, 1986 11940840

Pettinati HM, Stephens SM, Willis KM, et al: Evidence for less improvement in depression in patients taking benzodiazepines during unilateral ECT. Am J Psychiatry 147(8):1029–1035, 1990 2375437

Phutane VH, Thirthalli J, Muralidharan K, et al: Double-blind randomized controlled study showing symptomatic and cognitive superiority of bifrontal over bitemporal electrode placement during electroconvulsive therapy for schizophrenia. Brain Stimul 6(2):210–217, 2013 22560048

Pigot M, Andrade C, Loo C: Pharmacological attenuation of electroconvulsive therapy—induced cognitive deficits: theoretical background and clinical findings. J ECT 24(1):57–67, 2008 18379337

Pisvejc J, Hyrman V, Sikora J, et al: A comparison of brief and ultrabrief pulse stimuli in unilateral ECT. J ECT 14(2):68–75, 1998 9641801

Pluijms EM, Birkenhäger TK, Mulder PG, et al: Influence of episode duration of major depressive disorder on response to electroconvulsive therapy. J Affect Disord 90(2–3):233–237, 2006 16376432

Popeo D, Kellner CH: ECT for Parkinson's disease (editorial). Med Hypotheses 73(4):468–469, 2009 19660875

Poreisz C, Boros K, Antal A, et al: Safety aspects of transcranial direct current stimulation concerning healthy subjects and patients. Brain Res Bull 72(4–6):208–214, 2007 17452283

Porquez JM, Thompson TR, McDonald WM: Administration of ECT in a patient with an inoperable abdominal aortic aneurysm: serial imaging of the aorta during maintenance. J ECT 19(2):118–120, 2003 12792463

Postolache TT, Londono JH, Halem RG, et al: Electroconvulsive therapy in tardive dystonia. Convuls Ther 11(4):275–279, 1995 8919581

Prakash J, Kotwal A, Prabhu H: Therapeutic and prophylactic utility of the memory-enhancing drug donepezil hydrochloride on cognition of patients undergoing electroconvulsive therapy: a randomized controlled trial. J ECT 22(3):163–168, 2006 16957530

Price TRP, Levin R: The effects of electroconvulsive therapy on tardive dyskinesia. Am J Psychiatry 135(8):991–993, 1978 665856

Pridmore S, Pollard C: Electroconvulsive therapy in Parkinson's disease: 30 month follow up (letter). J Neurol Neurosurg Psychiatry 60(6):693, 1996 8648342

Pridmore S, Yeo PT, Pasha MI: Electroconvulsive therapy for the physical signs of Parkinson's disease without depressive disorder (letter). J Neurol Neurosurg Psychiatry 58(5):641–642, 1995 7745424

Prudic J, Sackeim HA, Devanand DP: Medication resistance and clinical response to electroconvulsive therapy. Psychiatry Res 31(3):287–296, 1990 1970656

Prudic J, Haskett RF, Mulsant B, et al: Resistance to antidepressant medications and short-term clinical response to ECT. Am J Psychiatry 153(8):985–992, 1996

Prudic J, Fitzsimons L, Nobler MS, et al: Naloxone in the prevention of the adverse cognitive effects of ECT: a within-subject, placebo controlled study. Neuropsychopharmacology 21(2):285–293, 1999 10432476

Prudic J, Peyser S, Sackeim HA: Subjective memory complaints: a review of patient self-assessment of memory after electroconvulsive therapy. J ECT 16(2):121–132, 2000 10868322

Prudic J, Olfson M, Marcus SC, et al: Effectiveness of electroconvulsive therapy in community settings. Biol Psychiatry 55(3):301–312, 2004 14744473

Prudic J, Haskett RF, McCall WV, et al: Pharmacological strategies in the prevention of relapse after electroconvulsive therapy. J ECT 29(1):3–12, 2013 23303417

Pullen SJ, Rasmussen KG, Angstman ER, et al: The safety of electroconvulsive therapy in patients with prolonged QTc intervals on the electrocardiogram. J ECT 27(3):192–200, 2011 21681107

Quante A, Luborzewski A, Brakemeier E-L, et al: Effects of 3 different stimulus intensities of ultrabrief stimuli in right unilateral electroconvulsive therapy in major depression: a randomized, double-blind pilot study. J Psychiatr Res 45(2):174–178, 2011 20728093

Rabheru K: Maintenance electroconvulsive therapy (M-ECT) after acute response: examining the evidence for who, what, when, and how? J ECT 28(1):39–47, 2012 22330700

Rabheru K, Persad E: A review of continuation and maintenance electroconvulsive therapy. Can J Psychiatry 42(5):476–484, 1997 9220110

Raes F, Sienaert P, Demyttenaere K, et al: Overgeneral memory predicts stability of short-term outcome of electroconvulsive therapy for depression. J ECT 24(1):81–83, 2008 18379339

Rahman R: A review of treatment of 176 schizophrenic patients in the mental hospital Pabna. Br J Psychiatry 114(511):775–777, 1968 5665962

Rami-González L, Salamero M, Boget T, et al: Pattern of cognitive dysfunction in depressive patients during maintenance electroconvulsive therapy. Psychol Med 33(2):345–350, 2003 12622313

Ranjkesh F, Barekatain M, Akuchakian S: Bifrontal versus right unilateral and bitemporal electroconvulsive therapy in major depressive disorder. J ECT 21(4):207–210, 2005 16301878

Rao V, Lyketsos CG: The benefits and risks of ECT for patients with primary dementia who also suffer from depression. Int J Geriatr Psychiatry 15(8):729–735, 2000 10960885

Rapinesi C, Kotzalidis GD, Serata D, et al: Prevention of relapse with maintenance electroconvulsive therapy in elderly patients with major depressive episode. J ECT 29(1):61–64, 2013 23011573

Rasmussen KG: Electroconvulsive therapy in patients with aortic stenosis. Convuls Ther 13(3):196–199, 1997 9342136

Rasmussen KG: The role of electroconvulsive therapy in chronic pain. Rev Analg 7(1):1–8, 2003

Rasmussen KG: Evidence for electroconvulsive therapy efficacy in mood disorders, in Electroconvulsive and Neuromodulation Therapies. Edited by Swartz C. Cambridge, UK, Cambridge University Press, 2009a, pp 109–123

Rasmussen KG: Sham electroconvulsive therapy studies in depressive illness: a review of the literature and consideration of the placebo phenomenon in electroconvulsive therapy practice. J ECT 25(1):54–59, 2009b 18580816

Rasmussen KG: Electroconvulsive therapy and melancholia: review of the literature and suggestions for further study. J ECT 27(4):315–322, 2011a 21673591

Rasmussen KG: Some considerations in choosing electroconvulsive therapy versus transcranial magnetic stimulation for depression. J ECT 27(1):51–54, 2011b 21343711

Rasmussen KG: A randomized controlled trial of ketorolac for prevention of headache related to electroconvulsive therapy. Pain Studies and Treatment 1(2):5–8, 2013

Rasmussen KG: Propofol for ECT anesthesia: a review of the literature. J ECT 30(3):210–215, 2014 24820943

Rasmussen KG: Do patients with personality disorders respond differentially to electroconvulsive therapy? A review of the literature and consideration of conceptual issues. J ECT 31(1):6–12, 2015a 25054362

Rasmussen KG: Improving ECT efficacy and decreasing cognitive side effects, in Brain Stimulation: Methodologies and Interventions. Edited by Reti I. Hoboken, NJ, Wiley-Blackwell, 2015b, pp 83–106

Rasmussen KG: Recall of paralysis after the seizure with right unilateral ultrabrief technique (letter). J ECT 31(2):e26, 2015c 25621544

Rasmussen KG: What type of cognitive testing should be part of routine electroconvulsive therapy practice? J ECT 32(1):7–12, 2016 26075697

Rasmussen K, Abrams R: Treatment of Parkinson's disease with electroconvulsive therapy. Psychiatr Clin North Am 14(4):925–933, 1991 1771154

Rasmussen KG, Flemming KD: Electroconvulsive therapy in patients with cavernous hemangiomas. J ECT 22(4):272–273, 2006 17143161

Rasmussen KG, Keegan BM: Electroconvulsive therapy in patients with multiple sclerosis. J ECT 23(3):179–180, 2007 17804994

Rasmussen KG, Lineberry TW: Patients who inappropriately demand electroconvulsive therapy. J ECT 23(2):109–113, 2007 17548983

Rasmussen KG, Lunde ME: Patients who develop epilepsy during extended treatment with electroconvulsive therapy. Seizure 16(3):266–270, 2007 17185006

Rasmussen KG, Ritter MJ: Anesthetic-induced pain on injection in electroconvulsive therapy: review of the literature and suggestions for prevention. J ECT 30(3):203–209, 2014a 24820946

Rasmussen KG, Ritter MJ: Some considerations of the tolerability of ketamine for ECT anesthesia: a case series and review of the literature. J ECT 30(4):283–286, 2014b 24820945

Rasmussen KG, Rummans TA: Electroconvulsive therapy for phantom limb pain. Pain 85(1–2):297–299, 2000 10692632

Rasmussen KG, Rummans TA: Electroconvulsive therapy in the management of chronic pain. Curr Pain Headache Rep 6(1):17–22, 2002 11749873

Rasmussen KG, Ryan DA: The effect of electroconvulsive therapy treatments on blood sugar in nondiabetic patients. J ECT 21(4):232–234, 2005 16301883

Rasmussen KG, Zorumski CF: Electroconvulsive therapy in patients taking theophylline. J Clin Psychiatry 54(11):427–431, 1993 8270586

Rasmussen KG, Zorumski CF, Jarvis MR: Electroconvulsive therapy in patients with cerebral palsy. Convuls Ther 9:205–208, 1993 11941214

Rasmussen KG, Jarvis MR, Zorumski CF: Ketamine anesthesia in electroconvulsive therapy. Convuls Ther 12(4):217–223, 1996 9034696

Rasmussen KG, Jarvis MR, Zorumski CF, et al: Low-dose atropine in electroconvulsive therapy. J ECT 15(3):213–221, 1999 10492860

Rasmussen KG, Russell JC, Kung S, et al: Electroconvulsive therapy for patients with major depression and probable Lewy body dementia. J ECT 19(2):103–109, 2003 12792460

Rasmussen KG, Karpyak VM, Hammill SC: Lack of effect of ECT on Holter monitor recordings before and after treatment. J ECT 20(1):45–47, 2004 15087997

Rasmussen KG, Spackman TN, Hooten WM: The clinical utility of inhalational anesthesia with sevoflurane in electroconvulsive therapy. J ECT 21(4):239–242, 2005 16301885

Rasmussen KG, Mueller M, Kellner CH, et al; CORE group: Patterns of psychotropic medication use among patients with severe depression referred for electroconvulsive therapy: data from the Consortium for Research on Electroconvulsive Therapy. J ECT 22(2):116–123, 2006a 16801827

Rasmussen KG, Ryan DA, Mueller PS: Blood glucose before and after ECT treatments in type 2 diabetic patients. J ECT 22(2):124–126, 2006b 16801828

Rasmussen KG, Hooten WM, Dodd ML, et al: QTc dispersion on the baseline ECG predicts arrhythmias during electroconvulsive therapy. Acta Cardiol 62(4):345–347, 2007a 17824294

Rasmussen KG, Laurila DR, Brady BM, et al: Anesthesia outcomes in a randomized double-blind trial of sevoflurane and thiopental for induction of general anesthesia in electroconvulsive therapy. J ECT 23(4):236–238, 2007b 18090695

Rasmussen KG, Mohan A, Stevens SR: Serum sodium does not correlate with seizure length or seizure threshold in electroconvulsive therapy. J ECT 23(3):175–176, 2007c 17804992

Rasmussen KG, Perry CL, Sutor B, et al: ECT in patients with intracranial masses. J Neuropsychiatry Clin Neurosci 19(2):191–193, 2007d 17431067

Rasmussen KG, Varghese R, Stevens SR, et al: Electrode placement and ictal EEG indices in electroconvulsive therapy. J Neuropsychiatry Clin Neurosci 19(4):453–457, 2007e 18070850

Rasmussen KG, Albin SM, Mueller PS, et al: Electroconvulsive therapy in patients taking steroid medication: should supplemental doses be given on the days of treatment? J ECT 24(2):128–130, 2008a 18580555

Rasmussen KG, Hart DA, Lineberry TW: ECT in patients with psychopathology related to acute neurologic illness. Psychosomatics 49(1):67–72, 2008b 18212179

Rasmussen KG, Leise AD, Stevens SR: Orthostatic hemodynamic changes after electroconvulsive therapy treatments. J ECT 24(2):134–136, 2008c 18580557

Rasmussen KG, Petersen KN, Sticka JL, et al: Correlates of myalgia in electroconvulsive therapy. J ECT 24(1):84–87, 2008d 18379340

Rasmussen KG, Imig MW, Varghese R: Remifentanil/thiopental combination and seizure length in electroconvulsive therapy. J ECT 25(1):31–33, 2009a 18665101

Rasmussen KG, Mueller M, Rummans TA, et al: Is baseline medication resistance associated with potential for relapse after successful remission of a depressive episode with ECT? Data from the Consortium for Research on Electroconvulsive Therapy (CORE). J Clin Psychiatry 70(2):232–237, 2009b 19192459

Rasmussen KG, Lineberry TW, Galardy CW, et al: Serial infusions of low-dose ketamine for major depression. J Psychopharmacol 27(5):444–450, 2013 23428794

Rasmussen KG, Kung S, Lapid MI, et al: A randomized comparison of ketamine versus methohexital anesthesia in electroconvulsive therapy. Psychiatry Res 215(2):362–365, 2014 24388729

Rasmussen KG, Johnson EK, Kung S, et al: An open-label, pilot study of daily right unilateral ultrabrief pulse electroconvulsive therapy. J ECT 32(1):33–37, 2016 26172059

Rau A, Grossheinrich N, Palm U, et al: Transcranial and deep brain stimulation approaches as treatment for depression. Clin EEG Neurosci 38(2):105–115, 2007 17515176

Ray I: Side effects from lithium (letter). Can Med Assoc J 112(4):417–418, 419, 1975 1111885

Ray SD: Relative efficacy of electroconvulsive therapy and chlorpromazine in schizophrenia. J Indian Med Assoc 38(7):332–333, 1962 14490710

Regenold WT, Weintraub D, Taller A: Electroconvulsive therapy for epilepsy and major depression. Am J Geriatr Psychiatry 6(2):180–183, 1998 9581214

Rehor G, Conca A, Schlotter W, et al: Rückfallraten innerhalb von 6 Monaten nach erfolgreicher EKT. Neuropsychiatrie (Deisenhofen) 23(3):157–163, 2009

Reid WH, Keller S, Leatherman M, et al: ECT in Texas: 19 months of mandatory reporting. J Clin Psychiatry 59(1):8–13, 1998 9491059

Remick RA: Acute brain syndrome associated with ECT and lithium (letter). Can Psychiatr Assoc J 23(2):129–130, 1978 647602

Ren J, Li H, Palaniyappan L, et al: Repetitive transcranial magnetic stimulation versus electroconvulsive therapy for major depression: a systematic review and meta-analysis. Prog Neuropsychopharmacol Biol Psychiatry 51:181–189, 2014 24556538

Rice EH, Sombrotto LB, Markowitz JC, et al: Cardiovascular morbidity in high-risk patients during ECT. Am J Psychiatry 151(11):1637–1641, 1994 7943453

Rikher KV, Johnson R, Kamal M: Cortical blindness after electroconvulsive therapy. J Am Board Fam Pract 10(2):141–143, 1997 9071696

Rivera FA, Lapid MI, Sampson S, et al: Safety of electroconvulsive therapy in patients with a history of heart failure and decreased left ventricular systolic heart function. J ECT 27(3):207–213, 2011 21865957

Roberts JM: Prognostic factors in the electroshock treatment of depressive states, I: clinical features from history and examination. J Ment Sci 105:693–702, 1959 14437823

Robin A, de Tissera S: A double-blind controlled comparison of the therapeutic effects of low and high energy electroconvulsive therapies. Br J Psychiatry 141:357–366, 1982 6756529

Robin AA, Harris JA: A controlled comparison of imipramine and electroplexy. J Ment Sci 108:217–219, 1962 14492854

Robinson M, Lighthall G: Asystole during successive electroconvulsive therapy sessions: a report of two cases. J Clin Anesth 16(3):210–213, 2004 15217662

Roccaforte WH, Wengel SP, Burke WJ: ECT for screaming in dementia (letter). Am J Geriatr Psychiatry 8(2):177, 2000 10804080

Rodriguez-Jimenez R, Bagney A, Torio I, et al: Clinical usefulness and economic implications of continuation/maintenance electroconvulsive therapy in a Spanish National Health System public hospital: a case series. Rev Psiquiatr Salud Ment 8(2):75–82, 2015 25618779

Roepke S, Luborzewski A, Schindler F, et al: Stimulus pulse-frequency-dependent efficacy and cognitive adverse effects of ultrabrief-pulse electroconvulsive therapy in patients with major depression. J ECT 27(2):109–113, 2011 20938351

Rowny SB, Cycowicz YM, McClintock SM, et al: Differential heart rate response to magnetic seizure therapy (MST) relative to electroconvulsive therapy: a nonhuman primate model. Neuroimage 47(3):1086–1091, 2009 19497373

Rubner P, Koppi S, Conca A: Frequency of and rationales for the combined use of electroconvulsive therapy and antiepileptic drugs in Austria and the literature. World J Biol Psychiatry 10(4 Pt 3):836–845, 2009 19995220

Rudorfer MV, Linnoila M, Potter WZ: Combined lithium and electroconvulsive therapy: pharmacokinetic and pharmacodynamic interactions. Convuls Ther 3(1):40–45, 1987a 11940888

Rudorfer MV, Linnoila M, Potter WZ: A reply to El-Mallakh (letter). Convuls Ther 3(4):309–310, 1987b 11940936

Rush AJ, George MS, Sackeim HA, et al: Vagus nerve stimulation (VNS) for treatment-resistant depressions: a multicenter study. Biol Psychiatry 47(4):276–286, 2000 10686262

Rush AJ, Marangell LB, Sackeim HA, et al: Vagus nerve stimulation for treatment-resistant depression: a randomized, controlled acute phase trial. Biol Psychiatry 58(5):347–354, 2005a 16139580

Rush AJ, Sackeim HA, Marangell LB, et al: Effects of 12 months of vagus nerve stimulation in treatment-resistant depression: a naturalistic study. Biol Psychiatry 58(5):355–363, 2005b 16139581

Russell JC, Rasmussen KG, O'Connor MK, et al: Long-term maintenance ECT: a retrospective review of efficacy and cognitive outcome. J ECT 19(1):4–9, 2003 12621270

Ruwitch JF, Perez JE, Miller TR, et al: Myocardial ischemia introduced by electroconvulsive therapy (abstract 2034). Circulation 90 (suppl 4), 1994

Sackeim HA: The anticonvulsant hypothesis of the mechanisms of action of ECT: current status. J ECT 15(1):5–26, 1999 10189616

Sackeim HA, Portnoy S, Neeley P, et al: Cognitive consequences of low-dosage electroconvulsive therapy. Ann N Y Acad Sci 462:326–340, 1986 3458413

Sackeim HA, Decina P, Kanzler M, et al: Effects of electrode placement on the efficacy of titrated, low-dose ECT. Am J Psychiatry 144(11):1449–1455, 1987a 3314538

Sackeim HA, Decina P, Portnoy S, et al: Studies of dosage, seizure threshold, and seizure duration in ECT. Biol Psychiatry 22(3):249–268, 1987b 3814678

Sackeim HA, Prudic J, Devanand DP, et al: The impact of medication resistance and continuation pharmacotherapy on relapse following response to electroconvulsive therapy in major depression. J Clin Psychopharmacol 10(2):96–104, 1990 2341598

Sackeim HA, Devanand DP, Prudic J: Stimulus intensity, seizure threshold, and seizure duration: impact on the efficacy and safety of electroconvulsive therapy. Psychiatr Clin North Am 14(4):803–843, 1991 1771150

Sackeim HA, Prudic J, Devanand DP, et al: Effects of stimulus intensity and electrode placement on the efficacy and cognitive effects of electroconvulsive therapy. N Engl J Med 328(12):839–846, 1993 8441428

Sackeim HA, Prudic J, Devanand DP, et al: A prospective, randomized, double-blind comparison of bilateral and right unilateral electroconvulsive therapy at different stimulus intensities. Arch Gen Psychiatry 57(5):425–434, 2000 10807482

Sackeim HA, Haskett RF, Mulsant BH, et al: Continuation pharmacotherapy in the prevention of relapse following electroconvulsive therapy: a randomized controlled trial. JAMA 285(10):1299–1307, 2001 11255384

Sackeim HA, Prudic J, Fuller R, et al: The cognitive effects of electroconvulsive therapy in community settings. Neuropsychopharmacology 32(1):244–254, 2007 16936712

Sackeim HA, Prudic J, Nobler MS, et al: Effects of pulse width and electrode placement on the efficacy and cognitive effects of electroconvulsive therapy. Brain Stimul 1(2):71–83, 2008 19756236

Sackeim HA, Dillingham EM, Prudic J, et al: Effect of concomitant pharmacotherapy on electroconvulsive therapy outcomes: short-term efficacy and adverse effects. Arch Gen Psychiatry 66(7):729–737, 2009 19581564

Sahlem GL, Short EB, Kerns S, et al: Expanded safety and efficacy data for a new method of performing electroconvulsive therapy: focal electrically administered seizure therapy. J ECT 32(3):197–203, 2016 27379790

Sajatovic M, Meltzer HY: The effect of short-term electroconvulsive treatment plus neuroleptics in treatment-resistant schizophrenia and schizoaffective disorder. Convuls Ther 9(3):167–175, 1993 11941209

Salzman C: The use of ECT in the treatment of schizophrenia. Am J Psychiatry 137(9):1032–1041, 1980 6107048

Sanacora G, Mason GF, Rothman DL, et al: Increased cortical GABA concentrations in depressed patients receiving ECT. Am J Psychiatry 160(3):577–579, 2003 12611844

Sands DE: Electro-convulsion therapy in 301 patients in a general hospital, with special reference to selection of cases and response to treatment. BMJ 2:289–293, 1946 20996122

Sandyk R: The relationship between ECT responsiveness and subtypes of tardive dyskinesia in bipolar patients. Int J Neurosci 54(3–4):315–319, 1990 2265982

Sareen J, Enns MW, Guertin JE: The impact of clinically diagnosed personality disorders on acute and one-year outcomes of electroconvulsive therapy. J ECT 16(1):43–51, 2000 10735331

Sartorius A, Wolf J, Henn FA: Lithium and ECT—concurrent use still demands attention: three case reports. World J Biol Psychiatry 6(2):121–124, 2005 16156485

Sartorius A, Kiening KL, Kirsch P, et al: Remission of major depression under deep brain stimulation of the lateral habenula in a therapy-refractory patient. Biol Psychiatry 67(2):e9–e11, 2010 19846068

Sartorius A, Aksay SS, Bumb JM, et al: Psychomimetic adverse effects of S-ketamine as an anesthetic for electroconvulsive therapy are related to low doses and not to Axis I diagnosis (letter). J ECT 31(1):73–74, 2015 25422919

Schak KM, Mueller PS, Barnes RD, et al: The safety of ECT in patients with chronic obstructive pulmonary disease. Psychosomatics 49(3):208–211, 2008 18448774

Schiele BC, Schneider RA: The selective use of electroconvulsive therapy in manic patients. Dis Nerv Syst 10(10):291–297, 1949 18142973

Schildkraut JJ: The catecholamine hypothesis of affective disorders: a review of supporting evidence. Am J Psychiatry 122(5):509–522, 1965 5319766

Schlaepfer TE: Deep brain stimulation for major depression—steps on a long and winding road. Biol Psychiatry 78(4):218–219, 2015 26195174

Schlaepfer TE, Cohen MX, Frick C, et al: Deep brain stimulation to reward circuitry alleviates anhedonia in refractory major depression. Neuropsychopharmacology 33(2):368–377, 2008 17429407

Schnur DB, Mukherjee S, Sackeim HA, et al: Symptomatic predictors of ECT response in medication-nonresponsive manic patients. J Clin Psychiatry 53(2):63–66, 1992 1347293

Schoeyen HK, Kessler U, Andreassen OA, et al: Treatment-resistant bipolar depression: a randomized controlled trial of electroconvulsive therapy versus algorithm-based pharmacological treatment. Am J Psychiatry 172(1):41–51, 2015 25219389

Schou M: Lithium and electroconvulsive therapy: adversaries, competitors, allies? Acta Psychiatr Scand 84(5):435–438, 1991 1776496

Schwartz M, Silver H, Tal I, et al: Tardive dyskinesia in northern Israel: preliminary study. Eur Neurol 33(3):264–266, 1993 8096816

Schwarz T, Loewenstein J, Isenberg KE: Maintenance ECT: indications and outcome. Convuls Ther 11(1):14–23, 1995 7796063

Seager CP, Bird RL: Imipramine with electrical treatment in depression—a controlled trial. J Ment Sci 108:704–707, 1962 13987497

Semkovska M, McLoughlin DM: Objective cognitive performance associated with electroconvulsive therapy for depression: a systematic review and meta-analysis. Biol Psychiatry 68(6):568–577, 2010 20673880

Semkovska M, McLoughlin DM: Measuring retrograde autobiographical amnesia following electroconvulsive therapy: historical perspective and current issues. J ECT 29(2):127–133, 2013 23303426

Semkovska M, Keane D, Babalola O, et al: Unilateral brief-pulse electroconvulsive therapy and cognition: effects of electrode placement, stimulus dosage and time. J Psychiatr Res 45(6):770–780, 2011 21109254

Semkovska M, Noone M, Carton M, et al: Measuring consistency of autobiographical memory recall in depression. Psychiatry Res 197(1–2):41–48, 2012 22397910

Semkovska M, Landau S, Dunne R, et al: Bitemporal versus high-dose unilateral twice-weekly electroconvulsive therapy for depression (EFFECT-Dep): a pragmatic, randomized, non-inferiority trial. Am J Psychiatry 173(4):408–417, 2016 26892939

Serra M, Gastó C, Navarro V, et al: Maintenance electroconvulsive therapy in elderly psychotic unipolar depression [in Spanish]. Med Clin (Barc) 126(13):491–492, 2006 16624227

Shapira B, Gorfine M, Lerer B: A prospective study of lithium continuation therapy in depressed patients who have responded to electroconvulsive therapy. Convuls Ther 11(2):80–85, 1995 7552058

Shapira B, Tubi N, Drexler H, et al: Cost and benefit in the choice of ECT schedule: twice versus three times weekly ECT. Br J Psychiatry 172:44–48, 1998 9534831

Sharma A, Hammer S, Egbert M, et al: Electroconvulsive therapy and ocular dystonia. J ECT 23(3):181–182, 2007 17804995

Shelef A, Mazeh D, Berger U, et al: Acute electroconvulsive therapy followed by maintenance electroconvulsive therapy decreases hospital re-admission rates of older patients with severe mental illness. J ECT 31(2):125–128, 2015 25373561

Shiozawa P, Fregni F, Benseñor IM, et al: Transcranial direct current stimulation for major depression: an updated systematic review and meta-analysis (Erratum appears in Int J Neuropsychopharmacol 2014; Sep;17(9):1539). Int J Neuropsychopharmacol 17(9):1443–1452, 2014 24713139

Shorter E, Fink M: Endocrine Psychiatry. New York, Oxford University Press, 2010

Shorter E, Healy D: Shock Therapy. New Brunswick, NJ, Rutgers University Press, 2007

Shrestha S, Shrestha BR, Thapa C, et al: Comparative study of esmolol and labetalol to attenuate haemodynamic responses after electroconvulsive therapy. Kathmandu Univ Med J (KUMJ) 5(3):318–323, 2007 18604047

Sienaert P, Peuskens J: Remission of tardive dystonia (blepharospasm) after electroconvulsive therapy in a patient with treatment-refractory schizophrenia. J ECT 21(2):132–134, 2005 15905759

Sienaert P, Peuskens J: Anticonvulsants during electroconvulsive therapy: review and recommendations. J ECT 23(2):120–123, 2007 17548985

Sienaert P, Rooseleer J, Peuskens J: Uneventful electroconvulsive therapy in a patient with dopa-responsive dystonia (Segawa syndrome). J ECT 25(4):284–286, 2009a 19444136

Sienaert P, Vansteelandt K, Demyttenaere K, et al: Randomized comparison of ultrabrief bifrontal and unilateral electroconvulsive therapy for major depression: clinical efficacy. J Affect Disord 116(1–2):106–112, 2009b 19081638

Sienaert P, Vansteelandt K, Demyttenaere K, et al: Ultra-brief pulse ECT in bipolar and unipolar depressive disorder: differences in speed of response. Bipolar Disord 11(4):418–424, 2009c 19500095

Sienaert P, Vansteelandt K, Demyttenaere K, et al: Randomized comparison of ultrabrief bifrontal and unilateral electroconvulsive therapy for major depression: cognitive side-effects. J Affect Disord 122(1–2):60–67, 2010 19577808

Sienaert P, Roelens Y, Demunter H, et al: Concurrent use of lamotrigine and electroconvulsive therapy. J ECT 27(2):148–152, 2011 20562637

Sikdar S, Kulhara P, Avasthi A, et al: Combined chlorpromazine and electroconvulsive therapy in mania. Br J Psychiatry 164(6):806–810, 1994 7952988

Slade EP, Jahn DR, Regenold WT, et al: Association of electroconvulsive therapy with psychiatric readmissions in US hospitals. JAMA Psychiatry 74(8):798–804, 2017 28658489

Slotema CW, Blom JD, Hoek HW, et al: Should we expand the toolbox of psychiatric treatment methods to include repetitive transcranial magnetic stimulation (rTMS)? A meta-analysis of the efficacy of rTMS in psychiatric disorders. J Clin Psychiatry 71(7):873–884, 2010 20361902

Small JG: Efficacy of electroconvulsive therapy in schizophrenia, mania, and other disorders, I: schizophrenia. Convuls Ther 1(4):263–270, 1985 11940832

Small JG, Milstein V: Lithium interactions: lithium and electroconvulsive therapy. J Clin Psychopharmacol 10(5):346–350, 1990 2258451

Small JG, Kellams JJ, Milstein V, et al: Complications with electroconvulsive treatment combined with lithium. Biol Psychiatry 15(1):103–112, 1980 7357049

Small JG, Small IF, Milstein V, et al: Manic symptoms: an indication for bilateral ECT. Biol Psychiatry 20(2):125–134, 1985 3970993

Small JG, Klapper MH, Kellams JJ, et al: Electroconvulsive treatment compared with lithium in the management of manic states. Arch Gen Psychiatry 45(8):727–732, 1988a 2899425

Small JG, Milstein V, Miller MJ, et al: Clinical, neuropsychological, and EEG evidence for mechanisms of action of ECT. Convuls Ther 4(4):280–291, 1988b

Small JG, Milstein V, Small IF: Electroconvulsive therapy for mania. Psychiatr Clin North Am 14(4):887–903, 1991 1685234

Smith GE, Rasmussen KG Jr, Cullum CM, et al; CORE Investigators: A randomized controlled trial comparing the memory effects of continuation electroconvulsive therapy versus continuation pharmacotherapy: results from the Consortium for Research in ECT (CORE) study. J Clin Psychiatry 71(2):185–193, 2010

Smith K, Surphlis WR, Gynther MD, et al: ECT-chlorpromazine and chlorpromazine compared in the treatment of schizophrenia. J Nerv Ment Dis 144(4):284–290, 1967

Sobin C, Sackeim HA, Prudic J, et al: Predictors of retrograde amnesia following ECT. Am J Psychiatry 152(7):995–1001, 1995 7793470

Song G-M, Tian X, Shuai T, et al: Treatment of adults with treatment-resistant depression: electroconvulsive therapy plus antidepressant or electroconvulsive therapy alone? Evidence from an indirect comparison meta-analysis. Medicine (Baltimore) 94(26):e1052, 2015 26131818

Spaans H-P, Kho KH, Verwijk E, et al: Efficacy of ultrabrief pulse electroconvulsive therapy for depression: a systematic review. J Affect Disord 150(3):720–726, 2013a 23790557

Spaans H-P, Verwijk E, Comijs HC, et al: Efficacy and cognitive side effects after brief pulse and ultrabrief pulse right unilateral electroconvulsive therapy for major depression: a randomized, double-blind, controlled study. J Clin Psychiatry 74(11):e1029–e1036, 2013b 24330903

Spellman T, McClintock SM, Terrace H, et al: Differential effects of high-dose magnetic seizure therapy and electroconvulsive shock on cognitive function. Biol Psychiatry 63(12):1163–1170, 2008 18262171

Spellman T, Peterchev AV, Lisanby SH: Focal electrically administered seizure therapy: a novel form of ECT illustrates the roles of current directionality, polarity, and electrode configuration in seizure induction. Neuropsychopharmacology 34(8):2002–2010, 2009 19225453 (Erratum appears in Neuropsychopharmacology 37[4]:1077, 2012)

Spiker DG, Stein J, Rich CL: Delusional depression and electroconvulsive therapy: one year later. Convuls Ther 1(3):167–172, 1985 11940820

Squire LB, Chace PM, Slater PC: Retrograde amnesia following electroconvulsive therapy. Nature 260(5554):775–777, 1976 1264252

Squire LR: Amnesia for remote events following electroconvulsive therapy. Behav Biol 12(1):119–125, 1974 4429508

Squire LR: A stable impairment in remote memory following electroconvulsive therapy. Neuropsychologia 13(1):51–58, 1975 1109461

Squire LR, Chace PM: Memory functions six to nine months after electroconvulsive therapy. Arch Gen Psychiatry 32(12):1557–1564, 1975 1200774

Squire LR, Cohen N: Memory and amnesia: resistance to disruption develops for years after learning. Behav Neural Biol 25(1):115–125, 1979 454335

Squire LR, Miller PL: Diminution of anterograde amnesia following electroconvulsive therapy. Br J Psychiatry 125:490–495, 1974 4477729

Squire LR, Slater PC: Forgetting in very long-term memory as assessed by an improved questionnaire technique. J Exp Psychol Hum Learn 104(1):50–54, 1975

Squire LR, Slater PC: Electroconvulsive therapy and complaints of memory dysfunction: a prospective three-year follow-up study. Br J Psychiatry 142:1–8, 1983 6831121

Squire LR, Chace PM, Slater PC: Assessment of memory for remote events. Psychol Rep 37:223–234, 1975a

Squire LR, Slater PC, Chace PM: Retrograde amnesia: temporal gradient in very long term memory following electroconvulsive therapy. Science 187(4171):77–79, 1975b 1109228

Squire LR, Wetzel CD, Slater PC: Memory complaint after electroconvulsive therapy: assessment with a new self-rating instrument. Biol Psychiatry 14(5):791–801, 1979 497304

Squire LR, Slater PC, Miller PL: Retrograde amnesia and bilateral electroconvulsive therapy: long-term follow-up. Arch Gen Psychiatry 38(1):89–95, 1981 7458573

Squire SR, Slater PC: Bilateral and unilateral ECT: effects on verbal and nonverbal memory. Am J Psychiatry 135(11):1316–1320, 1978 707628

Stern L, Hirschmann S, Grunhaus L: ECT in patients with major depressive disorder and low cardiac output. Convuls Ther 13(2):68–73, 1997 9253526

Stern RA, Nevels CT, Shelhorse ME, et al: Antidepressant and memory effects of combined thyroid hormone treatment and electroconvulsive therapy: preliminary findings. Biol Psychiatry 30(6):623–627, 1991 1932410

Stern R, Legendre S, Thorner A, et al: Exogenous thyroid hormone diminishes the amnestic side effects of electroconvulsive therapy. J Int Neuropsychol Soc 6:235, 2000

Stevenson GH, Geoghegan JJ: Prophylactic electroshock: a five year study. Am J Psychiatry 107(10):743–748, 1951 14819368

Stewart JT: Lithium and maintenance ECT. J ECT 16(3):300–301, 2000 11005054

Stiebel VG: Maintenance electroconvulsive therapy for chronic mentally ill patients: a case series. Psychiatr Serv 46(3):265–268, 1995 7796215

Stieper DR, Williams M, Duncan CP: Changes in impersonal and personal memory following electro-convulsive therapy. J Clin Psychol 7(4):361–366, 1951 14888718

Stoppe A, Louzã M, Rosa M, et al: Fixed high-dose electroconvulsive therapy in the elderly with depression: a double-blind, randomized comparison of efficacy and tolerability between unilateral and bilateral electrode placement. J ECT 22(2):92–99, 2006 16801822

Stoudemire A, Hill CD, Marquardt M, et al: Recovery and relapse in geriatric depression after treatment with antidepressants and ECT in a medical-psychiatric population. Gen Hosp Psychiatry 20(3):170–174, 1998 9650035

Strain JJ, Brunschwig L, Duffy JP, et al: Comparison of therapeutic effects and memory changes with bilateral and unilateral ECT. Am J Psychiatry 125(3):50–60, 1968 4875384

Strawn JR, Keck PE Jr, Caroff SN: Neuroleptic malignant syndrome. Am J Psychiatry 164(6):870–876, 2007 17541044

Strömgren LS: Therapeutic results in brief-interval unilateral ECT. Acta Psychiatr Scand 52(4):246–255, 1975 1189955

Strömgren LS: Electroconvulsive therapy in Aarhus, Denmark, in 1984: its application in nondepressive disorders. Convuls Ther 4(4):306–313, 1988 11940980

Strömgren LS, Christensen AL, Fromholt P: The effects of unilateral brief-interval ECT on memory. Acta Psychiatr Scand 54(5):336–346, 1976 1007937

Struve FA: Five-year prospective study of clinical EEG, neuropsychological, and demographic risk variables for persistent tardive dyskinesia, in Chronic Treatments in Neuropsychiatry. Edited by Kemali D, Racagni G. New York, Raven Press, 1985, pp 33–36

Sutor B, Rasmussen KG: Electroconvulsive therapy for agitation in Alzheimer disease: a case series. J ECT 24(3):239–241, 2008 18562945

Sutor B: Rasmussen K: Long-term maintenance electroconvulsive therapy in the treatment of schizophrenia and schizoaffective disorder-A case series. Clin Schizophr Relat Psychoses 2(4):326–330, 2009

Sutor B, Mueller PS, Rasmussen KG: Bradycardia and hypotension in a patient with severe aortic stenosis receiving electroconvulsive therapy dose titration for treatment of depression. J ECT 24(4):281–282, 2008 18580693

Suzuki K, Awata S, Matsuoka H: One-year outcome after response to ECT in middle-aged and elderly patients with intractable catatonic schizophrenia. J ECT 20(2):99–106, 2004 15167426

Suzuki K, Awata S, Takano T, et al: Adjusting the frequency of continuation and maintenance electroconvulsive therapy to prevent relapse of catatonic schizophrenia in middle-aged and elderly patients who are relapse-prone. Psychiatry Clin Neurosci 60(4):486–492, 2006 16884452

Swoboda E, Conca A, König P, et al: Maintenance electroconvulsive therapy in affective and schizoaffective disorder. Neuropsychobiology 43(1):23–28, 2001 11150895

Takahashi S, Mizukami K, Yasuno F, et al: Depression associated with dementia with Lewy bodies (DLB) and the effect of somatotherapy. Psychogeriatrics 9(2):56–61, 2009 19604326

Tang WK, Ungvari GS, Leung HCM: Effect of piracetam on ECT-induced cognitive disturbances: a randomized, placebo-controlled, double-blind study. J ECT 18(3):130–137, 2002 12394531

Taylor MA, Fink M: Melancholia: The Diagnosis, Pathophysiology, and Treatment of Depressive Illness. Cambridge, UK, Cambridge University Press, 2006

Taylor P, Fleminger JJ: ECT for schizophrenia. Lancet 1(8183):1380–1382, 1980 6104172

Tendolkar I, van Beek M, van Oostrom I, et al: Electroconvulsive therapy increases hippocampal and amygdala volume in therapy refractory depression: a longitudinal pilot study. Psychiatry Res 214(3):197–203, 2013 24090511

Tess AV, Smetana GW: Medical evaluation of patients undergoing electroconvulsive therapy. N Engl J Med 360(14):1437–1444, 2009 19339723

Tew JD Jr, Mulsant BH, Haskett RF, et al: Acute efficacy of ECT in the treatment of major depression in the old-old. Am J Psychiatry 156(12):1865–1870, 1999 10588398

Tew JD Jr, Mulsant BH, Haskett RF, et al: Relapse during continuation pharmacotherapy after acute response to ECT: a comparison of usual care versus protocolized treatment. Ann Clin Psychiatry 19(1):1–4, 2007 17453654

Tharyan P, Adams CE: Electroconvulsive therapy for schizophrenia. Cochrane Database Syst Rev 18(2):CD000076, 2005 15846598

Thenon J: Electrochoque monolateral. Acta Neuropsiquiatrica Argentina 2:292–296, 1956

Thienhaus OJ, Margletta S, Bennett JA: A study of the clinical efficacy of maintenance ECT. J Clin Psychiatry 51(4):141–144, 1990 2324077

Thirthalli J, Kumar CN, Bangalore RP, et al: Speed of response to threshold and suprathreshold bilateral ECT in depression, mania and schizophrenia. J Affect Disord 117(1–2):104–107, 2009a 19157566

Thirthalli J, Phutane VH, Muralidharan K, et al: Does catatonic schizophrenia improve faster with electroconvulsive therapy than other subtypes of schizophrenia? World J Biol Psychiatry 10(4 Pt 3):772–777, 2009b 19225955

Thirthalli J, Harish T, Gangadhar BN: A prospective comparative study of interaction between lithium and modified electroconvulsive therapy. World J Biol Psychiatry 12(2):149–155, 2011 20645670

Thomas J, Reddy B: The treatment of mania: a retrospective evaluation of the effects of ECT, chlorpromazine, and lithium. J Affect Disord 4(2):85–92, 1982 6213694

Thornton JE, Mulsant BH, Dealy R, et al: A retrospective study of maintenance electroconvulsive therapy in a university-based psychiatric practice. Convuls Ther 6(2):121–129, 1990 11941053

Toprak HI, Gedik E, Begeç Z, et al: Sevoflurane as an alternative anaesthetic for electroconvulsive therapy. J ECT 21(2):108–110, 2005 15905753

Tor P-C, Bautovich A, Wang M-J, et al: A systematic review and meta-analysis of brief versus ultrabrief right unilateral electroconvulsive therapy for depression. J Clin Psychiatry 76(9):e1092–e1098, 2015 26213985

Trevino K, McClintock SM, Husain MM: A review of continuation electroconvulsive therapy: application, safety, and efficacy. J ECT 26(3):186–195, 2010 20805727

Treynor W, Gonzalez R, Nolan-Hoeksema S: Rumination reconsidered: a psychometric analysis. Cognit Ther Res 27:247–259, 2003

Trollor JN, Sachdev PS: Electroconvulsive treatment of neuroleptic malignant syndrome: a review and report of cases. Aust N Z J Psychiatry 33(5):650–659, 1999

Tsao CI, Jain S, Gibson RH, et al: Maintenance ECT for recurrent medication-refractory mania. J ECT 20(2):118–119, 2004 15167429

UK ECT Review Group: Efficacy and safety of electroconvulsive therapy in depressive disorders: a systematic review and meta-analysis. Lancet 361(9360):799–808, 2003 12642045

Vaidya NA, Mahableshwarkar AR, Shahid R: Continuation and maintenance ECT in treatment-resistant bipolar disorder. J ECT 19(1):10–16, 2003 12621271

Vamos M: The cognitive side effects of modern ECT: patient experience or objective measurement? J ECT 24(1):18–24, 2008 18379330

van Beusekom BS, van den Broek WW, Birkenhäger TK: Long-term follow-up after successful electroconvulsive therapy for depression: a 4- to 8-year naturalistic follow-up study. J ECT 23(1):17–20, 2007 17435567

van den Broek WW, Leentjens AF, Mulder PG, et al: Low-dose esmolol bolus reduces seizure duration during electroconvulsive therapy: a double-blind, placebo-controlled study. Br J Anaesth 83(2):271–274, 1999 10618942

van den Broek WW, Groenland THN, Kusuma A, et al: Double-blind placebo controlled study of the effects of etomidate-alfentanil anesthesia in electroconvulsive therapy. J ECT 20(2):107–111, 2004 15167427

van den Broek WW, Birkenhäger TK, Mulder PG, et al: Imipramine is effective in preventing relapse in electroconvulsive therapy-responsive depressed inpatients with prior pharmacotherapy treatment failure: a randomized, placebo-controlled trial. J Clin Psychiatry 67(2):263–268, 2006 16566622

Vanelle J-M, Loo H, Galinowski A, et al: Maintenance ECT in intractable manic-depressive disorders. Convuls Ther 10(3):195–205, 1994 7834256

van Schaik AM, Comijs HC, Sonnenberg CM, et al: Efficacy and safety of continuation and maintenance electroconvulsive therapy in depressed elderly patients: a systematic review. Am J Geriatr Psychiatry 20(1):5–17, 2012 22183009

Van Valkenburg C, Clayton PJ: Electroconvulsive therapy and schizophrenia (editorial). Biol Psychiatry 20(7):699–700, 1985 2860929

van Waarde JA, Tuerlings JH, Verwey B, et al: Electroconvulsive therapy for catatonia: treatment characteristics and outcomes in 27 patients. J ECT 26(4):248–252, 2010a 19935090

van Waarde JA, Wielaard D, Wijkstra J, et al: Retrospective study of continuation electroconvulsive therapy in 50 patients. J ECT 26(4):299–303, 2010b 20357668

Verwijk E, Comijs HC, Kok RM, et al: Neurocognitive effects after brief pulse and ultrabrief pulse unilateral electroconvulsive therapy for major depression: a review. J Affect Disord 140(3):233–243, 2012 22595374

Verwijk E, Comijs HC, Kok RM, et al: Short- and long-term neurocognitive functioning after electroconvulsive therapy in depressed elderly: a prospective naturalistic study. Int Psychogeriatr 26(2):315–324, 2014 24280446

Verwijk E, Spaans HP, Comijs HC, et al: Relapse and long-term cognitive performance after brief pulse or ultrabrief pulse right unilateral electroconvulsive therapy: a multicenter naturalistic follow up. J Affect Disord 184:137–144, 2015 26093032

Vieweg R, Shawcross CR: A trial to determine any difference between two and three times a week ECT in the rate of recovery from depression. J Ment Health 7(4):403–409, 1998 29052474

Vishne T, Aronov S, Amiaz R, et al: Remifentanil supplementation of propofol during electroconvulsive therapy: effect on seizure duration and cardiovascular stability. J ECT 21(4):235–238, 2005 16301884

Vlissides DN, Lee CR, Hill SE: Lithium, anaesthesia and ECT (letter). Br J Anaesth 51(6):574, 1979 465275

Volpe FM, Tavares AR Jr: Lithium plus ECT for mania in 90 cases: safety issues (letter). J Neuropsychiatry Clin Neurosci 24(4):E33, 2012 23224476

Volpe FM, Tavares A, Correa H: Naturalistic evaluation of inpatient treatment of mania in a private Brazilian psychiatric hospital. Braz J Psychiatr 25(2):72–77, 2003 12975702

Vothknecht S, Kho KH, van Schaick HW, et al: Effects of maintenance electroconvulsive therapy on cognitive functions. J ECT 19(3):151–157, 2003 12972985

Wajima Z, Shiga T, Yoshikawa T, et al: Propofol alone, sevoflurane alone, and combined propofol-sevoflurane anaesthesia in electroconvulsive therapy. Anaesth Intensive Care 31(4):396–400, 2003 12973963

Walter G, Rey JM: Has the practice and outcome of ECT in adolescents changed? Findings from a whole-population study. J ECT 19(2):84–87, 2003 12792456

Wang N, Wang XH, Lu J, et al: The effect of repeated etomidate anesthesia on adrenocortical function during a course of electroconvulsive therapy. J ECT 27(4):281–285, 2011 22080238

Wang X, Chen Y, Zhou X, et al: Effects of propofol and ketamine as combined anesthesia for electroconvulsive therapy in patients with depressive disorder. J ECT 28(2):128–132, 2012 22622291

Ward C, Stern GM, Pratt RTC, et al: Electroconvulsive therapy in parkinsonian patients with the "on-off" syndrome. J Neural Transm (Vienna) 49(1–2):133–135, 1980 7441236

Watts BV, Groft A, Bagian JP, et al: An examination of mortality and other adverse events related to electroconvulsive therapy using a national adverse event report system. J ECT 27(2):105–108, 2011 20966769

Weeks D, Freeman CPL, Kendell RE: ECT, III: enduring cognitive deficits? Br J Psychiatry 137:26–37, 1980 7459537

Weeks HR III, Tadler SC, Smith KW, et al: Antidepressant and neurocognitive effects of isoflurane anesthesia versus electroconvulsive therapy in refractory depression. PLoS One 8(7):e69809, 2013 23922809

Weiner RD, Whanger AD, Erwin CW, et al: Prolonged confusional state and EEG seizure activity following concurrent ECT and lithium use. Am J Psychiatry 137(11):1452–1453, 1980 7435687

Weiner RD, Rogers HJ, Davidson J, Miller RD: Evaluation of the central nervous system risks of ECT. Psychopharmacol Bull 18:29–31, 1982

Weiner RD, Rogers HJ, Davidson JRT, et al: Effects of stimulus parameters on cognitive side effects. Ann N Y Acad Sci 462:315–325, 1986 3458412

Weiner RD, Coffey CE, Krystal AD: The monitoring and management of electrically induced seizures. Psychiatr Clin North Am 14(4):845–869, 1991 1771151

Weinger MB, Partridge BL, Hauger R, et al: Prevention of the cardiovascular and neuroendocrine response to electroconvulsive therapy, I: effectiveness of pretreatment regimens on hemodynamics. Anesth Analg 73(5):556–562, 1991 1952135

Weinstein MR, Fischer A: Combined treatment with ECT and antipsychotic drugs in schizophrenia. Dis Nerv Syst 32(12):801–808, 1971 5139202

Weintraub D, Lippmann SB: Electroconvulsive therapy in the acute poststroke period. J ECT 16(4):415–418, 2000 11314880

Weisberg LA, Elliott D, Mielke D: Intracerebral hemorrhage following electroconvulsive therapy (letter). Neurology 41(11):1849, 1991 1944925

Wells DG, Zelcer J, Treadrae C: ECT-induced asystole from a sub-convulsive shock. Anaesth Intensive Care 16(3):368–371, 1988 3056091

Wengel SP, Burke WJ, Pfeiffer RF, et al: Maintenance electroconvulsive therapy for intractable Parkinson's disease. Am J Geriatr Psychiatry 6(3):263–269, 1998 9659959

West ED: Electric convulsion therapy in depression: a double-blind controlled trial. Br Med J (Clin Res Ed) 282(6261):355–357, 1981 6780021

White PF, Amos Q, Zhang Y, et al: Anesthetic considerations for magnetic seizure therapy: a novel therapy for severe depression. Anesth Analg 103(1):76–80, 2006 16790630

Wijkstra J, Nolen WA, Algra A, et al: Relapse prevention in major depressive disorder after successful ECT: a literature review and a naturalistic case series. Acta Psychiatr Scand 102(6):454–460, 2000 11142436

Wild B, Eschweiler GW, Bartels M: Electroconvulsive therapy dosage in continuation/maintenance electroconvulsive therapy: when is a new threshold titration necessary? J ECT 20(4):200–203, 2004 15591850

Williams JB: Standardizing the Hamilton Depression Rating Scale: past, present, and future. Eur Arch Psychiatry Clin Neurosci 251 (suppl 2):II6–II12, 2001 11824839

Williams KM, Iacono WG, Remick RA, Greenwood P: Dichotic perception and memory following electroconvulsive treatment for depression. Br J Psychiatry 157:366–372, 1990 2245266

Williams MD, Rummans T, Sampson S, et al: Outcome of electroconvulsive therapy by race in the Consortium for Research on Electroconvulsive Therapy multisite study. J ECT 24(2):117–121, 2008 18580553

Williams MJ, Holliday K, Holly R: Maintenance electroconvulsive therapy versus pharmacological management in patients with major depressive disorder with successful induction ECT. Presented at the 2010 Southeastern Residency Conference, the Classic Center, Athens, Georgia, April 28–29, 2010

Winokur G, Kadrmas A: Convulsive therapy and the course of bipolar illness, 1940–1949. Convuls Ther 4(2):126–132, 1988 11940952

Winokur G, Coryell W, Keller M, et al: Relationship of electroconvulsive therapy to course in affective illness: a collaborative study. Eur Arch Psychiatry Clin Neurosci 240(1):54–59, 1990 2147905

Witton K: Efficacy of ECT following prolonged use of psychotropic drugs. Am J Psychiatry 119:79–80, 1962 14007787

Wolff GE: Results of four-year active therapy for chronic mental patients and the value of an individual maintenance dose of ECT. Am J Psychiatry 114(5):453–456, 1957 13470118

Wu Q, Prentice G, Campbell JJ: ECT treatment for two cases of dementia-related aggressive behavior. J Neuropsychiatry Clin Neurosci 22(2):E10–E11, 2010 20463126

Wulfson HD, Askanazi J, Finck AD: Propranolol prior to ECT associated with asystole. Anesthesiology 60(3):255–256, 1984 6364891

Yen T, Khafaja M, Lam N, et al: Post-electroconvulsive therapy recovery and reorientation time with methohexital and ketamine: a randomized, longitudinal, crossover design trial. J ECT 31(1):20–25, 2015 24755722

Yildiz A, Mantar A, Simsek S, et al: Combination of pharmacotherapy with electroconvulsive therapy in prevention of depressive relapse: a pilot controlled trial. J ECT 26(2):104–110, 2010 19935091

Youssef NA, McCall WV: Relapse prevention after index electroconvulsive therapy in treatment-resistant depression. Ann Clin Psychiatry 26(4):288–296, 2014 25401716

Zachrisson OCG, Balldin J, Ekman R, et al: No evident neuronal damage after electroconvulsive therapy. Psychiatry Res 96(2):157–165, 2000 11063788

Zarate CA Jr, Tohen M, Baraibar G: Combined valproate or carbamazepine and electroconvulsive therapy. Ann Clin Psychiatry 9(1):19–25, 1997 9167833

Zervas IM, Fink M: ECT for refractory Parkinson's disease (letter). Convuls Ther 7(3):222–223, 1991 11941126

Zervas IM, Pehlivanidis AA, Papakostas YG, et al: Effects of TRH administration on orientation time and recall after ECT. J ECT 14(4):236–240, 1998 9871843

Zielinski RJ, Roose SP, Devanand DP, et al: Cardiovascular complications of ECT in depressed patients with cardiac disease. Am J Psychiatry 150(6):904–909, 1993 8494067

Zimmerman M, Coryell W, Pfohl B, et al: ECT response in depressed patients with and without a DSM-III personality disorder. Am J Psychiatry 143(8):1030–1032, 1986 3728718

Zisselman MH, Rosenquist PB, Curlik SM: Long-term weekly continuation electroconvulsive therapy: a case series. J ECT 23(4):274–277, 2007 18090702

Zornberg GL, Pope HG Jr: Treatment of depression in bipolar disorder: new directions for research. J Clin Psychopharmacol 13(6):397–408, 1993 8120153

Zorumski CF, Rutherford JL, Burke WJ, et al: ECT in primary and secondary depression. J Clin Psychiatry 47(6):298–300, 1986 3711027

Zvara DA, Brooker RF, McCall WV, et al: The effect of esmolol on ST-segment depression and arrhythmias after electroconvulsive therapy. Convuls Ther 13(3):165–174, 1997 9342132

Zyss T, Zieba A, Hese RT, et al: Magnetic seizure therapy (MST)—a safer method for evoking seizure activity than current therapy with a confirmed antidepressant efficacy. NeuroEndocrinol Lett 31(4):425–437, 2010 20802450

Index

Page numbers printed in **boldface** type refer to tables or figures.